T0348415

Perioperative and Consultative Medicine

Editor

EFRÉN C. MANJARREZ

MEDICAL CLINICS
OF NORTH AMERICA

www.medical.theclinics.com

Consulting Editor
DANIEL D. DRESSLER

November 2024 • Volume 108 • Number 6

ELSEVIER

1600 John F. Kennedy Boulevard • Suite 1800 • Philadelphia, Pennsylvania, 19103-2899

http://www.theclinics.com

MEDICAL CLINICS OF NORTH AMERICA Volume 108, Number 6
November 2024 ISSN 0025-7125, ISBN-13: 978-0-443-31364-6

Editor: Taylor Hayes
Developmental Editor: Malvika Shah

Medical Clinics of North America (ISSN 0025-7125) is published bimonthly by Elsevier Inc., 360 Park Avenue South, New York, NY 10010-1710. Months of publication are January, March, May, July, September, and November. Business and editorial offices: 1600 John F. Kennedy Boulevard, Suite 1800, Philadelphia, PA 19103-2899. Periodicals postage paid at New York, NY, and additional mailing offices. Subscription prices are USD $336.00 per year (US individuals), $100.00 per year (US Students), $433.00 per year (Canadian individuals), $200.00 per year for (foreign students), $100.00 per year for (Canadian students), $479.00 per year (foreign individuals). For institutional access pricing please contact Customer Service via the contact information below. To receive student/resident rate, orders must be accompanied by name of affiliated institution, date of term, and the signature of program/residency coordinator on institution letterhead. Orders will be billed at individual rate until proof of status is received. Foreign air speed delivery is included in all Clinics' subscription prices. All prices are subject to change without notice. Orders, claims, and journal inquiries: Please visit our Support Hub page https://service.elsevier.com for assistance.

Reprints. For copies of 100 or more of articles in this publication, please contact the Commercial Reprints Department, Elsevier Inc., 360 Park Avenue South, New York, NY 10010-1710. Tel.: 212-633-3874; Fax: 212-633-3820; E-mail: reprints@elsevier.com.

Medical Clinics of North America is also published in Spanish by McGraw-Hill Interamericana Editores S. A., P.O. Box 5-237, 06500 Mexico, D.F., Mexico.

Medical Clinics of North America is covered in MEDLINE/PubMed (Index Medicus), Current Contents, ASCA, Excerpta Medica, Science Citation Index, and ISI/BIOMED.

JOURNAL TITLE: Medical Clinics of North America
ISSUE: 108.6

PROGRAM OBJECTIVE
The goal of the *Medical Clinics of North America* is to keep practicing physicians up to date with current clinical practice by providing timely articles reviewing the state of the art in patient care.

TARGET AUDIENCE
All practicing physicians and other healthcare professionals.

LEARNING OBJECTIVES
Upon completion of this activity, participants will be able to:
1. Review the pros and cons of preoperative medical evaluation.
2. Explain how to prevent and treat postoperative complications optimally.
3. Discuss perioperative care for heart failure, arrhythmias, valvular heart disease, and cancer.

ACCREDITATION
The Elsevier Office of Continuing Medical Education (EOCME) is accredited by the Accreditation Council for Continuing Medical Education (ACCME) to provide continuing medical education for physicians.

The EOCME designates this journal-based CME activity for a maximum of 14 *AMA PRA Category 1 Credit*(s)™. Physicians should claim only the credit commensurate with the extent of their participation in the activity.

All other healthcare professionals requesting continuing education credit for this enduring material will be issued a certificate of participation.

DISCLOSURE OF RELEVANT FINANCIAL RELATIONSHIPS
The EOCME evaluates the relevancy of financial relationships with its instructors, faculty, planners, and other individuals who are in a position to control the content of CME activities. The EOCME will review all identified disclosures and mitigate financial relationships with ineligible companies, as applicable. An ineligible company is any entity whose primary business is producing, marketing, selling, re-selling, or distributing healthcare products used by or on patients. For specific examples of ineligible companies visit accme.org/standards. EOCME is committed to providing its learners with CME activities that promote improvements or quality in healthcare and not a specific proprietary business or a commercial interest.

The authors and editors listed below have identified no financial relationships or relationships to products or devices they have with ineligible companies related to the content of this CME activity:
Lily L. Ackermann, MD, ScM, FHM, FACP; Andrew D. Auerbach, MD, MPH, MHM; Win M. Aung, MD, DM, MBA, FRCP, FACP; Moises Auron, MD; Furheen Baig, MD; Rebecca C. Engels, MD, MPH; Leonard S. Feldman, MD; Elizabeth Mahanna Gabrielli, MD, MSCTI; David Gelovani, MD, MS; Paul J. Grant, MD, SFHM, FACP; Zeina Hannoush, MD; Catriona M. Harrop, MD, SFHM, FACP; Andrew Hawrylak, MD; Kay M. Johnson, MD, MPH; Babar Junaidi, MD; Smita K. Kalra, MD; Efrén C. Manjarrez, MD, SFHM, FACP; Carlos E. Mendez, MD; Heather E. Nye, MD, PhD, SFHM, FACP; Avital Y. O'Glasser, MD, FACP, SFHM, DFPM; Merlin Packiam; Matthew A. Pappas, MD, MPH, FHM; Preethi Patel, MD; Alejandra Razzeto, MD; Jeffrey W. Redinger, MD; Michael D. Rudy, MD; Sunil K. Sahai, MD, FACP, FAAP, SFHM; Edie Shen, MD, FHM, DFPM; Jason F. Shiffermiller, MD, MPH; Barbara A. Slawski, MD, MS; Marcio Rotta Soares, MD; Anna Von, MD; Christopher Whinney, MD, FACP, SFHM; Steven J. Wilson, MD

The authors and editors listed below have identified financial relationships or relationships to products or devices they have with ineligible companies related to the content of this CME activity:
Scott Kaatz, DO, MSc, FACP, SFHM: *Researcher*: Bayer; Consultant: Anthos Therapeutics, Bayer, Bristol-Myers Squibb, Gilead, Janssen, Pfizer

Roop Kaw, MD: *Consultant*: Medtronic

Alana Sigmund, MD: *Stock Ownership*: Bristol-Myers Squibb, Pfizer

The Clinics staff listed below have identified no financial relationships or relationships to products or devices they have with ineligible companies related to the content of this CME activity:
Taylor Hayes; Michelle Littlejohn; Patrick J. Manley; Merlin Packiam; Malvika Shah

UNAPPROVED/OFF-LABEL USE DISCLOSURE

The EOCME requires CME faculty to disclose to the participants;

1. When products or procedures being discussed are off-label, unlabelled, experimental, and/or investigational (not US Food and Drug Administration [FDA] approved); and
2. Any limitations on the information presented, such as data that are preliminary or that represent ongoing research, interim analyses, and/or unsupported opinions. Faculty may discuss information about pharmaceutical agents that is outside of FDA-approved labelling. This information is intended solely for CME and is not intended to promote off-label use of these medications. If you have any questions, contact the medical affairs department of the manufacturer for the most recent prescribing information.

TO ENROLL

To enroll in the *Medical Clinics of North America* Continuing Medical Education program, call customer service at 1-800-654-2452 or sign up online at http://www.theclinics.com/home/cme. The CME program is available to subscribers for an additional annual fee of USD 319.00.

METHOD OF PARTICIPATION

In order to claim credit, participants must complete the following:

1. Complete enrolment as indicated above.
2. Read the activity.
3. Complete the CME Test and Evaluation. Participants must achieve a score of 70% on the test. All CME Tests and Evaluations must be completed online.

CME INQUIRIES/SPECIAL NEEDS

For all CME inquiries or special needs, please contact elsevierCME@elsevier.com.

MEDICAL CLINICS OF NORTH AMERICA

Perioperative and Consultative Medicine

MEDICAL CLINICS OF NORTH AMERICA

Contributors

CONSULTING EDITOR

DANIEL D. DRESSLER, MD, MSc, MHM, FACP
Professor of Medicine, Emory University School of Medicine, Atlanta, Georgia

EDITOR

EFRÉN C. MANJARREZ, MD, SFHM, FACP
Associate Professor of Clinical Medicine, Division of Hospital Medicine, Department of Medicine, University of Miami Miller School of Medicine, Miami, Florida

AUTHORS

LILY L. ACKERMANN, MD, ScM, FHM, FACP
Associate Professor, Department of Medicine, Sidney Kimmel Medical College at Thomas Jefferson University, Philadelphia, Pennsylvania

ANDREW D. AUERBACH, MD, MPH, MHM
Professor, Department of Hospital Medicine, University of California, San Francisco, California

WIN M. AUNG, MD, DM, MBA, FRCP, FACP
Assistant Clinical Professor, Department of Medicine, University of Florida School of Medicine, UF Health, Jacksonville, Florida

MOISES AURON, MD
Professor, Department of Hospital Medicine, Cleveland Clinic, Cleveland, Ohio

FURHEEN BAIG, MD
Clinical Instructor, Division of General Internal Medicine, University of Washington, Hospital Medicine, Seattle, Washington

REBECCA C. ENGELS, MD, MPH
Assistant Professor, Department of Medicine, The Johns Hopkins University School of Medicine, Baltimore, Maryland

LEONARD S. FELDMAN, MD
Associate Professor, Division of Hospital Medicine, Departments of Medicine and Pediatrics, Johns Hopkins Hospital, Baltimore, Maryland

DAVID GELOVANI, MD, MS
Chief Medical Resident, Department of Internal Medicine, Henry Ford Health, Detroit, Michigan

PAUL J. GRANT, MD, SFHM, FACP
Professor of Medicine, Division of Hospital Medicine, Department of Internal Medicine, Michigan Medicine, University of Michigan Medical School, Ann Arbor, Michigan

ZEINA HANNOUSH, MD
Associate Professor of Clinical Medicine, Division of Endocrinology, Diabetes and Metabolism, Department of Internal Medicine, University of Miami, Miller School of Medicine, Miami, Florida

CATRIONA M. HARROP, MD, SFHM, FACP
Associate Professor, Department of Medicine, Sidney Kimmel Medical College at Thomas Jefferson University, Philadelphia, Pennsylvania

ANDREW HAWRYLAK, MD
Assistant Professor of Medicine, Baylor Scott & White Health, Baylor College of Medicine, Temple, Texas

KAY M. JOHNSON, MD, MPH
Associate Professor, Division of General Internal Medicine, Department of Medicine, University of Washington School of Medicine, Hospital and Specialty Medicine, VA Puget Sound Healthcare System, Seattle, Washington

BABAR JUNAIDI, MD
Associate Site Director of Hospital Medicine Service at Emory University Orthopedic and Spine Hospital, Assistant Professor, Division of Hospital Medicine, Department of Medicine, Emory University Hospital, Johns Creek, Georgia

SCOTT KAATZ, DO, MSc, FACP, SFHM
Professor of Medicine, Department of Internal Medicine, Henry Ford Health, Detroit, Michigan

SMITA K. KALRA, MD
Associate Professor, Department of Medicine, UCI Hospitalist Program, University of California Irvine Medical Center, Orange, California

ROOP KAW, MD
Professor of Medicine, Department of Hospital Medicine, Outcomes Research Consortium, Department of Anesthesiology, Cleveland Clinic, Cleveland, Ohio

ELIZABETH MAHANNA GABRIELLI, MD, MSCTI
Associate Professor of Anesthesiology, Perioperative Medicine, and Pain Management, Division Neuroanesthesiology, Critical Care Medicine, Neurocritical Care and Geriatric Anesthesiology, University of Miami Miller School of Medicine, Miami, Florida

EFRÉN C. MANJARREZ, MD, SFHM, FACP
Associate Professor of Clinical Medicine, Division of Hospital Medicine, Department of Medicine, University of Miami Miller School of Medicine, Miami, Florida

CARLOS E. MENDEZ, MD
Associate Professor of Medicine, Division of General Internal Medicine, Medical College of Wisconsin, Milwaukee, Wisconsin

HEATHER E. NYE, MD, PhD, SFHM, FACP
Professor, SFVAHCS Department of Medicine, University of California, San Francisco, Associate Chief of Medicine, San Francisco VA Health Care System Hospital Medicine, San Francisco, California

AVITAL Y. O'GLASSER, MD, FACP, SFHM, DFPM
Professor, Division of Hospital Medicine, Department of Medicine, Department of Anesthesiology and Perioperative Medicine, Oregon Health and Science University, Portland, Oregon

MATTHEW A. PAPPAS, MD, MPH, FHM
Assistant Professor, Research Investigator, Cleveland Clinic Center for Value-Based Care Research, Staff Physician, Department of Hospital Medicine, Cleveland Clinic, Outcomes Research Consortium, Cleveland, Ohio

PREETHI PATEL, MD
Assistant Professor of Medicine, Department of Hospital Medicine, Cleveland Clinic, Cleveland Clinic Lerner College of Medicine, Integrated Hospital Care Institute, Cleveland, Ohio

ALEJANDRA RAZZETO, MD
Resident Physician, Division of Endocrinology, Diabetes and Metabolism, Department of Internal Medicine, University of Miami, Miller School of Medicine, Miami, Florida

JEFFREY W. REDINGER, MD
Assistant Professor, Division of General Internal Medicine, Department of Medicine, University of Washington School of Medicine, Hospital and Specialty Medicine, VA Puget Sound Healthcare System, Seattle, Washington

MICHAEL D. RUDY, MD
Assistant Professor of Medicine, Division of Hospital Medicine, Department of Internal Medicine, Director of Inpatient Medicine Consults and Co-Management Services, University of Michigan Medical School, Ann Arbor, Michigan

SUNIL K. SAHAI, MD, FACP, FAAP, SFHM
Professor and Division Chief, Division of General Internal Medicine, Department of Medicine, The University of Texas Medical Branch, Galveston, Texas

EDIE P. SHEN, MD, FHM, DFPM
Clinical Associate Professor, Division of General Internal Medicine, University of Washington, Hospital Medicine, Seattle, Washington

JASON F. SHIFFERMILLER, MD, MPH
Associate Professor, Division of Hospital Medicine, Department of Internal Medicine, University of Nebraska Medical Center, Omaha, Nebraska

ALANA SIGMUND, MD
Assistant Professor of Clinical Medicine, Weill Medical College of Cornell University, Medical Director, Arthroplasty Hospital for Special Surgery, New York, New York

BARBARA A. SLAWSKI, MD, MS
Professor, Chief of Hospital Medicine, Division of General Internal Medicine, Department of Medicine, Medical College of Wisconsin, The Hub for Collaborative Medicine, Milwaukee, Wisconsin

MARCIO ROTTA SOARES, MD
Assistant Professor of Clinical Medicine, Division Chief of Geriatrics, Palliative and Hospital Medicine, University of Miami Miller School of Medicine, Miami, Florida

ANNA VON, MD
Assistant Professor of Medicine, Department of Internal Medicine, Emory University School of Medicine, Atlanta, Georgia

CHRISTOPHER WHINNEY, MD, FACP, SFHM
Clinical Assistant Professor of Medicine, Department of Hospital Medicine, Cleveland Clinic Lerner College of Medicine, Integrated Hospital Care Institute, Cleveland Clinic, Cleveland, Ohio

STEVEN J. WILSON, MD
Assistant Professor of Medicine, Department of Internal Medicine, University of Michigan Medical School, Ann Arbor, Michigan

Contents

antithrombotic options available, an appropriate prophylaxis strategy can be employed.

For patients considering surgery, the preoperative evaluation allows physicians to identify and treat acute cardiac conditions before less-urgent surgery, predict the benefits and harms of a proposed surgery, and make temporary management changes to reduce operative risk. Multiple risk prediction tools are reasonable for use in estimating perioperative cardiac risk, but management changes to reduce risk have proven elusive. For all but the most urgent surgical procedures, patients with active coronary syndromes or decompensated heart failure should have surgery postponed.

Frequently, the question of whether or not a patient is stable for surgery boils down to the question, "Does this patient need a preoperative stress test?" However, coronary artery disease and ischemic heart disease are only some of the many cardiac conditions that patients present with preoperatively—and that can negatively impact their intraoperative management and postoperative outcomes. This article will explore the evidence based, patient centered best practices surrounding the perioperative evaluation and management of heart failure, arrhythmias, and valvular heart disease.

Peri-operative anemia is a common condition encountered in adult surgical patients. It is increasingly recognized as a predictor of post-operative morbidity and mortality. Evaluation and treatment of anemia pre-operatively can reduce transfusion needs and potentially improve outcomes in surgical patients. This article discusses anemia optimization strategies in peri-operative setting with special focus on use of intravenous iron therapy. Additionally, the authors describe the role of transfusion medicine and best practices around red blood cell, platelet, and plasma transfusions.

Pulmonary complications are very common after noncardiac surgery and can be easily overlooked. If not properly screened for or evaluated these can in many instances lead to postoperative respiratory failure or even death. Decisions regarding ambulatory versus inpatient surgery, modality of anesthesia, protective ventilation and method of weaning, type of analgesia, and postoperative monitoring can be crucial to avoid such complications.

Historically and for ease of classification, the geriatric patient has received a chronologic definition of a person 65 years and older. Chronologic age remains an independent risk of postoperative complications and adverse surgical outcomes. Frailty is an expression of an individual's biological age and as such a more reliable determination of their vulnerabilities or re-silience to stress. The concept of prehabilitation has shown promise as a proactive approach to optimize a patient's functional, cognitive, nutri-tional, and emotional in preparation for surgical interventions. Postopera-tive delirium is the most common neuropsychological complication after surgery.

Perioperative risks associated with acute hepatitis, cirrhosis, and chronic kidney disease are substantial and prevalence of underlying chronic kid-ney or liver disease is rising; surgeries in these populations have accord-ingly become more common. Optimal perioperative management in both cases is paramount; this article focuses on understanding disease patho-physiology, a targeted preoperative evaluation, accurate estimation of perioperative risk, and anticipation and management of common postop-erative complications.

Medication management in the perioperative period is a critical part of the decision-making prior to surgery. While randomized trial levels of evidence in this space are scant, retrospective data and expert consensus provide practical guidance for these decisions. Clinicians must understand risks and benefits of withholding versus continuing medications, stop medica-tions based on pharmacokinetics and effect on primary disease and surgi-cal risk, and resume medications after surgery in a timely manner. Knowing alternate routes of medication administration can help keep chronic dis-ease processes stable through surgery.

Hip fractures are a frequent cause of hospitalization in the elderly popula-tion and can lead to significant morbidity and mortality. As the population continues to age, the incidence of hip fractures is expected to increase. The internist/hospitalist plays a critical role in the care of this population as many patients have multiple medical comorbidities. Management of the fragility hip fracture patient requires knowledge of several perioperative topics including preoperative risk assessment, risk reduction strategies, the optimal timing of surgical repair, venous thromboembolism prevention, and postoperative care considerations such as early mobilization with physical therapy, and osteoporosis treatment.

Win M. Aung and Sunil K. Sahai

The preoperative care of patients with cancer plays a pivotal role in ensuring optimal outcomes and enhancing the overall quality of life for individuals undergoing surgical interventions. This review aims to provide a comprehensive overview of the key considerations, challenges, and strategies involved in the preoperative management of oncology patients. We delve into the multidisciplinary approach required to address the unique needs of this patient population, emphasizing the importance of collaboration among surgeons, oncologists, anesthesiologists, primary care physicians, hospitalists, and other health care professionals.

Carlos E. Mendez, Jason F. Shiffermiller, Alejandra Razzeto, and Zeina Hannoush

Patients with hyperglycemia, thyroid dysfunction, and adrenal insufficiency face increased perioperative risk, which may be mitigated by appropriate management. This review addresses preoperative glycemic control, makes evidence-based recommendations for the increasingly complex perioperative management of noninsulin diabetes medications, and provides guideline-supported strategies for the perioperative management of insulin, including suggested indications for continuous intravenous insulin. The authors propose a strategy for determining when surgery should be delayed in patients with thyroid dysfunction and present a matrix for managing perioperative stress dose corticosteroids based on the limited evidence available.

Heather E. Nye, Edie P. Shen, and Furheen Baig

Surgery under anesthesia poses a significant stress to the body, and postoperative complications occur in up to 20% of cases. An understanding of postoperative complications, including assessment of patients at risk, risk mitigation, early recognition, and evidence-based treatment, is essential to provide high-value health care. Common postoperative complications reviewed in this article include fever, cerebrovascular accident, nausea and vomiting, ileus, and urinary retention, including discussion of pathophysiology, prevention, and treatment.

Foreword

Perioperative and Consultative Medicine: A Religious Experience

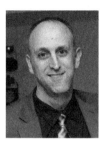

Daniel D. Dressler, MD, MSc, MHM, FACP
Consulting Editor

It has been more than 40 years since Goldman and Rudd[1] introduced the original "Ten Commandments for Effective Consultation" and almost 20 years since an update in these items.[2] For primary care physicians, hospitalists, and subspecialty physicians, most of those tenets have stood the test of time (**Table 1**) and have led to greater communication between surgeons and consulting physicians, collaborative care and care comanagement, and highly valuable research and quality improvement initiatives that have improved patient care and outcomes in the perioperative setting.

Over this last half-century, we have come a long way in reducing unnecessary preoperative testing and using patient-centered approaches to target necessary testing. Nevertheless, there is still opportunity to reduce testing variation across the country.[3] We now use evidence to reduce unnecessary bridging of anticoagulation when we stop those medications preprocedure.[4,5] We now save lives and reduce postoperative morbidity by limiting transfusions when expected blood loss occurs; however, some types of surgery or patients with active acute coronary syndromes might dictate nuanced approaches.[6] We can more effectively reduce postoperative delirium in elderly patients and other patients with frailty.[7] We emulate our leaders and pioneers in perioperative care comanagement.[8] We optimize care and mitigate risk in patients with individualized needs, including those with medical conditions that might otherwise preclude surgical care.

Dr Manjarrez and his esteemed colleagues have assembled a world-class summary of the key aspects of medical consultation and the comanagement of clinical care in the perioperative setting. They have made this care a religious experience. Our surgical colleagues, their patients, and our patients will benefit from the expertise and resources included within this compendium.

Med Clin N Am 108 (2024) xv–xvii
https://doi.org/10.1016/j.mcna.2024.08.005
0025-7125/24/© 2024 Published by Elsevier Inc.

Table 1
Ten tenets of medical consultation (modified for 2025)

Original Tenet[1,2,a]	2025 Consultant Action
Determine the question	• Clarify the question(s) being posed. Respond to specific questions when asked
Establish urgency	• Determine whether the requested consultation is emergent, urgent, or elective and respond within an appropriate timeframe based on the request
Look for yourself	• Gather data independently of what is reported by primary team(s)
Be as brief as appropriate	• The consultant should document relevant data for decision making and recommendations but need not exhaustively repeat all data previously recorded
Be specific and thorough	• Leave specific recommendations to answer the question(s) posed by the primary team and do not ignore relevant items that might not have been asked • Leave a prioritized list of recommendations
Provide contingency plans	• Anticipate potential problems and document contingency plans • Maintain availability to assist with carrying out the recommended plans, when needed or requested
Comanage when appropriate or requested[a]	• Comanage aspects of patient care when a primary physician requests, and offer to take responsibility to manage aspects of care within the consultant's realm of expertise that falls clearly outside of the requesting physician's realm of expertise • Open communication and discussion between consultant and primary clinicians should delineate clearly who is managing which aspects of care
Teach with tact and pragmatism	• Consultants can actively share their expertise and (when appropriate) literature evidence supporting their recommendations with requesting clinicians • Use judgment to tailor the communication strategy (eg, verbal vs electronic messaging vs chart documentation vs offering references, and so forth) based on various relevant factors (eg, urgency of consultation, and requesting clinician's specialty and level of training)
Talk is cheap, effective, and essential	• There is no substitute for direct personal contact with the primary clinician. Prioritize verbal communication whenever possible, even when the consultant has already clearly documented recommendations in the electronic record or transmitted them by other electronic means
Follow up with appropriate frequency	• Follow up as frequently as appropriate, as dictated by the clinical situation (which might be multiple times per day; daily; or less frequently) • Document each follow-up interaction • Clearly delineate in the chart when your next follow-up will occur, especially if it is not anticipated to be at least daily • When the patient's problems that prompted the consultation request are no longer active, the consultant can sign off (at times with discussion with the primary team), document the sign off in the medical record, and remain available for reconsultation if/when needed

[a] With some slight modifications.

We define religion as an institutionalized system of attitudes, beliefs, and practices. We as medical consultants will practice the religion of perioperative consultation and comanagement, based on high-quality literature evidence—and not just beliefs—that will help us support optimal outcomes for so many patients in this sometimes-high-risk clinical setting.

Daniel D. Dressler, MD, MSc, MHM, FACP
Emory University Hospital
1364 Clifton Road Northeast
Atlanta, GA 30322, USA

E-mail address:
ddressl@emory.edu

REFERENCES

1. Goldman L, Lee T, Rudd P. Ten commandments for effective consultations. Arch Intern Med 1983;143(9):1753–5.
2. Salerno SM, Hurst FP, Halvorson S, et al. Principles of effective consultation: an update for the 21st-century consultant. Arch Intern Med 2007;167:271–5.
3. Columbo JA, Scali ST, Neal D, et al. Increased preoperative stress test utilization is not associated with reduced adverse cardiac events in current US surgical practice. Ann Surg 2023;278:621.
4. Douketis JD, Spyropoulos AC, Murad MH, et al. Executive summary. Perioperative management of antithrombotic therapy: an American College of Chest Physicians clinical practice guideline. Chest 2022;162:1127–39.
5. Douketis JD, Spyropoulos AC, Murad MH, et al. Perioperative management of antithrombotic therapy: an American College of Chest Physicians clinical practice guideline. Chest 2022;162:e207–43.
6. Hovaguimian F, Myles PS. Restrictive versus liberal transfusion strategy in the perioperative and acute care settings: a context-specific systematic review and meta-analysis of randomized controlled trials. Anesthesiology 2016;125:46–61.
7. Kim DH, Lee SB, Park CM, et al. Comparative safety analysis of oral antipsychotics for in-hospital adverse clinical events in older adults after major surgery: a nationwide cohort study. Ann Intern Med 2023;176:1153–62.
8. Huddleston JM, Long KH, Naessens JM, et al. Medical and surgical comanagement after elective hip and knee arthroplasty: a randomized, controlled trial. Ann Intern Med 2004;141(1):28–38.

Preface

Perioperative Medicine Front and Center

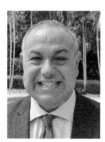

Efrén C. Manjarrez, MD, SFHM, FACP
Editor

Worldwide, there are over 200 million noncardiac surgeries performed annually.[1] Since the landmark article by Goldman and colleagues[2] in the late 1970s to characterize cardiac risk associated with noncardiac surgery, researchers have made significant gains to identify vulnerable patients and minimize perioperative risk. The American College of Cardiology (ACC) has subsequently given us multiple editions of perioperative cardiac guidelines.[3] The field of perioperative medicine was born, and the research has blossomed to encompass many other organ systems. Office-based internists and hospitalists have noticed. At the Society of Hospital Medicine CONVERGE Annual Meetings, perioperative medicine lectures are among the most well attended. Along with cardiologists, surgeons, and anesthesiologists, hospitalists and office-based internists also have become many of the scholars of this field. Many are contributors to this issue.

Despite innovations in surgical technique (now minimally invasive, robotic, and ambulatory), anesthesia, risk assessment, risk reduction, state-of-the-art perioperative monitoring, and innovations in care, like Enhanced Recovery After Surgery (ERAS) bundles,[4,5] surgery is still associated with significant morbidity and mortality for at-risk patients.

In this issue, senior leaders in the field of perioperative medicine collaborate with emerging authors. The purpose is to bring office-based internists, hospitalists, advanced practice providers, resident physicians, and the entire perioperative team up-to-date with current best practices in perioperative care in a streamlined manner. All authors supplement their articles with tables, diagrams, and algorithms to facilitate learning and streamline clinical care. The issue covers perioperative medicine by organ system. The issue walks readers through elements of excellent preoperative consults and targeted preoperative testing. Other articles include updated practice guidelines, risk predictors by organ systems, and risk reduction strategies, prophylaxis, nuances

Med Clin N Am 108 (2024) xix–xx
https://doi.org/10.1016/j.mcna.2024.07.002
0025-7125/24/© 2024 Published by Elsevier Inc.

of perioperative medication management, frailty and prehabilitation, and selected postoperative complications. We include a unique discussion of two special patient populations with unique needs—the hip fracture patient and the cancer patient going for surgery. New to readers may be how to rethink how we assess preoperative functional capacity (eg, the DASI score) and implications for perioperative risk assessment and Myocardial Injury after Noncardiac Surgery (MINS).

This issue is not meant to be a comprehensive textbook. Rather, it serves to give focused, targeted advice to the reader in high-yield relevant topics impacting care in 2024. Importantly, this issue does not include a discussion on the emerging aspects of perioperative care of COVID-19, nor could it incorporate the recommendations of the forthcoming ACC's Guideline on Perioperative Evaluation and Management of Noncardiac Surgery, whose publication was delayed until late 2024. Rather, specific to cardiology, authors took the prior ACC guidelines of 2014, the more recent Canadian and European guidelines, and reported on the high-yield research since published for guidance on risk assessment and risk reduction. Readers are advised to stay tuned to the ACC guidelines still in press.

It is my hope that this issue guides the reader and the entire perioperative team to achieve high-quality perioperative care with superior outcomes.

FUNDING

No Funding.

Efrén C. Manjarrez, MD, SFHM, FACP
Division of Hospital Medicine
University of Miami
Miller School of Medicine
Miami, FL 33136, USA

E-mail address:
emanjarrez@med.miami.edu

REFERENCES

1. Weiser TG, Haynes AB, Molina G, et al. Estimate of the global volume of surgery in 2012: an assessment supporting improved health outcomes. Lancet 2015; 385(Suppl 2):S11.
2. Goldman L, Caldera DL, Nussbaum SR, et al. Multifactorial index of cardiac risk in noncardiac surgical procedures. N Engl J Med 1977;297(16):845–50.
3. Fleisher LA, Fleischmann KE, Auerbach AD, et al. 2014 ACC/AHA guideline on perioperative cardiovascular evaluation and management of patients undergoing noncardiac surgery: a report of the American College of Cardiology/American Heart Association Task Force on practice guidelines. J Am Coll Cardiol 2014; 64(22):e77–137.
4. Wainwright TW, Gill M, McDonald DA, et al. Consensus statement for perioperative care in total hip replacement and total knee replacement surgery: Enhanced Recovery After Surgery (ERAS®) Society recommendations. Acta Orthop 2020; 91(1):3–19.
5. Frassanito L, Vergari A, Nestorini R, et al. Enhanced recovery after surgery (ERAS) in hip and knee replacement surgery: description of a multidisciplinary program to improve management of the patients undergoing major orthopedic surgery. Musculoskelet Surg 2020;104(1):87–92.

Medical Consultation and Comanagement

Rebecca C. Engels, MD, MPH[a,*], Catriona M. Harrop, MD, SFHM[b],
Lily L. Ackermann, MD[c]

KEYWORDS

- Consultative medicine • Surgical comanagement • Medical comanagement

KEY POINTS

- Effective medical consultations involve determining the question asked, establishing the urgency of the consultation, gathering primary data, communicating as briefly as appropriate, making specific recommendations, providing contingency plans, understanding one's role in the process, offering educational information, communicating recommendations directly to the requesting physician, and providing appropriate follow-up.
- Comanagement shifts the dynamic to more of a shared responsibility and accountability for patient care across specialties and can involve a more proactive approach to patient care as opposed to a reactive approach.
- With the rise in popularity of hospitalists and the recognition of improved outcomes associated with their care, surgical comanagement models have increased.
- Successful comanagement models have clear champions and stakeholders from each service involved in the arrangement to identify service-specific obstacles and challenges, clarify roles and responsibilities, address financial issues with help from hospital leadership, decide on metrics for quality improvement and performance measurement, and engage other stakeholders such as physical therapy, nutrition, nursing, other subspecialists, and hospital leadership.

INTRODUCTION

One of the most complex periods in a patient's hospital stay is the perioperative period. It is the time before, during, and after a given surgical procedure.[1] It is defined in 3 phases: preoperative, operative, and postoperative. Both the Accreditation Council for Graduate Medical Education (ACGME) and the American Board of Internal Medicine (ABIM) require training in perioperative medicine.[2] In many settings nationally, hospitalists run perioperative programs that consist of an evaluation prior to a

a Department of Medicine, The Johns Hopkins University School of Medicine, 600 North Wolfe Street, Meyer 8-134D, Baltimore, MD 21247, USA; b Department of Medicine, Sidney Kimmel Medical College at Thomas Jefferson University, 1101 Market Street, Suite 19069, Philadelphia, PA 19107, USA; c Department of Medicine, Sidney Kimmel Medical College at Thomas Jefferson University, 1025 Walnut Street, Suite 801 College Building, Philadelphia, PA 19107, USA
* Corresponding author. 600 North Wolfe Street, Meyer 8, Baltimore, MD 21287.
E-mail address: rengels2@jh.edu

Med Clin N Am 108 (2024) 993–1004
https://doi.org/10.1016/j.mcna.2024.04.012   medical.theclinics.com

procedure as well as providing postoperative care alongside the surgical team. Perioperative care has become such an integral part of hospital medicine that since 2006, it is considered a core competency by the Society of Hospital Medicine (SHM). In its latest update, the SHM stated, "Optimal care for the surgical patient is realized with a team approach that coordinates the hospitalist and the surgical team's expertise."[3]

The coordination of care between the surgeon, anesthesiologist, primary care provider, and hospitalist during the perioperative period is the basis of comanagement and is rooted in the fundamental skill of medical consultation.

DISCUSSION
Medical Consultation

In 1983, Goldman and colleagues[4] proposed the first framework for medical consultation entitled "Ten Commandments for Effective Consultations." In brief, the commandments for best practices are to determine the question asked, establish the urgency of the consultation, gather primary data, communicate as briefly as appropriate, make specific recommendations, provide contingency plans, understand one's role in the process, offer educational information, communicate recommendations directly to the requesting physician, and provide appropriate follow-up.[5]

However, since these guidelines were published, there has been an exponential growth in the complexity of medical decision-making, testing, and treatment. As our population ages, patients are living longer with an increasing number of comorbidities. These complex medical issues require an active role in the comprehensive care of the patient, a comanager, rather than the more passive consultant role.[6] Surgeons have increased productivity demands, and there is a high projected cost of surgery and surgical-related complications.[6–8]

Based on the changing landscape, survey responses from both internists and surgeons resulted in an update published in 2007.[6] Updated recommendations included increased verbal communication, asking how the referring physician can help rather than trying to define a specific question and defining if there is a need for comanagement relationship rather than if a specific question is desired.[6,9] Since the 1983, editorial subsequent literature outlined that establishing the reason for consultation can encompass a variety of topics such as seeking medical optimization, commenting on surgical risk, or seeking management of medical issues in the perioperative period.[6,10] Ideally, direct closed-loop verbal communication between the requesting service to clarify the question and scope of involvement is considered best practice.[10]

There has been a paradigm shift in place of a request for surgical "clearance" instead addresses an overall global preoperative evaluation to identify factors that place patients at a high risk for the procedure.[5,6,10] The consult should comment on patient's overall risk for the specific surgery, if there are any further treatment or tests to help mitigate perioperative risk, prevention of complications such as thromboembolism or infection, perioperative medication management, and any specific medical comorbidities that should be discussed with the anesthesiologist.[10] In general, office-based internists and hospitalists should discuss any anesthetic concerns, such as cardiac or pulmonary with the anesthesiologist rather than commenting on the specific anesthetic plan given this is beyond the scope of an internist.[5,10] Most importantly, especially for patients at increased risk, the overall medical risks and measures to help reduce those risks should be discussed with the patient, other consultants involved, the surgeon, and the anesthesiologist preferably in a multidisciplinary discussion.[5,10] The focus of the pre-op visit should be on time-sensitive medical optimization for the surgical procedure and mitigation of perioperative risk while avoiding unnecessary testing.[10]

Make recommendations brief. Compliance with recommendations is also thought to be one measure of the effectiveness of a consultation.[5,10] A multivariate analysis demonstrated increased adherence to consultant recommendations when there were 5 or fewer recommendations, increased severity of patient illness, and recommendations involving medication management.[5,10,11]

The medical consultant should establish the urgency of the consultation from the beginning. All consults should be performed within 24 hours and all urgent consults should be seen as soon as possible.[5,10] Other elements that make a consultation successful include a brief response time, specific, focused and definitive recommendations, specifying which recommendations were critical, and verbally communicated recommendations were felt to improve compliance.[5,10–15]

A more patient-centered approach to the original 10 commandments of consultation (**Table 1**) is provided by Nye and includes not only determining why a consult is called but also identifying ways and preemptively acting to prevent patient deterioration.[9] Best practices include not only establishing the team's urgency, but once a chart has been reviewed, the consultant should also establish their own urgency as the surgical team may not have identified other active issues.[9] Once it is determined that action needs to be taken more quickly, and it is incumbent as a consultant to act.

Key elements

1. Contingency plans with both written and verbal communication should be provided and documented in the chart.[5,9,10]

Table 1 Ten commandments of consultation	
Revised Commandments of Consultation	**Comments**
Determine the question	Still go the extra mile and look at the patient as a whole
Establish surgical team urgency	Always look in the chart to establish your urgency
Be specific	Discrete instructions, specify exact dose, timing
Provide contingency plans, if/then statements	Be clear with instructions
Relay recommendations	Use written and verbal communication, reach out to the attending and reach out to other consultants
Explain your thinking	Make your consult a teachable moment to empower the consulting teams
Follow-up, comment on any studies/ laboratories you have recommended	Ask the team why recommendations were not followed if they were not
Leave daily notes, even if brief	A daily note can help teams know that you are active in care
Be clear when signing off	Let the team know you are signing off, leave a number to call for quest ions
Arrange outpatient follow-up	Subspecialty care follow-up can be difficult, work with other consultants to arrange this, and arrange follow-up with primary care providers

Adapted from Salerno et al, Arch Intern Med. 2007;167(3):271-275. 2007, Nye H. "Hospitalists as Consultants", ACP 2023 Internal Medicine Meeting.

2. Ensure that any critical information is communicated directly to an attending, and it is important to have direct communication especially if concerns are not being relayed.[9]

3. The thought process should be explained and consults should be made into teachable moments by empowering those consulting you to know the first few steps to help build an appreciation of what to do when a consultant is not readily available.[9]

4. Consistent daily progress notes and comment on all recommended diagnostics—even if laboratories are normal—are an important part of building a relationship with the consulting service.[5,9,10]

5. Leave 24/7 contact information when rotating off service and help arrange for outpatient follow-up.

Poor communication harms the consult relationship and ultimately patient outcomes. Consults fail where there is noncontiguous care and unclear lines of responsibility. Care is provided at various times during the day with limited opportunity for synchronous interaction. In a 10 year survey of malpractice claims, closed-loop communication failures were found to be the root of 70% of sentinel events.[16] Claims with communication failures were significantly less likely to be dropped, denied, or dismissed than claims without (54% vs 67%, $P = .015$). Nearly 47% of claims involved provider–provider miscommunication. The information types most frequently miscommunicated were contingency plans, diagnosis, and illness severity. Forty percent of communication failures involved a failed handoff; the majority could potentially have been averted by using a handoff tool (77%). Mean total costs for cases involving communication failures were higher ($237,600 vs $154,100, $P = .005$).[16] Another retrospective review of 498 malpractice claims from 2001 to 2011 identified communication failures in 49% of claims, with about 53% due to failure to communicate to the patient, 47% due to provider to provider miscommunications, and 40% occurring during handoffs.[17] Claims with communication failures cost more and were significantly less likely to be dropped, denied, or dismissed, and contingency plans, diagnosis, and illness severity were the most common miscommunications.[17] Given the large number of communications in hospital medicine, strategic and specific tools to mitigate communication failures are included later (**Table 2**).[18–20]

Collaboration with Anesthesia

Internists and hospitalists need to consider anesthesia as a partner and direct customer when performing their preoperative medical consultation. The specialty of perioperative medicine can involve anesthesiologists, hospitalists, surgeons, primary care physicians, medical subspecialists, or geriatricians. It is important to recognize the partnership with anesthesiologists as perioperative physicians who specialize in the preoperative, intraoperative, and postoperative care of patients undergoing

Table 2 Communication strategies and tools	
Strategies	**Specific Tools**
Clear delineation of responsibility	Checklists
Service agreements on expectations	Structured handoff tools (SBAR, IPASS)
Continuity of care providers	
Multidisciplinary rounds	
Set an expectation for direct communication	

Adapted from Nye H. "Hospitalists as Consultants", ACP 2023 Internal Medicine Meeting.

surgery.[21] Anesthesiologists have expertise in critical care, pain medicine, intraoperative care, and immediate postoperative recovery and care. They have led advances in enhanced recovery protocols and regional pain management techniques that have allowed multiple surgical procedures to be performed in ambulatory settings where in the past patients required inpatient stays.[22] While anesthesiologists have dramatically improved the intraoperative and immediate postoperative care outcomes, the preoperative period has traditionally belonged to internists and increasing hospitalists who are running more and more preoperative clinics.[22] Anesthesiologists rely on internist's preoperative evaluation to help optimize a patient's underlying chronic medical conditions as this falls outside of the anesthesia scope of practice. For example, anesthesiologists are not trained in titrating oral agents. They rely on internal medicine to titrate all oral medicines, such as diabetes pills, preoperatively.

Preoperative clinics involve comprehensive medical optimization with coordinated care between internists, hospitalists, anesthesiologists, and surgeons. Several studies have demonstrated the impact of optimization pathways and clinics on surgical outcomes with models involving both anesthesiologists, internists, and hospitalists.[23] Perioperative medicine is a relatively new specialty that focuses on the care of the patient before and after surgery with a multidisciplinary team that involves all physicians who are involved in the medical management of the patient during this specific time period.[24] **Box 1** outlines the recommendations for useful information to include in a preoperative evaluation.[25] Internists provide great value to the entire multidisciplinary team when a preoperative evaluation contains key information that helps inform the surgical and anesthetic plan.

Enhanced Recovery Pathway

The Enhanced Recovery After Surgery protocol was developed by a group of academic surgeons in Europe in 2001 to develop a multidisciplinary team to improve recovery postoperatively. Emphasis is on a multimodal, multidisciplinary approach to the surgical patient with a team consisting of surgeons, anesthetists, and other physicians involved in surgical care. Office-based internists and hospitalists would do well to familiarize themselves with these quality metrics on which surgeons focus. Key elements (**Table 3**) include evidence-based changes such as overnight fasting to carbohydrate drinks 2 hours before surgery, minimally invasive, careful management of fluids to maintain balance rather than large volumes of intravenous fluids, avoidance of or early removal of drains and tubes, early mobilization, and oral intake the day of the operation. Enhanced recovery protocols have resulted in a 30% to 50% reduced length of stay and complications, while readmissions and costs are reduced.[26,27]

Medical Consultation Versus Comanagement

As outlined earlier, in the traditional medical consult model, a service will ask a hospitalist a specific question, such as preoperative evaluations or how to manage hyponatremia. Identifying appropriate patients for medical consultation as well as the scope of involvement of the internist remains the responsibility of the primary service. The hospitalist has the responsibility of making sure it is an effective consult, but the requesting service essentially maintains all components of a patient's care, including placing the orders as recommended by the consultant. However, in a paradigm shift, a study of 323 physicians at 3 academic medical centers demonstrated a divergence of opinion between surgeons and internists.[6] Surgeons desired more involvement from internists with a comanagement relationship and consults that are not limited to a specific question. This differed from internists' opinions where they felt consultants should not be writing orders and that curbside consults were acceptable. This is a new

---

Box 1
Useful information to include in preoperative consults

Useful Information to Include in Preoperative Consults[a]

How to preoperatively optimize function of an unhealthy organ system

Guidance on managing oral drug regimens:
- First-line and second-line agents
- Initial dosage and titration; recommended combinations
- How to manage side effects

Expected time until patient is optimized for the procedure if abovementioned management is followed

Tests that might be indicated preoperatively to direct therapy to optimize function

Additional interventions indicated by the patient's disease, and appropriate timing (preoperatively, intraoperatively, and postoperatively)
- Include assurance that consultant will follow up with specified nonurgent postoperative care without prompting

Current pertinent anticoagulation recommendations

Details on coronary stents—when placed, where placed, and type (drug-eluting or bare metal)

Focused information on cardiac defibrillators and other implanted devices, specifically
- Whether patient is pacer-dependent
- Effect of magnet placement
- Has battery recently been checked?

Recommendations on intraoperative /perioperative management of
- Rare diseases
- Blood disorders, especially coagulation abnormalities
- Brittle diabetes (loading doses, optimal makeup of infusions, treatment targets)
- Endocrine disorders (eg, perioperative dosing of thyroid drugs)

Newer recommendations/data (<5 year old) on acute medical management, especially in patients with complex comorbidities

Explanations/references when recommendations deviate from accepted guidelines

Legible contact information, including an emergency phone number to ensure access prior to early morning procedures

[a] In all cases, be as specific as possible and favor quantitative over qualitative.

Adapted from Lubarsky D, Candiotti K. Giving anesthesiologists what they want: How to write a useful preoperative consult. CCJM. 2009;76(10 suppl 4):S32-S36. https://doi.org/10.3949/ccjm. 76.s4.06.

---

discovery of the value that surgeons have, where they are seeking a deeper comanagement relationship with internists and hospitalists.[9]

Comanagement shifts the dynamic to more of a shared responsibility and accountability for patient care across specialties.[28] **Table 4** outlines the main differences between consults and comanagement. Surgical comanagement models evolved primarily due to the increasing medical complexity of surgical patients considering the changing demography and prevalence of the aging population.[29]

The SHM defines comanagement as "an arrangement between a hospital medicine team and a medical subspecialty, or surgical specialty team to jointly share responsibility for the patient while hospitalized."[30] SHM published a White Paper on a guide to comanagement that outlines the key processes that are needed to ensure the successful formation of comanagement agreements.[31] Successful comanagement models have clear champions and stakeholders from each service involved in the arrangement to identify

Table 3
Elements of enhanced recovery pathway

Preoperative	Intraoperative	Postoperative
Preadmission education	Regional and epidural anesthesia	Early nutrition
Fluid and carbohydrate loading	Careful fluid balance	Multimodal pain control, avoidance of opioids, nonopioid analgesia, NSAIDs
Reduced time for fasting	Maintain normal temperature, active warming	Early mobilization
Selective bowel preparation	Short-acting anesthetics	Early catheter removal
Administer venous thromboembolism prophylaxis	Avoiding opioids	Goal for moving toward discharge
No premedication	Pain and nausea management	Avoid nasogastric tubes
Early discharge planning		Stimulate gut motility

Adapted from Ljungqvist O, Scott M, Fearon KC. Enhanced recovery after surgery: a review. JAMA Surg 2017;152(3):292. Wainwright TW, Gill M, McDonald DA, et al. Consensus statement for perioperative care in total hip replacement and total knee replacement surgery: Enhanced Recovery After Surgery (ERAS) Society recommendations. Acta Orthop 2020;91(1):3–19.

service-specific obstacles and challenges, clarify roles and responsibilities, address financial issues with help from hospital leadership, decide on metrics for quality improvement and performance measurement, set meeting timelines to monitor comanagement progress, and engage other stakeholders such as physical therapy, nutrition, nursing, other subspecialists, and hospital leadership.[28,31,32] Transparency is key in comanagement. A shared written agreement that clearly outlines the roles, responsibilities, and scope of practice of each service within the patient's care is negotiated. Clear inclusion criteria on which patients would be included in the comanagement model is also key. Provider satisfaction is also a measurable metric. Finally, a clear process for feedback needs to be in place to allow the service to evolve as inevitably will occur.

CURRENT EVIDENCE OF BENEFITS TO MEDICAL COMANAGEMENT
Surgical Comanagement

The hospitalists' model of care has demonstrated reductions in length of stay, cost, and improvement in quality metrics and is evident in both models of hospitalists as

Table 4
Comanagement and consultation

	Comanagement	Consultation
Relationship with surgery	Negotiated formal agreement	Informal, as needed
Focus	Comprehensive, prevent pre-op complications	One question, often sign off when answered
Implementation	Agreement about orders, expectation for direct verbal communication	No expectation, just recommendations
Patient selection	Predetermined criteria, pre-op clinic, screening of patients	Referral by surgery
Discharge planning	Shared	Solely surgical team

Adapted from Nye H. "Hospitalists as Consultants", ACP 2023 Internal Medicine Meeting., Cohn S. Decision Making in Perioperative Medicine: Clinical Pearls 1st edition 2022. McGraw Hill. New York.

comanagers and as the primary attending.[33] In a surgical comanagement model, advantages include prevention of complications, early diagnosis, and management of medical complications both preoperative and postoperative.[33,34] Over time on a comanagement service, hospitalists gain specialized knowledge of the patients, procedures, and expected postoperative complications and form a partnership with surgeons.[33,34] For example, with intricate knowledge of procedures and close communication with the surgical team, hospitalists can effectively manage complex anticoagulation questions in the perioperative period, individualize pain control in those at high risk of delirium, and effectively manage complications such as anemia and effective fluid management in perioperative heart and renal failure.[33,34]

Hospitalists in a comanagement arrangement may recognize, predict, and mitigate problems associated with medical comorbidities unrecognized by the surgical team. They can offer advice on preoperative optimization andif surgery should be delayed for further treatment of active medical comorbidities.[33] More importantly, in those with significant comorbidities, they are able to help facilitate a discussion in a shared decision-making process to discuss the benefits and risks of surgery in relation to patient goals.[33,34] At a hospital level, hospitalists are able to implement evidence-based guidelines such as establishing order sets for medical issues to ensure best practices, coordinate other specialist consultations, contribute to multidisciplinary quality improvement, and identify and address barriers to discharge.[29,31,35,36] Hospitalists are able to work effectively with nursing, physical and occupational therapy, and social work to provide proactive care coordination to reduce length of stay.[29,31,35]

Surgical Comanagement Studies with Benefits

Multiple studies have shown a benefit in comanagement models across surgical fields (**Table 5**). Orthopedic surgery was the first surgical specialty to embrace proactive physician involvement in routine care and has a significant number of studies demonstrating benefit.[37] A 2015 meta-analysis of randomized clinical trials for patients with hip fracture concluded that a comprehensive geriatric care model was associated with greater functional improvement and an increased proportion of patients discharged back to their prior place of residence but found no significant difference in mortality or length of stay.[37]

Surgical Comanagement Studies Without Benefit

In contrast, the evidence supporting hospitalist involvement in the routine perioperative care of adults undergoing surgery, including younger adults, is limited (**Table 6**).

Table 5 Studies with benefits	
Surgery Type	**Studies with Benefit**
Orthopedic surgery (hip fracture and neurosurgery spine, geriatric populations)	Decreased time to consultation, decreased time to surgery, decreased length of stay, decreased hospital cost, fewer numbers of consultants, decreased complications, fewer rapid response calls[25,32,37–39,45,46]
Vascular surgery	Decreased rates of complications, decreased pain, decreased mortality[40]
Colorectal surgery	Decreased length of stay, decreased ICU transfers, decreased medical consultation[41]
Otolaryngology	Reduction in length of stay and cost[42]

Table 6 Studies without benefits	
Surgery Type	**Studies Without Benefit**
General surgical patients	No benefit[30,33,34,43,44]
Orthopedic surgery Neurosurgery	No benefit[37,47]
Geriatric hip fracture	Higher morbidity and mortality, but many not in a dedicated hip fracture program[48]

Patient selection for comanagement is important and when selecting a comanagement service, identifying high-risk patient groups to intervene on with a comanagement model likely will show the greatest impact.[28] Two different studies of hospitalist surgical comanagement models at the same institution demonstrated different outcomes based on the patient population.[28] Hospitalist comanagement in healthier elective joint surgery patients reduced minor complications (such as incidence of urinary tract infections, fever, and hyponatremia) but had no effect on moderate or major complications such as myocardial infarction, pulmonary embolism, or pneumonia.[38] However, in geriatric hip fracture patients who have a greater number of comorbidities, higher operative risk, and require urgent surgical procedures have a greater benefit from comanagement. Hospitalist comanagement of hip fracture patients decreased time to surgery and lowered length of stay by 2.2 days.[39]

SUMMARY

Hospital medicine grew exponentially since its inception given the pressures office-based internists faced, and with it came a group of providers that excelled at providing safe, high-value, and high-quality care in the perioperative setting. Overall, consultative medicine aims to answer specific questions regarding certain aspects of a patient's care. Consultative medicine represented a more reactive approach to care, responding to issues as they arose. As patients undergoing surgeries became on average older and more medically complex, the paradigm shifted from simple consultation to comanagement models evolved to provide a more thorough and proactive approach to patient care. Hospitalists made an ideal partner for office-based internists, surgeons, and anesthesiologists in caring for these patients. Outcomes of comanagement services are mixed, likely related to the variability with how they can be structured. A successful comanagement model involves a thoughtful and detailed approach involving multiple stakeholders and appropriate delineation of roles and responsibilities as they relate to patient care.

CLINICS CARE POINTS

- Effective medical consultation involves a patient-centered approach with clear and consistent communication.

- Preoperative evaluations should comment on a patient's optimization for a procedure rather than clearance for a procedure, and anesthesiology should be viewed as a key partner in these consults.

- Comanagement services create a shared responsibility for patient care between internists and surgical specialties to help better predict and mitigate adverse outcomes related to medical comorbidities.

DISCLOSURES

The authors have nothing to disclose.

REFERENCES

1. Davrieux CF, Palermo M, Serra E, et al. Stages and factors of the "perioperative process": points in common with the aeronautical industry. ABCD, arq bras cir dig 2019;32(1):e1423.
2. Raslau D, Kasten MJ, Kebede E, et al. Developing a comprehensive perioperative education curriculum for internal medicine residency training. J Educ Perioper Med 2017;19(3):E608.
3. Nichani S, Brooks ME, Fitterman N, et al. The core competencies in hospital medicine—clinical conditions 2023 update. J Hosp Med 2023;18(S2).
4. Goldman L, Lee T, Rudd P. Ten commandments for effective consultations. Arch Intern Med 1983;143(9):1753–5.
5. Cohn SL, editor. Decision making in perioperative medicine: clinical Pearls. New York: McGraw Hill; 2021.
6. Salerno SM, Hurst FP, Halvorson S, et al. Principles of effective consultation: an update for the 21st-century consultant. Arch Intern Med 2007;167(3):271–5.
7. Whinney C, Michota F. Surgical comanagement: A natural evolution of hospitalist practice. J Hosp Med 2008;3(5):394–7.
8. Jaffer AK, Michota F. Why perioperative medicine matters more than ever. Cleve Clin J Med 2006;73(Supplement 1):S1.
9. Nye H. Hospitalists as consultants: best communication practices in a team-based care approach. San Diego, CA: Presented at: American College of Physicians Conference; 2023.
10. Cohn SL. Overview of the principles of medical consultation and perioperative medicine. In: Post T, editor. Wolters Kluwer.
11. Ballard WP, Gold JP, Charlson ME. Compliance with the recommendations of medical consultants. J Gen Intern Med 1986;1(4):220–4.
12. Pupa LE, Coventry JA, Hanley JF, et al. Factors affecting compliance for general medicine consultations to non-internists. Am J Med 1986;81(3):508–14.
13. Ferguson RP, Rubinstien E. Preoperative medical consultations in a community hospital. J Gen Intern Med 1987;2(2):89–92.
14. Sears CL, Charlson ME. The effectiveness of a consultation. Compliance with initial recommendations. Am J Med 1983;74(5):870–6.
15. Lee T, Pappius EM, Goldman L. Impact of inter-physician communication on the effectiveness of medical consultations. Am J Med 1983;74(1):106–12.
16. Zwarenstein M, Reeves S. Working together but apart: barriers and routes to nurse–physician collaboration. Jt Comm J Qual Improv 2002;28(5):242–7, 209.
17. Humphrey KE, Sundberg M, Milliren CE, et al. Frequency and nature of communication and handoff failures in medical malpractice claims. J Patient Saf 2022; 18(2):130–7.
18. Nagpal K, Vats A, Ahmed K, et al. A systematic quantitative assessment of risks associated with poor communication in surgical care. Arch Surg 2010;145(6): 582–8.
19. Bougeard AM, Watkins B. Transitions of care in the perioperative period - a review. Clin Med 2019;19(6):446–9.
20. Starmer AJ, Spector ND, O'Toole JK, et al. Implementation of the I PASS handoff program in diverse clinical environments: A multicenter prospective effectiveness implementation study. J Hosp Med 2023;18(1):5–14.

21. Pfeifer K, Ahn K, Kain ZN. Anesthesiologists and hospitalists in perioperative care: together we are stronger. Anesth Analg 2022;134(3):463–5.
22. Hepner D, Harrop CM, Whinney C, et al. Pro-con debate: anesthesiologist- versus hospitalist- run preoperative clinics and perioperative care. Anesth Analg 2022;134(3):466–74.
23. Kain ZN, Vakharia S, Garson L, et al. The perioperative surgical home as a future perioperative practice model. Anesth Analg 2014;118(5):1126–30.
24. Al-Shammari L, Douglas D, Gunaratnam G, et al. Perioperative medicine: a new model of care? Br J Hosp Med 2017;78(11):628–32.
25. Lubarsky D, Candiotti K. Giving anesthesiologists what they want: How to write a useful preoperative consult. CCJM 2009;76(10 suppl 4):S32–6.
26. Ljungqvist O, Scott M, Fearon KC. Enhanced recovery after surgery: a review. JAMA Surg 2017;152(3):292.
27. Wainwright TW, Gill M, McDonald DA, et al. Consensus statement for periopera- tive care in total hip replacement and total knee replacement surgery: Enhanced Recovery After Surgery (ERAS ®) Society recommendations. Acta Orthop 2020; 91(1):3–19.
28. Siegal EM. Just because you can, doesn't mean that you should: A call for the rational application of hospitalist comanagement. J Hosp Med 2008;3(5): 398–402.
29. Fierbințeanu-Braticevici C, Raspe M, Preda AL, et al. Medical and surgical co- management – A strategy of improving the quality and outcomes of perioperative care. Eur J Intern Med 2019;61:44–7.
30. *Society of* Hospital Medicine's State of Hospital Medicine Report. Philadelphia, PA: Society of Hospital Medicine; 2023.
31. Thompson RE, Pfeifer K, Grant PJ, et al. Hospital medicine and perioperative care: a framework for high-quality, high-value collaborative care. J Hosp Med 2017;12(4):277–82.
32. Auerbach AD. Surgical comanagement. In: Post T, editor. Wolters Kluwer.
33. Rohatgi N, Schulman K, Ahuja N. Comanagement by hospitalists: why it makes clinical and fiscal sense. Am J Med 2020;133(3):257–8.
34. Rohatgi N, Loftus P, Grujic O, et al. Surgical comanagement by hospitalists im- proves patient outcomes: a propensity score analysis. Ann Surg 2016;264(2): 275–82.
35. Shaw M, Pelecanos AM, Mudge AM. Evaluation of internal medicine physician or multidisciplinary team comanagement of surgical patients and clinical outcomes: a systematic review and meta-analysis. JAMA Netw Open 2020;3(5):e204088.
36. Sharma G, Kuo YF, Freeman J, et al. Comanagement of hospitalized surgical pa- tients by medicine physicians in the United States. Arch Intern Med 2010;170(4): 363–8.
37. Swart E, Kates S, McGee S, et al. The case for comanagement and care path- ways for osteoporotic patients with a hip fracture. J Bone Joint Surg 2018; 100(15):1343–50.
38. Huddleston JM, Long KH, Naessens JM, et al. Medical and surgical comanage- ment after elective hip and knee arthroplasty: a randomized, controlled trial. Ann Intern Med 2004;141(1):28–38.
39. Phy MP, Vanness DJ, Melton LJ, et al. Effects of a hospitalist model on elderly pa- tients with hip fracture. Arch Intern Med 2005;165(7):796–801.
40. Iberti CT, Briones A, Gabriel E, Dunn AS. Hospitalist-vascular surgery comanage- ment: effects on complications and mortality. Hosp Pract (1995) 2016;44(5): 233–6.

41. Rohatgi N, Wei PH, Grujic O, Ahuja N. Surgical Comanagement by Hospitalists in Colorectal Surgery. J Am Coll Surg 2018;227(4):404–10.e5.
42. Montero Ruiz E, Rebollar Merino Á, Rivera Rodríguez T, et al. Effect of comanagement with internal medicine on hospital stay of patients admitted to the Service of Otolaryngology. Acta Otorrinolaringol Esp 2015;66(5):264–8.
43. Auerbach AD, Rasic MA, Sehgal N, et al. Opportunity missed: medical consultation, resource use, and quality of care of patients undergoing major surgery. Arch Intern Med 2007;167(21):2338–44.
44. Sharma G. Medical consultation for surgical cases in the era of value-based care. JAMA Intern Med 2014;174(9):1477–8.
45. Mazzarello S, McIsaac DI, Montroy J, et al. Postoperative shared-care for patients undergoing non-cardiac surgery: a systematic review and meta-analysis. Can J Anaesth 2019;66(9):1095–105.
46. Batsis JA, Phy MP, Melton LJ 3rd, et al. Effects of a hospitalist care model on mortality of elderly patients with hip fractures. J Hosp Med 2007;2(4):219–25.
47. Auerbach AD, Wachter RM, Cheng HQ, et al. Comanagement of surgical patients between neurosurgeons and hospitalists. Arch Intern Med 2010;170(22):2004–10.
48. Maxwell BG, Mirza A. Medical comanagement of hip fracture patients is not associated with superior perioperative outcomes: a propensity score-matched retrospective cohort analysis of the National Surgical Quality Improvement Project. J Hosp Med 2020;15(8):468–74.

Preoperative Testing

Alana Sigmund, MD[a,b,*], Matthew A. Pappas, MD, MPH, FHM[c,d,e],
Jason F. Shiffermiller, MD, MPH[f]

KEYWORDS

- Preoperative care • Preoperative testing • Surgery • Value-based care

KEY POINTS

- Preoperative blood tests, including coagulation studies, blood counts, and serum chemistries, should not be routinely performed. Selective testing should be based on comorbidity, medication history, and the planned procedure.
- Routine preoperative screening for urinary tract infection is not indicated except in patients undergoing urologic procedures.
- Preoperative pregnancy testing should be performed in all patients who have the ability to become pregnant.
- Preoperative pulmonary function testing and chest radiograph should not be performed in patients with stable lung disease but are indicated in patients with symptoms suggestive of an undiagnosed cardiopulmonary condition.
- Reconciling published guidelines with the current evidence for preoperative cardiac stress testing is challenging. The role of preoperative stress testing has not been precisely determined but it is most clearly indicated in patients with symptoms consistent with coronary artery disease.

Preoperative medical evaluation can quantify and manage a patient's surgical risk in a way that minimizes inefficiencies and improves outcomes.[1–3] Judicious use of preoperative testing aids in that effort. Indiscriminate testing, conversely, can undermine the value of preoperative medical evaluation by adding cost and resulting in unnecessary care. Here, we review common preoperative tests and assess their role in the preoperative medical evaluation. **Table 1** summarizes the indications and evidence for each preoperative test.

---

[a] Weill Medical College of Cornell University; [b] Arthroplasty Hospital for Special Surgery, 541 East 71st Street, New York, NY 10021, USA; [c] Department of Hospital Medicine, Cleveland Clinic, 9500 Euclid Avenue, Mail Stop G-10, Cleveland, OH 44195, USA; [d] Center for Value-based Care Research, Cleveland Clinic, Cleveland, OH, USA; [e] Outcomes Research Consortium, Cleveland, OH, USA; [f] Division of Hospital Medicine, Department of Internal Medicine, University of Nebraska Medical Center, 986435 Nebraska Medical Center, Omaha, NE 68198-6435, USA
* Corresponding author. 535 East 70th Street, New York, NY 10021.
E-mail address: sigmunda@HSS.EDU

Med Clin N Am 108 (2024) 1005–1016
https://doi.org/10.1016/j.mcna.2024.04.010
0025-7125/24/© 2024 Elsevier Inc. All rights reserved.

medical.theclinics.com

Table 1
Preoperative testing

Preoperative Test	Indications	Evidence
Laboratory Testing		
Coagulation studies	• Medical history suggestive of bleeding diathesis • Warfarin therapy	Abstracted multicenter cohort data from the National Surgical Quality Improvement Program (NSQIP) demonstrating limited diagnostic potential
Complete blood count	• Surgery with risk of substantial blood loss • Moderate or higher probability of anemia	Retrospective data demonstrating association between anemia and worse postoperative outcomes
Creatinine	• Chronic kidney disease • Diabetes mellitus • Hypertension • Current or planned use of nephrotoxic medications • Cardiac risk stratification	Large retrospective studies, pooled data from cohort studies, one prospective study, one meta-analysis
Electrolytes	• Diuretic use or other suspicion for hyponatremia	Large retrospective studies, pooled data from cohort studies
Glucose and HgA1c	• Diabetes mellitus	Meta-analysis of cohort studies, systematic review of cohort studies
Liver panel	• Known or suspected liver disease • Assessment of nutritional status	Large retrospective and prospective studies, pooled data from cohort studies
Urinalysis	• Urologic surgeries	Small study prospective data
Pregnancy testing	• All surgeries for eligible patients	Retrospective large study
Procedures		
Stress testing	• Symptoms that would otherwise prompt workup of new obstructive coronary disease where coronary computed tomography angiography (CTA) is unavailable or contraindicated • Known coronary disease with symptoms potentially consistent with an alternate cause, such that stress testing would rule in or rule out an acute cardiac condition	Large single-center cohort study of patients considering a wide variety of noncardiac surgeries
Electrocardiography	• High risk of a perioperative coronary event	Small prospective cohort studies
Pulmonary function testing	• Symptoms suggestive of undiagnosed pulmonary disease • Prior to pulmonary surgery	Small to medium-sized retrospective studies and a single prospective cohort study
Chest radiograph	• Signs or symptoms suggestive of undiagnosed cardiopulmonary disease	Pooled data from cohort studies

Abbreviation: HbA1c, hemoglobin A1c.

HEMATOLOGY
Coagulation Studies

Patients taking anticoagulants and patients with severe liver disease are discussed elsewhere in this issue. For other patients, preoperative coagulation testing is intended to uncover bleeding disorders. Fortunately, the risk of a previously undiscovered bleeding disorder is low: in a structured assessment of patients presenting to outpatient physicians' offices, fewer than 1 in 1,000 patients had von Willebrand disease, the most common inherited bleeding disorder.[4,5] Unfortunately, because the pretest probability of a bleeding disorder is low and coagulation studies are imperfectly related to the risk of bleeding, neither PT/INR nor PTT are useful in identifying patients without heightened suspicion based on history.[4] Medical history, including family history, remains the most useful tool to interrogate the risk of a bleeding disorder.

Complete Blood Count

As with coagulation studies, measurement of platelet count has little utility as the probability of undiscovered thrombocytopenia is low: in NHANES, around 239 of 240 persons will have a platelet count above 100,000, and studies in the preoperative setting have found low yield.[6] And there is little reason to think that screening for leukopenia or leukocytosis would be useful. Therefore, although at many centers a complete blood count (CBC) is no more expensive than isolated measurement of hemoglobin or hematocrit, and the CBC is built into clinical workflow, the key factor in whether to obtain a CBC is the value of preoperative hemoglobin measurement.

Anemia is both relatively common among patients considering surgery and significant for patient care in multiple ways. First, preoperative anemia is clearly associated with perioperative risk.[7–9] Second, anemia is clearly associated with transfusion; because multiple randomized trials have found higher risk of death in patients assigned to more liberal transfusion strategies, presumably each unit of packed red blood cells confers some marginal risk.[10–13] Third, anemia can be consequent to multiple etiologies, some of which require further workup and investigation and some of which are likely associated with elevated perioperative risk. Although the causal pathways underlying these associations remain uncertain, and interventional studies are lacking, identifying anemia could plausibly lead to better patient outcomes.[14]

Therefore, hemoglobin measurement may be indicated either before a surgery whose expected blood loss is substantial or (as in the outpatient setting) when history is suggestive of anemia. Advancing age may be the clearest single predictor of anemia,[15] but providers performing preoperative evaluations are likely to see a wide variety of individually uncommon conditions associated with anemia, including inflammatory conditions, bleeding of obscure source, and malignancies. Comprehensive rules that capture all such conditions would be intractable, but thoughtful clinicians in this setting will likely identify many persons at intermediate probability of anemia. For those patients and for patients before surgeries with substantial expected blood loss, hemoglobin measurement would be reasonable.

SERUM CHEMISTRIES
Creatinine

Elevation in serum creatinine is an independent risk factor for postoperative complications and is a component of some commonly used cardiac risk stratification tools.[16–20] The criteria for preoperative creatinine measurement should capture patients at higher risk for chronic kidney disease and those at higher risk for postoperative cardiac complications. The exact criteria, however, have not been established by evidence.

Age more than 50 years has been suggested as a criterion for testing but when evaluated in patients aged 70 years or more, preoperative creatinine was not independently associated with postoperative adverse outcomes.[21,22] It would be reasonable to measure preoperative serum creatinine in patients with chronic kidney disease stage 3 or higher, diabetes mellitus, hypertension, and possibly other conditions associated with chronic kidney disease such as congestive heart failure and systemic lupus erythematosus. Similarly, preoperative measurement is reasonable in patients taking diuretics, angiotensin-converting enzyme inhibitors, angiotensin receptor blockers, nonsteroidal anti-inflammatories, or other potentially nephrotoxic medications, and in those who will be exposed to potentially nephrotoxic agents in the perioperative period.

Electrolytes

Preoperative hyponatremia and hypernatremia, even at values near the normal range, are independently associated with postoperative mortality.[23–25] It has been recommended that serum sodium be measured preoperatively in patients with previous hyponatremia and in patients taking diuretics, but it is unknown whether preoperative sodium correction results in improved outcomes. Preoperative abnormalities in potassium and other electrolytes have not been associated with perioperative adverse events.[21] However, in patients with risk factors for hyperkalemia, such as those taking aldosterone antagonists, angiotensin-converting enzyme inhibitors, or angiotensin receptor blockers, it is reasonable to measure the potassium preoperatively.

Glucose

In patients with diabetes mellitus, there is evidence from a meta-analysis of cohort data that good preoperative glycemic control is associated with a lower risk for perioperative complications, particularly infections.[26] Consensus guidelines recommend preoperative measurement of HgA1c and glucose in patients with diabetes.[27] In patients without diabetes, the data on preoperative glucose or HgA1c testing are mixed. A systematic review of cohort data found some evidence for an association between preoperative hyperglycemia and increased risk for postoperative adverse events in patients without diabetes who underwent orthopedic, spine, or vascular surgeries.[28] In patients without diabetes who are undergoing other surgeries, routine preoperative glucose and HgA1c measurement are not recommended.

Liver Panel

The liver panel typically includes transaminases, alkaline phosphatase, total bilirubin, albumin, and protein. In patients without a clear indication for testing, a preoperative liver panel is unlikely to reveal abnormalities and exceedingly unlikely to result in a change in management.[21] In patients with known or suspected liver disease, though, preoperative testing is strongly indicated. The risk of postoperative mortality is increased in patients with cirrhosis and is closely related to the severity of liver disease. For instance, in a study of patients with cirrhosis undergoing gastrointestinal, orthopedic, or cardiovascular surgery, mortality was 5.7% in patients with a Model for End-stage Liver Disease (MELD) score less than 8 compared to approximately 55% in patients with a MELD score greater than 20.[29] Bilirubin level is necessary for calculation of the MELD score. Both bilirubin and albumin are necessary for calculation of the Veterans Outcomes and Costs Associated with Liver disease–Penn score, which is equivalent to or better than the MELD score at predicting postoperative mortality in patients with cirrhosis.[30] Liver panel testing is also indicated to assess for preoperative malnutrition. Hypoalbuminemia, as a marker of nutritional status, has been independently associated with postoperative complications and mortality in a number of large studies including a variety of surgical populations.[31–34] Preoperative nutritional optimization in patients with hypoalbuminemia may be beneficial.[35]

UROLOGIC
Urinalysis

Urinalysis has been extensively investigated in orthopedic surgery both to reduce the rate of perioperative urinary tract infection and surgical-site infection.[36–39] In one retrospective study of 200 nonprosthetic knee procedures, urinalysis was found to increase the risk of unnecessary downstream testing[38] and in a systematic review, antibiotic treatment of asymptomatic bacteriuria prior to hip and knee arthroplasty was not supported by the evidence.[39] Urinalysis in asymptomatic patients prior to neurosurgical procedures and outpatient general surgery procedures also failed to reduce the risk of complications.[40,41] The presence of albuminuria on urinalysis was noted to predict postoperative kidney injury in all-comer surgical patients in one retrospective study.[42] In a large retrospective study of NSQIP data, however, designed to develop a web-based prediction model for acute kidney injury after surgery, other measures such as preoperative serum creatinine, surgery type, and age were found to predict postoperative acute kidney injury, and so urinalysis may not be necessary to risk stratify a patient preoperatively.[43] Preoperative urinalysis has been found to have utility prior to some urologic procedures.[44] In general, urinalysis is not an effective tool to detect and treat urinary tract infections preoperatively or reduce the risk of postoperative wound infections and may be associated with low-value care. Urinalysis, therefore, is suggested prior to certain urologic procedures, and if further preoperative evaluation for renal failure risk is indicated.

Pregnancy Screening

Up to 2% of patients with pregnancy will undergo nonobstetric surgery per year.[45] Preoperative pregnancy screening positivity rates range between 0.15% and 2.2.%.[46,47] The American Society of Anesthesiologists (ASA) noted that pregnancy screening in premenopausal female patients led to "postponement, cancellations, or changes in management in 100.0% of the cases of pregnancy."[48] Patients with pregnancy undergoing nonobstetric surgery face risks of teratogenic effects due to anesthetics, spontaneous miscarriage, preterm labor, low birth weight, and adverse fetal effects from hypoxemia, hypercapnia, stress, and hypotension.[49–51] All patients who have the ability to become pregnant should be screened for pregnancy preoperatively.

CARDIAC TESTING
Cardiac Stress Testing

Current guidelines from the ACC/AHA, released in 2014, suggest consideration of preoperative cardiac stress testing if (1) a patient's risk of a major adverse cardiac event is 1% or greater; (2) the patient's functional status is poor or unknown; and (3) the results of stress testing would plausibly change management.[52]

However, in the decade since the release of those guidelines, scholarship has suggested several shortcomings in this approach. First, different risk assessment tools use different definitions of major adverse cardiac events and have poor concordance across the 1% risk threshold.[53] Moreover, the Revised Cardiac Risk Index (RCRI; perhaps the most widely used preoperative risk assessment tool) was not well calibrated to a contemporary Canadian cohort, where all patients—including those with an RCRI of 0—had a risk exceeding 1%.[54] Depending on the definition and cohort used, very different numbers of patients would exceed this arbitrary risk threshold.

Second, similar problems plague patient selection according to functional status. Third, preoperative cardiac stress testing likely increases the likelihood of further cardiac testing (a "care cascade") while decreasing the likelihood that a patient will complete the noncardiac surgery under consideration.[55] The results of preoperative stress testing will likely not improve predictions of the most significant postoperative complications, and most patients without angina—even those at high risk of a perioperative complication—have a pretest probability of obstructive coronary disease that is too low for functional stress testing to be diagnostically useful.7

Based on theory and older cohort data, some experts continue to recommend cardiac stress imaging prior to major vascular surgery.[56] However, surgical type is a predictor in all modern risk prediction tools, and a large randomized trial found no benefit to coronary revascularization before vascular surgery.[19,20,57,58] There is little reason to think that either the information provided by stress testing or the consequences of testing differ in persons considering vascular surgery as compared to persons considering other major noncardiac surgery.

The authors recommend obtaining preoperative cardiac stress testing rarely, and generally only in scenarios where functional stress testing would be indicated regardless of upcoming surgery. To our view, stress testing offers little in this setting otherwise.

Electrocardiography

By expert consensus and current guidelines, patients undergoing low-risk procedures do not require preoperative electrocardiography.[52,59] Among patients whose risk of a major adverse cardiac event exceeds 1%, ACC/AHA guidelines recommend a resting 12-lead electrocardiography (ECG) for patients with structural heart disease, coronary artery disease, significant arrhythmias, cerebrovascular disease, or peripheral arterial disease.[52]

In the largest cohort study of preoperative electrocardiography, the only ECG abnormalities associated with postoperative myocardial infarction (MI) were left and right bundle branch block. However, neither left nor right bundle branch blocks were independent predictors of postoperative MI in a model including RCRI criteria.[60] Therefore, in the absence of a suspected arrhythmia, it seems that the primary function of a preoperative ECG is to establish a baseline. In the setting of a perioperative coronary event, that baseline would allow MI to be distinguished from myocardial injury after noncardiac surgery. It seems reasonable to use preoperative ECG testing for evaluation of suspected arrhythmia and possibly to establish a baseline in patients at elevated risk for perioperative coronary events. A precise probability threshold would be difficult to establish, dependent on local resources, and require a well-calibrated model to implement. As such, the threshold that should be considered "elevated" will likely differ across different care teams.

PULMONARY TESTING

Postoperative pulmonary complications are common, even when the site of surgery is outside of the chest. Postoperative pulmonary complications can also be severe, accounting for over 20% of postoperative mortality.[61] Using preoperative pulmonary function tests (PFTs) or chest x-ray (CXR) to risk stratify patients for postoperative pulmonary complications, however, is generally not recommended.

Pulmonary Function Tests

Studies of preoperative PFTs have been conducted in patients at increased risk of postoperative pulmonary complications due to intra-abdominal surgery, chronic obstructive pulmonary disease (COPD) history, or both. While some studies found no independent association between any preoperative measure of pulmonary function and pulmonary complications,[62,63] others found that at least one measure of preoperative pulmonary function was independently associated with pulmonary complications. The predictive pulmonary function measures were FEV_1/FVC ratio 0.5 or less in one study,[64] FEV1, residual volume, and diffusion capacity as continuous variables in another,[65] and FEV1 less than 61% predicted in the third.[66] Even in the studies that found preoperative pulmonary function measures to be predictive of postoperative complications, clinical risk factors such as the type of surgery and the ASA classification, were generally stronger predictors of postoperative pulmonary complications than pulmonary function measures.

Based on this evidence, expert bodies recommend against the routine use of PFTs for preoperative risk stratification in patients undergoing extrathoracic surgery.[48,67] They also recommend against the use of PFTs to determine candidacy for extrathoracic surgery, citing a postoperative mortality risk of 6% in a study of patients with FEV1 less than 50% predicted.[34,62] There is no clear threshold for pulmonary function measures below which surgery should be canceled. There is, however, a potential role for preoperative PFTs in patients with unexplained respiratory symptoms. While there is no trial evidence to support this practice, it is reasonable to expect a lower risk of complications following diagnosis and treatment of the underlying condition in patients with unexplained respiratory symptoms. There is also a well-established role for PFTs in the evaluation of patients planning lung resection.[68]

Chest X-ray

Abnormal preoperative CXRs have been independently associated with postoperative pulmonary complications in multiple studies of patients at increased risk due to intra-abdominal surgery, COPD history, or smoking status.[62,63,69] Studies using pooled data have reported abnormal preoperative CXRs in 10% to 21% of patients, but only 0.1% to 3% of CXRs had an abnormality that resulted in a change in management.[21,70] Based on this evidence, expert bodies recommend against the routine use of CXRs for preoperative risk stratification.[48,67] The recommendation against routine use is strongest in patients younger than age 50 years, in whom fewer than 5% of preoperative CXRs are abnormal.[21] In older patients, preoperative CXR might be considered in patients with risk factors such as COPD, abdominal surgery, or thoracic surgery.[71] The criteria, however, have not been clearly established, and there are no trial data to guide the management of any abnormal results. Preoperative CXRs are clearly indicated if signs or symptoms of cardiac or pulmonary disease, such as cough, dyspnea, or adventitious breath sounds, are present in patients planning surgery. According to one study, abnormal CXRs can be expected in approximately 20% of patients with clinical predictors of cardiac or pulmonary disease compared to less than 1% of patients without clinical predictors.[72]

SUMMARY

In the testing reviewed here, no tests were universally indicated other than preoperative pregnancy testing, which is suggested in any patient planning surgery who could become pregnant. Some testing, such as urinalysis and PFTs are only suggested if otherwise indicated and may only play a role for organ-specific surgeries. Other common tests, such as CBC, creatinine, electrolytes, glucose, and HgA1c, are indicated based on a combination of patient-specific and surgery-specific factors. High-value preoperative cardiac testing remains an area of active research. In summary, judicious use of preoperative testing may allow the clinician to risk-stratify the patient, guide care, and avoid unnecessary downstream testing.

CLINICS CARE POINTS

- Personal and family history are the only adequate preoperative screening measures for detecting bleeding disorders. Coagulation studies are inadequate as they may be normal in patients with some bleeding disorders, such as von Willebrand disease.

- Preoperative anemia confers a substantial risk for perioperative complications, particularly if transfusion is required. While routine preoperative measurement of hemoglobin is not recommended, hemoglobin measurement will be commonly indicated in patients at higher risk of anemia due to medical comorbidity or the bleeding risk of the planned procedure.

- Preoperative risk stratification for patients with liver disease is important given the potential for mortality. Risk stratification should be based on a validated metric which will require measurement of serum chemistries.

- Except in patients undergoing pulmonary surgery, preoperative pulmonary function testing is not useful in patients with stable asthma or COPD and should not be used to determine candidacy for surgery.

- Applying the RCRI score to the 2014 ACC/AHA guidelines for preoperative cardiac risk stratification is problematic because, in some studies, the 1% risk threshold is exceeded by all patients, even those with a score of zero.

DISCLOSURE

Dr. M.A. Pappas reports funding from NIH, United States, (NHLBI, United States, K08HL141598). Dr. A. Sigmund reports ownership of common stock in CVS, Bristol Myers Squibb, Walgreen's, and Pfizer. Dr. J.F. Shiffermiller has nothing to disclose.

REFERENCES

1. Bierle DM, Raslau D, Regan DW, et al. Preoperative evaluation before noncardiac surgery. Mayo Clin Proc 2020;95(4):807–22.
2. Ferschl MB, Tung A, Sweitzer B, et al. Preoperative clinic visits reduce operating room cancellations and delays. Anesthesiology 2005;103(4):855–9.
3. Partridge JS, Harari D, Martin FC, et al. Randomized clinical trial of comprehensive geriatric assessment and optimization in vascular surgery. Br J Surg 2017; 104(6):679–87.
4. Seicean A, Schiltz NK, Seicean S, et al. Use and utility of preoperative hemostatic screening and patient history in adult neurosurgical patients. J Neurosurg 2012; 116(5):1097–105.
5. Bowman M, Hopman WM, Rapson D, et al. The prevalence of symptomatic von Willebrand disease in primary care practice. J Thromb Haemost 2010;8(1):213–6.
6. Kaplan EB, Sheiner LB, Boeckmann AJ, et al. The usefulness of preoperative laboratory screening. JAMA 1985;253(24):3576–81.
7. Pappas MA, Auerbach AD, Kattan MW, et al. Diagnostic and prognostic value of cardiac stress testing before major noncardiac surgery-A cohort study. J Clin Anesth 2023;90:111193.
8. Musallam KM, Tamim HM, Richards T, et al. Preoperative anaemia and postoperative outcomes in non-cardiac surgery: a retrospective cohort study. Lancet 2011;378(9800):1396–407.

9. Luo X, Li F, Hu H, et al. Anemia and perioperative mortality in non-cardiac surgery patients: a secondary analysis based on a single-center retrospective study. BMC Anesthesiol 2020;20(1):112.

10. Mazer CD, Whitlock RP, Fergusson DA, et al. Restrictive or liberal red-cell transfusion for cardiac surgery. N Engl J Med 2017;377(22):2133–44.

11. Carson JL, Terrin ML, Noveck H, et al. Liberal or restrictive transfusion in high-risk patients after hip surgery. N Engl J Med 2011;365(26):2453–62.

12. Hebert PC, Wells G, Blajchman MA, et al. A multicenter, randomized, controlled clinical trial of transfusion requirements in critical care. transfusion requirements in critical care investigators, canadian critical care trials group. N Engl J Med 1999;340(6):409–17.

13. Carson JL, Stanworth SJ, Dennis JA, et al. Transfusion thresholds for guiding red blood cell transfusion. Cochrane Database Syst Rev 2021;12(12):CD002042.

14. Frank SM, Cushing MM. Bleeding, anaemia, and transfusion: an ounce of prevention is worth a pound of cure. Br J Anaesth 2021;126(1):5–9.

15. Le CH. The prevalence of anemia and moderate-severe anemia in the US population (NHANES 2003-2012). PLoS One 2016;11(11):e0166635.

16. Mathew A, Devereaux PJ, O'Hare A, et al. Chronic kidney disease and postoperative mortality: a systematic review and meta-analysis. Kidney Int 2008;73(9): 1069–81.

17. Antoniak D, Are C, Vokoun C, et al. The relationship between age and chronic kidney disease in patients undergoing pancreatic resection. J Gastrointest Surg 2018;22(8):1376–84.

18. Antoniak DT, Benes BJ, Hartman CW, et al. Impact of chronic kidney disease in older adults undergoing hip or knee arthroplasty: a large database study. J Arthroplasty 2020;35(5):1214–1221 e1215.

19. Lee TH, Marcantonio ER, Mangione CM, et al. Derivation and prospective validation of a simple index for prediction of cardiac risk of major noncardiac surgery. Circulation 1999;100(10):1043–9.

20. Gupta PK, Gupta H, Sundaram A, et al. Development and validation of a risk calculator for prediction of cardiac risk after surgery. Circulation 2011;124(4): 381–7.

21. Smetana GW, Macpherson DS. The case against routine preoperative laboratory testing. Med Clin North Am 2003;87(1):7–40.

22. Dzankic S, Pastor D, Gonzalez C, et al. The prevalence and predictive value of abnormal preoperative laboratory tests in elderly surgical patients. Anesth Analg 2001;93(2):301–8, 302nd contents page.

23. Leung AA, McAlister FA, Rogers SO Jr, et al. Preoperative hyponatremia and perioperative complications. Arch Intern Med 2012;172(19):1474–81.

24. Mc Causland FR, Wright J, Waikar SS. Association of serum sodium with morbidity and mortality in hospitalized patients undergoing major orthopedic surgery. J Hosp Med 2014;9(5):297–302.

25. Cole JH, Highland KB, Hughey SB, et al. The association between borderline dysnatremia and perioperative morbidity and mortality: retrospective cohort study of the american college of surgeons national surgical quality improvement program database. JMIR Perioper Med 2023;6:e38462.

26. Seisa MO, Saadi S, Nayfeh T, et al. A systematic review supporting the endocrine society clinical practice guideline for the management of hyperglycemia in adults hospitalized for noncritical illness or undergoing elective surgical procedures. J Clin Endocrinol Metab 2022;107(8):2139–47.

27. Korytkowski MT, Muniyappa R, Antinori-Lent K, et al. Management of hyperglycemia in hospitalized adult patients in non-critical care settings: an endocrine society clinical practice guideline. J Clin Endocrinol Metab 2022;107(8):2101–28.

28. Bock M, Johansson T, Fritsch G, et al. The impact of preoperative testing for blood glucose concentration and haemoglobin A1c on mortality, changes in management and complications in noncardiac elective surgery: a systematic review. Eur J Anaesthesiol 2015;32(3):152–9.

29. Teh SH, Nagorney DM, Stevens SR, et al. Risk factors for mortality after surgery in patients with cirrhosis. Gastroenterology 2007;132(4):1261–9.

30. Mahmud N, Fricker Z, Panchal S, et al. External validation of the VOCAL-penn cirrhosis surgical risk score in 2 large, independent health systems. Liver Transpl 2021;27(7):961–70.

31. Gibbs J, Cull W, Henderson W, et al. Preoperative serum albumin level as a predictor of operative mortality and morbidity: results from the National VA Surgical Risk Study. Arch Surg 1999;134(1):36–42.

32. Chahrour MA, Kharroubi H, Al Tannir AH, et al. Hypoalbuminemia is associated with mortality in patients undergoing lower extremity amputation. Ann Vasc Surg 2021;77:138–45.

33. McLean C, Mocanu V, Birch DW, et al. Hypoalbuminemia predicts serious complications following elective bariatric surgery. Obes Surg 2021;31(10):4519–27.

34. Smetana GW, Lawrence VA, Cornell JE, et al. Preoperative pulmonary risk stratification for noncardiothoracic surgery: systematic review for the American College of Physicians. Ann Intern Med 2006;144(8):581–95.

35. Jie B, Jiang ZM, Nolan MT, et al. Impact of preoperative nutritional support on clinical outcome in abdominal surgical patients at nutritional risk. Nutrition 2012;28(10):1022–7.

36. Hollenbeck BL, Hoffman M, Fang CJ, et al. Elimination of routine urinalysis before elective orthopaedic surgery reduces antibiotic utilization without impacting catheter-associated urinary tract infection or surgical site infection rates. Hip Pelvis 2021;33(4):225–30.

37. Welch JM, Zhuang T, Shapiro LM, et al. Is low-value testing before low-risk hand surgery associated with increased downstream healthcare use and reimbursements? a national claims database analysis. Clin Orthop Relat Res 2022;480(10):1851–62.

38. Lawrence VA, Kroenke K. The unproven utility of preoperative urinalysis. Clinical use. Arch Intern Med 1988;148(6):1370–3.

39. Mayne AIW, Davies PSE, Simpson JM. Antibiotic treatment of asymptomatic bacteriuria prior to hip and knee arthroplasty; a systematic review of the literature. Surgeon 2018;16(3):176–82.

40. Wattsman TA, Davies RS. The utility of preoperative laboratory testing in general surgery patients for outpatient procedures. Am Surg 1997;63(1):81–90.

41. Haskell-Mendoza AP, Radhakrishnan S, Nardin AL, et al. Utility of routine preoperative urinalysis in the prevention of surgical site infections. World Neurosurg 2023;180:e449–59.

42. Park S, Lee S, Lee A, et al. Preoperative dipstick albuminuria and other urine abnormalities predict acute kidney injury and patient outcomes. Surgery 2018;163(5):1178–85.

43. Woo SH, Zavodnick J, Ackermann L, et al. Development and validation of a web-based prediction model for AKI after surgery. Kidney360 2021;2(2):215–23.

44. Lu ZH, Lin TY, Huang HS, et al. Preoperative urine analysis is an effective tool to predict fever after miniaturized percutaneous nephrolithotomy on large renal stones. Urol J 2021;18(6):600–7.

45. Crowhurst JA. Anaesthesia for non-obstetric surgery during pregnancy. Acta Anaesthesiol Belg 2002;53(4):295–7.
46. Kahn RL, Stanton MA, Tong-Ngork S, et al. One-year experience with day-of-surgery pregnancy testing before elective orthopedic procedures. Anesth Analg 2008;106(4):1127–31, table of contents.
47. Twersky RS, Singleton G. Preoperative pregnancy testing: "justice and testing for all". Anesth Analg 1996;83(2):438–9.
48. Committee on Standards and Practice Parameters, Apfelbaum JL, Connis RT, Nickinovich DG, et al. Practice advisory for preanesthesia evaluation: an updated report by the american society of anesthesiologists task force on preanesthesia evaluation. Anesthesiology 2012;116(3):522–38.
49. Duncan PG, Pope WD, Cohen MM, et al. Fetal risk of anesthesia and surgery during pregnancy. Anesthesiology 1986;64(6):790–4.
50. Webb MP, Helander EM, Meyn AR, et al. Preoperative assessment of the pregnant patient undergoing nonobstetric surgery. Anesthesiol Clin 2018;36(4):627–37.
51. Wingfield M, McMenamin M. Preoperative pregnancy testing. Br J Surg 2014; 101(12):1488–90.
52. Fleisher LA, Fleischmann KE, Auerbach AD, et al. 2014 ACC/AHA guideline on perioperative cardiovascular evaluation and management of patients undergoing noncardiac surgery: executive summary: a report of the American College of Cardiology/American Heart Association Task Force on Practice Guidelines. Circulation 2014;130(24):2215–45.
53. Pappas MA, Sessler DI, Rothberg MB. Anticipated rates and costs of guideline-concordant preoperative stress testing. Anesth Analg 2019;128(2):241–6.
54. Duceppe E, Parlow J, MacDonald P, et al. Canadian cardiovascular society guidelines on perioperative cardiac risk assessment and management for patients who undergo noncardiac surgery. Can J Cardiol 2017;33(1):17–32.
55. Pappas MA, Auerbach AD, Kattan MW, et al. Consequences of preoperative cardiac stress testing-A cohort study. J Clin Anesth 2023;90:111158.
56. Rihal CS, Eagle KA, Mickel MC, et al. Surgical therapy for coronary artery disease among patients with combined coronary artery and peripheral vascular disease. Circulation 1995;91(1):46–53.
57. Bilimoria KY, Liu Y, Paruch JL, et al. Development and evaluation of the universal ACS NSQIP surgical risk calculator: a decision aid and informed consent tool for patients and surgeons. J Am Coll Surg 2013;217(5):833–42, e831-833.
58. McFalls EO, Ward HB, Moritz TE, et al. Coronary-artery revascularization before elective major vascular surgery. N Engl J Med 2004;351(27):2795–804.
59. Halvorsen S, Mehilli J, Cassese S, et al. 2022 ESC Guidelines on cardiovascular assessment and management of patients undergoing non-cardiac surgery. Eur Heart J 2022;43(39):3826–924.
60. van Klei WA, Bryson GL, Yang H, et al. The value of routine preoperative electrocardiography in predicting myocardial infarction after noncardiac surgery. Ann Surg 2007;246(2):165–70.
61. Lakshminarasimhachar A, Smetana GW. Preoperative evaluation: estimation of pulmonary risk. Anesthesiol Clin 2016;34(1):71–88.
62. Kroenke K, Lawrence VA, Theroux JF, et al. Postoperative complications after thoracic and major abdominal surgery in patients with and without obstructive lung disease. Chest 1993;104(5):1445–51.
63. Lawrence VA, Dhanda R, Hilsenbeck SG, et al. Risk of pulmonary complications after elective abdominal surgery. Chest 1996;110(3):744–50.

64. Wong DH, Weber EC, Schell MJ, et al. Factors associated with postoperative pulmonary complications in patients with severe chronic obstructive pulmonary disease. Anesth Analg 1995;80(2):276–84.

65. Barisione G, Rovida S, Gazzaniga GM, et al. Upper abdominal surgery: does a lung function test exist to predict early severe postoperative respiratory complications? Eur Respir J 1997;10(6):1301–8.

66. Fuso L, Cisternino L, Di Napoli A, et al. Role of spirometric and arterial gas data in predicting pulmonary complications after abdominal surgery. Respir Med 2000; 94(12):1171–6.

67. Qaseem A, Snow V, Fitterman N, et al. Risk assessment for and strategies to reduce perioperative pulmonary complications for patients undergoing noncardiothoracic surgery: a guideline from the American College of Physicians. Ann Intern Med 2006;144(8):575–80.

68. Brunelli A, Kim AW, Berger KI, et al. Physiologic evaluation of the patient with lung cancer being considered for resectional surgery: diagnosis and management of lung cancer, 3rd ed. Chest 2013;143(5 Suppl):e166S–90S.

69. Bluman LG, Mosca L, Newman N, et al. Preoperative smoking habits and postoperative pulmonary complications. Chest 1998;113(4):883–9.

70. Archer C, Levy AR, McGregor M. Value of routine preoperative chest x-rays: a meta-analysis. Can J Anaesth 1993;40(11):1022–7.

71. Subramani Y, Nagappa M, Wong J, et al. Preoperative evaluation: estimation of pulmonary risk including obstructive sleep apnea impact. Anesthesiol Clin 2018;36(4): 523–38.

72. Rucker L, Frye EB, Staten MA. Usefulness of screening chest roentgenograms in preoperative patients. JAMA 1983;250(23):3209–11.

Medical Clinics of North America—Periprocedural Antithrombotics
Prophylaxis and Interruption

Steven J. Wilson, MD[a],*, David Gelovani, MD, MS[b], Anna Von, MD[c],
Scott Kaatz, DO, MSc, SFHM[b], Paul J. Grant, MD, SFHM[a]

KEYWORDS

- Anticoagulation management • Periprocedural care • Thromboembolic risk
- Bridging anticoagulation • Venous thromboembolism prophylaxis • Bleeding risk

KEY POINTS

- While there are validated scoring systems to assess venous thromboembolism risk, there are no standardized models to assess bleeding risk in surgical patients.
- Low molecular weight heparin and low-dose unfractionated heparin are the pharmacologic agents of choice for most nonorthopedic surgeries but direct oral anticoagulants (DOACs) and aspirin are oral options for total hip replacement and total knee replacement surgeries.
- Extended-duration prophylaxis is recommended for total hip arthroplasty and should be considered for high-risk patients undergoing other major orthopedic surgeries, major abdominal or pelvic surgery, thoracic surgery for cancer, or bariatric surgery.
- Periprocedural bridging is not necessary during interruption of DOACs and should be driven by patient-specific thrombotic risk factors during interruption of warfarin.
- While warfarin should be interrupted at least 5 days prior to moderate–high risk procedures, the procedural bleeding risk and patient renal function guide the duration of interruption of DOACs.

INTRODUCTION

Accurate assessment of both venous thromboembolism (VTE) and bleeding risk is critical in the periprocedural setting and must include consideration of individual patient

[a] Michigan Medicine, Department of Internal Medicine, 1500 E. Medical Center Drive, UH South, Unit 4, SPC 5220, Ann Arbor, MI 48109, USA; [b] Henry Ford Health, Department of Internal Medicine, 2799 W Grand Boulevard, Detroit, MI 48202, USA; [c] Emory University School of Medicine, Department of Internal Medicine, 1364 Clifton Road NE, Suite N-305, Atlanta, GA 30322, USA
* Corresponding author. Michigan Medicine, Department of Internal Medicine, 1500 E. Medical Center Drive, UH South, Unit 4, SPC 5220, Ann Arbor, MI 48109.
E-mail address: wilsonst@med.umich.edu

Med Clin N Am 108 (2024) 1017–1037
https://doi.org/10.1016/j.mcna.2024.04.005
0025-7125/24/© 2024 Elsevier Inc. All rights reserved.

characteristics and type of surgery. Historically, management was primarily focused on discontinuation of anticoagulation therapy (as applicable) to minimize bleeding risk, with the use of mechanical compression devices and heparin analogs for VTE prophylaxis in those without an indication for chronic anticoagulation. However, advances in surgical techniques and the emergence of novel pharmacologic agents have allowed providers to take a more nuanced approach by utilizing evidence-based strategies for periprocedural VTE prophylaxis and anticoagulation interruption.

PERIPROCEDURAL VENOUS THROMBOEMBOLISM PREVENTION

a. Epidemiology
   i. VTE is a well-recognized postprocedural complication that carries risk of significant morbidity and mortality. It is estimated that VTE may affect up to 25% of postsurgical patients, with the highest incidence seen in patients undergoing hip and knee surgery, as well as oncologic surgery.[1] However, risk varies considerably depending on the type of surgery and individual patient risk factors.
b. Risk assessment
   i. VTE risk assessment systems
      1. Validated scoring systems (ie, Caprini and Rogers scores) have been developed to help risk-stratify patients undergoing major surgery.[2,3] While both tools have some limitations, the Caprini score is generally accepted as the superior risk calculator given ease of use and overall improved discrimination between patient risk strata.[4]
   ii. Bleeding risk assessment
      1. Thromboprophylaxis-related bleeding risk is derived from both the type of surgery and individual patient factors. **Table 1** provides estimates of bleeding risk for most nonorthopedic surgeries, as well as for major orthopedic

Table 1	
Estimated bleeding risk by type of surgery	
Surgery Type	**Estimated Bleeding Risk**
Nonorthopedic	
General/abdominal/pelvic	0.7%–1.2%[a]
Bariatric	1.3%
Plastic/reconstructive	0.5%–1.8%
Vascular	1.2%
High-risk cardiac	4.7%
Thoracic	1%–5%
Neurosurgery/craniotomy	1.1%
Spinal column	< 0.5%
High-risk trauma	3.4%–4.7%
Orthopedic	
Major orthopedic surgery (TKA, THA, and HFS)	1.5%
Hip joint replacement	0.1%–3.1%[a]
Knee joint replacement	0.2%–1.4%[a]

Abbreviations: HFS, hip fracture surgery; THA, total hip arthroplasty; TKA, total knee arthroplasty.
[a] Denotes that studies from which bleeding rates were derived may have included patients already on VTE prophylaxis.
Adapted from: American College of Chest Physicians Evidence-Based Clinical Practice Guidelines,[5,6] The Journal of Thrombosis and Hemostasis,[7] and Digestive Diseases[8]

surgery. It is important to note that the strength of evidence is lower quality for nonorthopedic surgery.[5]

2. Several models assessing bleeding risk based on patient factors have been developed; however, these have been validated in patients receiving treatment anticoagulation dosing (ie, for atrial fibrillation or VTE).[9] At present, there are no standardized risk assessment tools to assess individual bleeding risk in surgical patients receiving prophylactic doses of anticoagulation.

c. VTE risk reduction

  i. Mechanical prophylaxis

    1. For patients undergoing major surgery, the American Society of Hematology (ASH) guideline panel conditionally recommends using pharmacologic or mechanical prophylaxis.[10] Mechanical prophylaxis may be used for patients at low risk for VTE, but in general, pharmacologic prophylaxis is preferred for most patients with at least moderate risk for VTE.[10] For patients at high risk for VTE, combined use of mechanical and pharmacologic prophylaxis is preferred over pharmacologic prophylaxis alone based on low-certainty evidence demonstrating a possible reduction in symptomatic PE.[11] For patients at high risk of bleeding that precludes the use of pharmacologic prophylaxis, ASH recommends the use of mechanical prophylaxis with intermittent compression devices preferred over graduated compression stockings.[10,12]

  ii. Pharmacologic prophylaxis

    1. **Table 2** outlines the various options for pharmacologic VTE prophylaxis.

  iii. Contraindications to pharmacologic prophylaxis

    1. Absolute contraindications to pharmacologic VTE prophylaxis are infrequent but may include major active bleeding, active peptic ulcer, presence of a high-risk bleeding disorder (ie, hemophilia or other significant bleeding disorder), thrombocytopenia (ie, platelet count $<50,000/\mu L$), coagulopathy (ie, significantly elevated international normalized ratio [INR]), and renal failure.[14,15]

  iv. Extended VTE prophylaxis

    1. The ASH recommends administering extended VTE prophylaxis (defined as beyond 3 weeks from surgery) in specific patient populations undergoing major surgery.[10] While there does not appear to be a mortality benefit, the available evidence suggests that extended prophylaxis likely reduces symptomatic PE, as well as proximal and distal DVT, without significantly increasing bleeding risk.[10]

    2. Extended prophylaxis has shown to reduce symptomatic VTE events in patients following abdominal surgery for cancer, total knee arthroplasty, total hip arthroplasty, and hip fracture surgery; however, it may increase the risk of minor bleeding following total hip arthroplasty.[6,16–18]

d. Surgery-specific VTE risk reduction

  i. Orthopedic surgery

    1. Pharmacologic prophylaxis (with mechanical prophylaxis during hospitalization) is recommended for major orthopedic surgeries. No single pharmacologic strategy has shown superiority in VTE risk reduction; therefore, it is important to consider the patient's individual risk factors for thrombosis and bleeding in choosing an agent.[19]

    2. For total hip and knee arthroplasty, direct oral anticoagulants (DOACs) are a first-line option for postprocedural prophylaxis. Aspirin is another widely used first-line option and the EPCAT II trial showed that aspirin prophylaxis

Table 2
Pharmacologic agents commonly used for venous thromboembolism prophylaxis after surgery

Agent	Delivery	Dosing	Considerations
LMWH	Subcutaneous	Enoxaparin • 40 mg daily • 30 mg every 12 h • 30 mg daily (if CrCl <30 mL/min) Dalteparin 5000 units daily	• Higher doses of enoxaparin can be used in patients with obesity • Less bleeding risk compared to UFH • LMWH has a lower incidence of HIT compared to unfractionated heparin (UFH)
UFH	Subcutaneous	5000 units every 8–12 h	• More frequent dosing over LMWH • Higher doses commonly used for patients with obesity (ie, 7500 units) • Higher bleeding risk compared to LMWH • No renal dosing adjustments needed
Fondaparinux	Subcutaneous	2.5 mg daily (1.25 mg daily if CrCl is 30–50mL/min)	• Contraindicated if CrCl <30 mL/min • FDA black box warning for epidural/spinal hematoma risk with neuraxial anesthesia
DOACs	Oral	Apixaban 2.5 mg twice daily Rivaroxaban 10 mg daily Dabigatran 110 mg initially followed by 220 mg once hemostasis achieved, then 220 mg daily maintenance	• Currently FDA-approved for VTE prophylaxis in only THA and TKA • Rivaroxaban: Avoid if CrCl <15 mL/min; avoid in Child-Pugh Class B and C liver disease • Apixaban: No renal adjustment for VTE prophylaxis; avoid in Child–Pugh Class C liver disease • Dabigatran: FDA-approved in THA, off-label for TKA
Warfarin	Oral	Titrate to INR goal of 2–3	• Can be used when extended VTE prophylaxis is indicated (ie, THA, TKA) but has fallen out of favor given preference for aspirin or DOACs • Contraindicated in pregnancy
Aspirin[a]	Oral	Variable; low-dose options advised (ie, 81 mg once daily)	• Frequently used for extended VTE prevention following orthopedic surgery (ie, THA, TKA)

Abbreviations: HIT, heparin-induced thrombocytopenia; DOAC, direct oral anticoagulant; THA, total hip arthroplasty; TKA, total knee arthroplasty; VTE, venous thromboembolism.

[a] Per the EPCAT II trial, a hybrid strategy with aspirin or rivaroxaban may be used for VTE prophylaxis in patients undergoing TKA or THA.[13]

upon discharge (after initial DOAC prophylaxis) was noninferior to postdischarge rivaroxaban. However, aspirin prophylaxis is recommended with very low certainty by ASH, and recent studies have suggested inferiority of aspirin over low molecular weight heparin (LMWH) for VTE prevention.[10,13,20] While LMWH has demonstrated to be highly effective in preventing VTE, the ASH guidelines favor DOACs over LMWH.[10] Furthermore, LMWH has fallen out of favor given the strong preference for using an oral agent for VTE prophylaxis.

3. For hip fracture surgery, LMWH is recommended. The preponderance of studies assessing VTE prophylaxis in hip fracture patients has focused on heparin; however, the use of oral options (ie, DOACs, aspirin) has been increasing. A recent multicenter randomized trial showed aspirin to be noninferior to LMWH in patients with a variety of fractures.[21]

4. Factor XI(a) inhibitors are a new class of anticoagulants. Although preliminary data appear promising for effective VTE prevention with low bleeding risk,[22] these agents remain investigational.

5. Prophylaxis should be continued 10 to 14 days after all major orthopedic surgeries with extended duration up to 35 days for total hip arthroplasty. There are limited data in total knee arthroplasty and hip fracture surgery, but extended prophylaxis is commonly administered depending on individualized risk factors.

6. Other orthopedic procedures such as nonarthroplasty knee surgery, foot and ankle surgery, and upper limb surgery generally carry a lower inherent risk of VTE. The American College of Chest Physicians (ACCP) guidelines do not recommend pharmacologic prophylaxis for lower limb immobilization or knee arthroscopy,[6] but more recent studies favor using LMWH for patients requiring lower limb immobilization in a cast or brace.[23] When patient-specific VTE risk factors are present, including anesthesia time greater than 90 minutes, pharmacologic prophylaxis should be considered.[24]

ii. General and abdominal and pelvic surgeries

1. The 2012 ACCP guidelines recommend a risk-assessment method approach to patients undergoing general or abdominal-pelvic surgeries, specifically including gastrointestinal (GI), urologic, gynecologic, bariatric, vascular, and plastic and reconstructive surgery, as shown in **Table 3**.[5] Note[25] that laparoscopic cholecystectomy does not benefit from pharmacologic prophylaxis, and other surgery-specific recommendations are highlighted in later discussion.[10]

2. For noncancer patients undergoing major abdominal and pelvic surgeries, extended duration ($\geq$14 days) of pharmacologic prophylaxis with LMWH significantly reduces VTE.[26] The ASH guidelines include a low-certainty recommendation for extended prophylaxis following any major surgery.[10]

iii Surgery in patients with cancer

1. Patients with cancer undergoing surgery are at an increased risk of postprocedural VTE. The best supported options for pharmacologic prophylaxis are LMWH and fondaparinux; however, the American Society of Clinical Oncology 2023 guidelines update broadens the options to include apixaban or rivaroxaban (after LMWH or low-dose unfractionated heparin [LDUH] in the early postprocedural period) based on a small number of studies.[27]

Table 3
Recommended thromboprophylaxis by risk level for general or abdominal-pelvic surgeries

	Risk of Major Bleeding Complications	
Risk of Symptomatic VTE[a]	Average Risk (~1%)	High-risk (~2%) or Severe Consequences
Very low (<0.5%)	No specific prophylaxis	
Low (~1.5%)	Mechanical prophylaxis	
Moderate (~3.0%)	LMWH, LDUH, or mechanical prophylaxis	Mechanical
High (~6.0%)	LMWH or LDUH plus mechanical prophylaxis	Mechanical, until pharmacologic can be added safely
High-risk cancer surgery	LMWH or LDUH plus mechanical prophylaxis and extended duration LMWH postdischarge	Mechanical, until pharmacologic can be added safely
High-risk when LDUH or LMWH contraindicated or unavailable	Fondaparinux or low-dose aspirin (160 mg) aspirin or mechanical prophylaxis or both	Mechanical, until pharmacologic can be added safely

Abbreviations: LDUH, low-dose unfractionated heparin; LMWH, low-molecular weight heparin.
[a] Risk estimates based on observed data from the population in the validation study for the Caprini score.[25]
Adapted from 2012 ACCP Guidelines.[5]

2. Pharmacologic prophylaxis should be given for 7 to 10 days during the postprocedural period. An extended duration of 4 weeks is recommended for abdominal and pelvic surgeries in high-risk patients and for patients undergoing thoracic surgery for cancer (ie, pneumonectomy, esophagectomy, and high-risk lobectomy/segmentectomy).[28] The addition of mechanical prophylaxis while inpatient is recommended.

iv. Bariatric surgery

1. Due to the inherent comorbidities often associated with bariatric surgery, many patients are at high risk of VTE. There are increasing data to suggest extended-duration prophylaxis (10–15 days) is beneficial in this population,[29] and the 2019 American Association of Clinical Endocrinologists (AACE)/The Obesity Society (TOS)/American Society for Metabolic and Bariatric Surgery (ASMBS)/Obesity Medicine Association (OMA)/American Society of Anesthesiologists (ASA) guidelines recommend consideration of extended prophylaxis in high-risk patients.[30]

2. Weight-based dosing adjustment of LMWH should be considered for patients with significant obesity.

v. Urologic surgery

1. The European Association of Urology provides many surgery-specific and patient-specific recommendations for postprocedural thromboprophylaxis.[31]

2. The 2019 ASH guidelines highlight that patients undergoing transurethral resection of the prostate (TURP) or radical prostatectomy without additional compelling risk factors (including surgery-specific factors such as extended node dissection and/or open radical prostatectomy) should not receive pharmacologic prophylaxis.[10]

vi. Gynecologic surgery

1. While the ASH Guidelines recommend pharmacologic prophylaxis for all major gynecologic surgeries, the 2021 ACOG guidelines recommend a

risk-assessment method approach as outlined in **Table 3** (with the main differences being mechanical prophylaxis only for low-risk patients, the option of mechanical prophylaxis only for moderate-risk patients, and fondaparinux favored for patients with high bleeding risk where LMWH and LDUH cannot be used and risk of bleeding has diminished in the postprocedural period).[32]

vii. Vascular surgery

1. Major vascular surgeries pose an increased risk of VTE. In many cases, postprocedural therapeutic anticoagulation is indicated depending on patient risk factors and the type of surgery.

2. The data regarding pharmacologic VTE prophylaxis are limited; however, the ASH guidelines allow for the option of using pharmacologic prophylaxis for patients at high risk for VTE. When employed, LMWH or LDUH is the agent of choice.

3. The 2018 National Institute of Health and Clinical Excellence guidelines suggest administering 7 days of LMWH if VTE risk is greater than the risk of bleeding (except for low-risk patients undergoing varicose vein surgery <90 minutes long).[23] Alternatively, mechanical prophylaxis is advised if bleeding risk is greater than VTE risk.[23] It should be noted that caution with mechanical prophylaxis is necessary in patients with peripheral arterial disease. Measuring the ankle-brachial-index before mechanical prophylaxis use may inform decision-making.[33]

viii. Cardiac surgery

1. The evidence for benefit of primary thromboprophylaxis in cardiac surgery patients is limited and controversial.[34,35] The 2019 ASH guidelines found only low-certainty evidence that did not clearly support pharmacologic prophylaxis.[10] However, pharmacologic prophylaxis should be considered for high-risk patients with the remainder of patients being assessed on a case-by-case basis.[10]

ix. Thoracic surgery

1. There are limited data and no recent guidelines for thromboprophylaxis in noncancer thoracic surgery patients.[36] The 2012 ACCP guidelines recommend the following:

    a. patients at high risk for VTE receive LMWH or LDUH combined with mechanical prophylaxis,

    b. patients at moderate risk receive LMWH, LDUH, or mechanical prophylaxis,

    c. patients at high risk of both VTE and bleeding use mechanical prophylaxis alone until pharmacologic prophylaxis can be added safely.[5]

x. Neurosurgery

1. Due to the severe consequences of bleeding complications, pharmacologic prophylaxis is generally not recommended in major neurosurgical procedures except for those at very high risk for VTE, such as patients undergoing craniotomy for malignancy.[6,10] Mechanical prophylaxis should be used until the bleeding risk declines at which time LMWH can be considered for high-risk patients who have prolonged immobilization.[5,10]

xi. Otolaryngology surgery

1. There are no recent guidelines for thromboprophylaxis in patients undergoing head and neck surgery. The otolaryngology literature favors a risk-stratification approach to pharmacologic prophylaxis using risk-assessment systems such as the Caprini score balanced against the risk of bleeding.[37,38]

xii. Trauma surgery
1. Trauma patients are at high risk of VTE but balancing the risk of bleeding with pharmacologic prophylaxis is challenging, especially for injuries with severe bleeding consequences such as traumatic brain injury, spinal cord injury, and solid organ trauma.
2. There is some variability in guideline recommendations but the AAST/American College of Surgeons (ACS) 2021 guidelines present a consensus approach for clinical implementation. LMWH is the pharmacologic agent of choice and should be started immediately for patients without high-risk injuries.[39] Twice-daily prophylactic dosing is generally recommended though it is not Food and Drug Administration (FDA)-approved for this indication. LDUH is recommended for patients with renal dysfunction.[39]
3. For traumatic brain injury, timing of initiation is based on bleeding risk stratification schemes such as the Berne-Norwood criteria. Otherwise, pharmacologic prophylaxis should be started within 48 hours unless there is evidence of ongoing solid organ hemorrhage.[39]
4. Prophylactic placement of an inferior vena cava filter is not recommended.[39]

PERIPROCEDURAL ANTICOAGULATION MANAGEMENT

Approximately one-fifth of patients prescribed a vitamin K antagonist (VKA) or DOAC will undergo surgery or invasive procedures each year.[40] The periprocedural management of anticoagulants poses a common clinical scenario as these medications have broad indications, including treatment and prophylaxis of VTE as well as prevention of arterial thromboembolism (ATE) in atrial fibrillation, mechanical heart valves, and peripheral arterial disease.[41,42] These diseases and their anticoagulation have become more prevalent in an aging population for which surgery or invasive procedures are more common, thus increasing the incidence of this clinical issue.[43,44] The decision to interrupt anticoagulation for elective surgery or invasive procedures should consider individualized risk stratification, including procedure-specific bleeding risk (**Table 4**) and patient-specific risk factors for periprocedural thromboembolism (**Table 5**) and bleeding.[45]

Procedural Bleeding Risk

Guidelines suggest continuing anticoagulation uninterrupted for minor procedures like cataract surgery, basal cell and squamous cell excision, and minor dental procedures including cleanings and tooth extractions. High bleeding risk procedures require anticoagulation interruption. This process involves communication between the proceduralist and the prescriber of the anticoagulant to balance bleeding and thromboembolic risks. Interruption intervals for spinal anesthesia and procedures have conflicting guidelines with anesthesia guidelines typically suggesting longer hold times.[46]

Periprocedural Thromboembolic Risk

Risk of periprocedural thromboembolism is empirically estimated within the 2022 ACCP guidelines (see **Table 5**).[40] This framework helps balance the timing of preprocedural and postprocedural anticoagulation interruption and whether unfractionated heparin or low molecular weight heparin (LMWH) bridging for patients taking warfarin is indicated. Of note, for patients with a new VTE within the past 3 months, it may be prudent to delay non-time-sensitive surgery as risk of VTE recurrence is very high during this timeframe.

Table 4
Bleeding risk classification by surgery/procedure

Minimal Bleeding Risk Procedures	Low–moderate Bleeding Risk Procedures	High Bleeding Risk Procedures
~0% risk of major bleed in 30 d	0%–2% risk of major bleed in 30 d	>2% risk of major bleed in 30 d
Minor dermatologic procedures (excision of basal and squamous cell skin cancers, actinic keratoses, and premalignant or cancerous skin nevi)	Arthroscopy	Major surgery with extensive tissue injury
Ophthalmologic procedures, such as cataract surgery	Cutaneous and/or lymph node biopsies	Cancer surgery including solid tumor resection
Minor dental procedures (dental extraction, restoration, prosthetics, endodontics), dental cleaning, and fillings	Hand/foot surgery	Major orthopedic surgery including shoulder replacement surgery
Pacemaker or cardioverter-defibrillator device implantation	Coronary angiography	Reconstructive plastic surgery
—	GI endoscopy and/or biopsy	Urologic or GI surgery, including anastomosis
—	Abdominal hysterectomy	Transurethral prostate resection, bladder resection, or tumor ablation
—	Laparoscopic cholecystectomy	Nephrectomy
—	Abdominal hernia repair	Colonic polyp resection
—	Hemorrhoidal surgery	Bowel resection
—	Bronchoscopy with or without biopsy	Percutaneous endoscopic gastrotomy placement
—	Epidural injection	Endoscopic retrograde cholangiopancreatography
—	—	Surgery or biopsy of highly vascular organs (kidneys, liver, and spleen)
—	—	Cardiac, intracranial, or spinal surgery
—	—	Any major operation with duration >45 min
—	—	Neuraxial anesthesia

Commonly accepted examples of minimal, low–moderate, and high bleeding risk procedures.
Adapted from the 2022 American College of Chest Physician Guidelines.[40,45]

Periprocedural Management of Warfarin

The decision to interrupt warfarin therapy should include stratification of procedural bleeding risk and the individual's risk of bleeding and thromboembolism. For minimal bleeding risk procedures, it is not necessary to withhold warfarin therapy as interruption with bridging may result in higher bleeding complications as was demonstrated in a randomized trial of patients undergoing pacemaker implantation.[47] Other

Table 5
Periprocedural thromboembolism risk stratification by patient-specific factors

Risk Category	Venous Thromboembolism	Atrial Fibrillation	Prosthetic Heart Valves
High risk (>10% annual risk of ATE or >10% monthly risk of VTE); Bridging suggested	VTE within the last 1–3 mo Severe thrombophilia (protein C, protein S, or antithrombin deficiency; homozygous factor V Leiden or prothrombin gene G20210 A mutation or double heterozygous for each mutation; multiple thrombophilias) Antiphospholipid antibodies Active cancer with associated high VTE risk	$CHA_2DS_2VASc \geq 7$ or $CHADS_2 \geq 5$ Stroke or transient ischemic event within the last 3 mo Rheumatic valvular heart disease	Bileaflet mechanical mitral valve with major risk factors for stroke Caged ball or tilting-disc mitral and/or aortic valve Stroke or transient ischemic event within the last 3 mo
Moderate risk (4%–10% annual risk of ATE or 4%–10% monthly risk of VTE); Preprocedural bridging suggested for prosthetic heart valves without postprocedural bridging. Bridging not suggested for atrial fibrillation or VTE risk	VTE within the last 3–12 mo Recurrent VTE Nonsevere thrombophilia (heterozygous factor V Leiden or prothrombin gene G20210 A mutation) Active cancer or history of cancer	CHA_2DS_2VASc 5–6 or $CHADS_2$ 3–4	Bileaflet mechanical mitral valve without major risk factors for stroke Bileaflet mechanical aortic valve with major risk factors for stroke
Low risk (<4% annual risk of ATE or <2% monthly risk of VTE); Bridging not suggested	VTE >12 mo ago	CHA_2DS_2VASc 1–4 or $CHADS_2$ 0–2 and no prior stroke or transient ischemic event	Bileaflet mechanical aortic valve without major risk factors for stroke Bioprosthetic mitral and aortic valves including TAVI

Suggested risk stratification for patient-specific periprocedural thromboembolism.[40,45,55]
Abbreviations: VTE, Venous thromboembolism; TAVI, Transcatheter aortic valve implantation.
Adapted from the 2022 American College of Chest Physician Guidelines and 2020 AHA/ACC Guidelines.

procedures that do not require warfarin interruption include cataract surgery, many dermatologic procedures (including Moh's surgery), simple dental procedures, and GI endoscopy without biopsy. Otherwise, warfarin is typically held prior to surgery, and the 2022 ACCP guidelines suggest discontinuation of warfarin therapy at least 5 days prior to low/moderate bleeding risk procedures.[40] For high bleeding risk procedures, a commonly utilized interruption protocol stops warfarin therapy at least 5 days prior to the procedure and restart within 24 hours following the procedure after ensuring the patient is tolerating oral intake, adequate hemostasis is achieved, and no other invasive procedures are planned.[48] More than 90% of patients will experience normalization of their INR to less than 1.3 or have a near normal INR of 1.3 to 1.4 after 5 days of warfarin interruption, thus routine INR testing is not necessary.[49] This interruption strategy for warfarin often results in up to 1 week of subtherapeutic anticoagulation and may place patients at an increased risk of thromboembolism in the periprocedural period.[50] Risk stratification of patient-specific risk factors for thromboembolism can guide the decision to bridge interrupted VKA therapy with heparin or LMWH (see **Table 5**). The aim of periprocedural bridging is to minimize the duration of subtherapeutic anticoagulation.

Venous Thromboembolism

There are virtually no randomized trials for periprocedural interruption of warfarin in patients with VTE. A systematic review of 27 cohort studies found no decrease in VTE with a trend toward greater bleeding with bridging.[51] Registry data found poor correlation with bridging use and adverse outcomes and guidelines suggest bridging is overused.[40,52]

Atrial Fibrillation

The BRIDGE trial demonstrated safety in forgoing preprocedural and postprocedural bridging for patients taking warfarin for atrial fibrillation.[53] This randomized trial interrupted warfarin therapy 5 days prior to procedure and restarted warfarin within 24 hours following the procedure. These patients had a mean $CHADS_2$ score of 2.3 with only 12.8% of patients having a $CHADS_2$ score of 4 or more. Bridging was associated with a 3 fold increase in major bleeding risk; forgoing bridging was noninferior compared to bridging with respective ATE events. This trial informed the 2022 ACCP guidelines, which do not suggest periprocedural bridging of warfarin therapy for low–moderate-risk patients with atrial fibrillation. It is important to note that bridging is reasonable for patients with atrial fibrillation at high-risk for thromboembolism, such as those with a CHA_2DS_2VASc score of 7 or more or $CHADS_2$ score of 5 or 6, or those who have experienced stroke or TIA within the last 3 months or have a history of periprocedural stroke (see **Table 5**).[40]

Mechanical Heart Valves

Guidelines have long recommended bridging for most patients with mechanical heart valves; however, the 2022 ACCP guidelines suggest against bridging for some patients. Patients with low-risk mechanical aortic valves like bileaflet or On-X (but not single titling disk or ball-cage valves) with no other risk factors are suggested to forgo bridging, consistent with their 2012 guidelines (see **Table 5**).[40] Furthermore, the latest guidelines suggest mechanical mitral valves with a similar low-risk category may also be managed without periprocedural bridging. An important caveat is to identify additional patient-specific risk factors which require bridging (see **Table 5**).

The PERIOP-2 trial informed the 2022 ACCP guidelines and demonstrated safety in forgoing postprocedural bridging for patients taking warfarin for atrial fibrillation or mechanical heart valves. This trial interrupted warfarin therapy 5 days prior to procedure and randomized patients to receive LMWH bridging or placebo during the postprocedural period. These patients had a mean $CHADS_2$ score of 2.4 with only 17.5% of patients having a $CHADS_2$ score of 4 or more. Three hundred five patients with prosthetic mechanical valves were included, 133 of which were mitral valves and 172 aortic valves. In patients with mechanical heart valves, there was no significant difference in major thromboembolism and bleeding between the postprocedural bridging and no bridging groups. It is important to note that all patients received bridging anticoagulation with dalteparin during the pre procedural period.[54]

Patients with supratherapeutic INR in the preprocedural period or a target INR 2.5 to 3.5, such as those with mechanical mitral valve replacement, may need interruption of warfarin therapy for more than 5 days.[55,56] In patients with INR greater than 2.0 requiring urgent or emergent surgery, warfarin reversal is achieved with a combination of a prothrombin complex concentrate and vitamin K supplementation.[57]

Warfarin may be safely resumed within 24 hours following the surgery regardless of the procedural bleeding risk after ensuring the patient is tolerating oral intake, adequate hemostasis is achieved, and no other invasive procedures are planned.[40] **Table 6** provides a summary of bridging strategies for patients with high thrombotic risk stratified by procedural bleeding risk.

Periprocedural Management of Direct Oral Anticoagulants

Apixaban, rivaroxaban, edoxaban, and dabigatran have approximately 10 to 14 hour elimination half-lives (18–28 hours for dabigatran in patients with estimated creatinine

Table 6
Bridging strategies for patients on warfarin with high thrombotic risk stratified by procedural bleeding risk

	Low-moderate Bleeding Risk Procedure	High Bleeding Risk Procedure
5 d prior to procedure	*Stop* warfarin	*Stop* warfarin
3 d prior to procedure	*Start* therapeutic dose bridge in high thrombotic risk patients (see **Table 5**)	*Start* therapeutic dose bridge in high thrombotic risk patients (see **Table 5**)
1 d prior to procedure	*Stop* bridge	*Stop* bridge
Within 24 h following procedure	Resume warfarin at double home dose if adequate hemostasis achieved	Resume warfarin at double home dose if adequate hemostasis achieved
1 d following procedure	Resume therapeutic dose bridge in high thrombotic risk patients; Adjust warfarin dose according to INR	Adjust warfarin dose according to INR
2–3 d following procedure	Continue bridge in high thrombotic risk patients; Adjust warfarin dose according to INR	Resume therapeutic dose bridge in high thrombotic risk patients; Adjust warfarin dose according to INR
Therapeutic INR achieved	*Stop* bridge if present	*Stop* bridge if present

Bridging strategies for patients on warfarin with high thrombotic risk stratified by procedural bleeding risk[40]
Abbreviations: INR, International normalized ratio.

clearance ≤50 mL/min) and onset of action within 1 to 4 hours after administration (**Table 7**).[58,59] As a result, the periprocedural management of DOACs can be standardized with consideration of patient-specific renal function in the case of dabigatran. The short elimination half-lives and rapid onset of action obviate periprocedural bridging, and forgoing periprocedural bridging has been demonstrated to be safe.[60]

Management Guided by Procedural Bleeding Risk

For minimal bleeding risk procedures, including cardiac device implantation and atrioventricular node ablation, it is not necessary to interrupt DOAC therapy.[61–64] It is also reasonable to continue DOAC therapy without interruption for the same procedures deemed acceptable with warfarin (ie, cataract surgery, many dermatologic procedures, and simple dental procedures).

The PAUSE study investigated the safety of a standardized periprocedural DOAC management protocol in patients with atrial fibrillation undergoing a nonurgent surgery or invasive procedure. Apixaban, rivaroxaban, and edoxaban may be interrupted as early as 1 day prior to low–moderate bleeding risk procedures and 2 days prior to high bleeding risk procedures. Given dabigatran is primarily renally eliminated, it may require longer preprocedural interruption for patients with renal impairment. DOACs may be safely resumed 24 hours (postprocedural day 1) following low–moderate bleeding risk surgery and 48 to 72 hours (postprocedural day 2–3) following procedures of high bleeding risk. These interruption strategies were associated with low periprocedural rates of thromboembolism and major bleeding and are summarized in **Table 8**.[65]

Although this data inform the 2022 ACCP guidelines, there remains discrepancy when comparing these guidelines to the 2018 American Society of Regional Anesthesia and Pain Medicine (ASRA) guidelines. The ASRA guidelines recommend shared decision-making in periprocedural management of DOACs for low-risk procedures with consideration of a 2 half-life interval interruption before the procedure. Importantly, the ASRA guidelines suggest holding DOACs for 3 days prior to neuraxial anesthesia given the concern for risk of paraspinal hematoma. Additionally, the 2018 ASRA guidelines suggest considering preprocedural bridging in patients with high risk for thromboembolism (**Table 9**).[46]

Measuring Serum Direct Oral Anticoagulant Levels

Although measuring serum DOAC levels for elective procedures is seldom indicated, there may be utility when considering DOAC reversal prior to emergent surgery (with andexanet-alpha for apixaban and rivaroxaban, and idarucizumab for dabigatran).[40] If the DOAC level is less than 50 ng/mL, it may be safe to proceed with most surgeries

Table 7					
Pharmacokinetics of direct oral anticoagulants					
	Apixaban	**Rivaroxaban**	**Dabigatran Creatinine Clearance ≥50**	**Dabigatran Creatinine Clearance ≤50**	**Edoxaban**
Time to C_{max}	2.5–4 h	2–4 h	~1.5 h	~1.5 h	1–2 h
Elimination half-life	12 h	11–13 h	12–14 h	18–28 h	10–14 h

A summary of pharmacokinetics of DOAC most commonly prescribed in the United States with respect to time to maximal serum concentration (C_{max}) and elimination half-life. Creatinine clearance is estimated by the Cockcroft–Gault method.[58,59,71]

Table 8
Direct oral anticoagulant interruption strategies used in the PAUSE management trial

	Apixaban	Rivaroxaban	Dabigatran Creatinine Clearance ≥50	Dabigatran Creatinine Clearance ≤50	Edoxaban
Preprocedural interruption	Days	Days	Days	Days	Not studied
Minimal bleeding risk procedure	No interruption	No interruption	No interruption	No interruption	—
Low-moderate bleeding risk procedure	1	1	1	2	—
High bleeding risk procedure	2	2	2	4	—
Postprocedural resumption	—	—	—	—	—
Low-moderate bleeding risk procedure	1	1	1	1	—
High bleeding risk procedure	2-3	2-3	2-3	2-3	—

A summary of direct oral anticoagulant periprocedural interruption used in the PAUSE management trial strategies stratified by procedural bleeding risk and, for dabigatran, estimated creatinine clearance. Creatinine clearance is estimated by the Cockcroft–Gault method.[65,71]

Table 9
Direct oral anticoagulant interruption strategies suggested by the 2018 American Society of Regional Anesthesia and Pain Medicine guidelines

	Apixaban	Rivaroxaban	Edoxaban	Dabigatran Creatinine Clearance ≥50	Dabigatran Creatinine Clearance <50
Preprocedural interruption					
Low bleeding risk procedure	No interruption or hold for 2 half-lives	No interruption or hold for 2 half-lives	No interruption or hold for 2 half-lives	No interruption or hold for 2 half-lives	No interruption or hold for 2 half-lives
Moderate and high bleeding risk procedure	75 h (3 d)	65 h (3 d)	70 h (3 d)	4 d	5–6 d
Postprocedural resumption					
VTE risk not very high	Full dose at least 24 h after procedure	Full dose at least 24 h after procedure	Full dose at least 24 h after procedure	Full dose at least 24 h after procedure	Full dose at least 24 h after procedure
Very high VTE risk	Full dose at least 12 h after procedure	Full dose at least 12 h after procedure	Full dose at least 12 h after procedure	Half dose at least 12 h after procedure	Half dose at least 12 h after procedure

A summary of direct oral anticoagulant periprocedural interruption suggested by the 2018 ASRA guidelines. Strategies stratified by procedural bleeding risk, patient risk for VTE, and, for dabigatran, estimated creatinine clearance. Creatinine clearance is estimated by the Cockcroft–Gault method.[46,71]

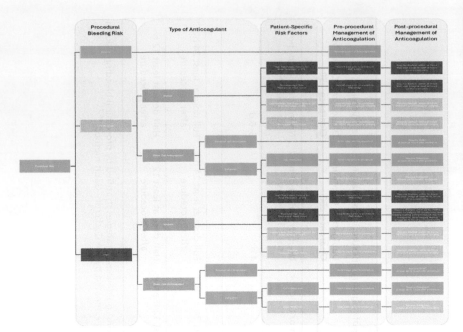

Fig. 1. A simplified algorithm to guide clinical decision-making in periprocedural interruption of anticoagulation.[72]

without reversal.[66,67] If the DOAC level is greater than 50 ng/mL or rapid DOAC testing is not available, DOAC reversal may be warranted prior to proceeding with emergent surgery.[68,69] Prothrombin complex concentrates may be given to overcome the anticoagulant effect of DOACs if reversal agents are unavailable or cost-prohibitive, but they do not actively reduce DOAC serum levels (**Fig. 1**).[40,70]

SUMMARY

Proficiency in the periprocedural management of antithrombotic agents is essential for the practicing provider given the high-risk nature of both thrombotic events and bleeding. For patients on long-term anticoagulation therapy, understanding if and when to hold the anticoagulant prior to surgery, as well as when to resume during the postprocedural period, is imperative for patient safety. Although rare, some patients on chronic warfarin therapy should receive anticoagulation bridging with a heparin product (ie, LMWH) during the periprocedural period. This differs from the DOACs where periprocedural bridging is essentially never indicated. All surgical patients require a thoughtful VTE risk assessment and bleeding risk assessment in order to implement safe and effective VTE prevention measures. In addition to knowing the several pharmacologic options available for VTE prophylaxis, the clinician must also understand their timing of periprocedural administration and duration of therapy postprocedurally.

CLINICS CARE POINTS

- Pharmacologic prophylaxis should be continued 10 to 14 days after all major orthopedic surgeries with extended duration up to 35 days for total hip arthroplasty.

- Pharmacologic prophylaxis is not recommended for patients undergoing laparoscopic cholecystectomy or TURP without other VTE risk factors.
- Mechanical prophylaxis alone should be used for most major neurosurgical procedures until the bleeding risk declines.
- Periprocedural bridging of warfarin for VTE is suggested only in patients who have had less than 3 months of therapy, and delay or rescheduling of the procedure is preferred.
- Preprocedural bridging of warfarin is suggested for patients with mechanical heart valves and moderate–high thrombotic risk factors; however, it is reasonable to forego postprocedural bridging in patients with low–moderate thrombotic risk factors.
- Although procedural bleeding risk guides the duration of periprocedural interruption of DOACs, the presence of renal dysfunction should also be considered for interruption of dabigatran.

REFERENCES

1. Gordon RJ, Lombard FW. Perioperative Venous Thromboembolism. Anesth Analg 2017;125(2):403–12.
2. Caprini JA. Thrombosis Risk Assessment as a Guide to Quality Patient Care. Disease-a-Month 2005;51(2–3):70–8.
3. Rogers SO, Kilaru RK, Hosokawa P, et al. Multivariable Predictors of Postoperative Venous Thromboembolic Events after General and Vascular Surgery: Results from the Patient Safety in Surgery Study. J Am Coll Surg 2007;204(6):1211–21.
4. Champagne B, Laryea J. Venous Thromboembolism Prophylaxis. Clin Colon Rectal Surg 2013;26(03):153–9.
5. Gould M, Garcia D, Wren S, et al. Prevention of VTE in Nonorthopedic Surgical Patients Antithrombotic Therapy and Prevention of Thrombosis, 9th ed: American College of Chest Physicians Evidence-Based Clinical Practice Guidelines. Chest 2012;141(2 Suppl):e227S–77S.
6. Falck-Ytter Y, Francis CW, Johanson NA, et al. Prevention of VTE in Orthopedic Surgery Patients: Antithrombotic Therapy and Prevention of Thrombosis, 9th ed: American College of Chest Physicians Evidence-Based Clinical Practice Guidelines. Chest 2012;141(2):e278Se325S.
7. DAHL OE, QUINLAN DJ, BERGQVIST D, et al. A critical appraisal of bleeding events reported in venous thromboembolism prevention trials of patients undergoing hip and knee arthroplasty. J Thromb Haemostasis 2010;8(9):1966–75.
8. Susmallian S, Danoch R, Raskin B, et al. Assessing Bleeding Risk in Bariatric Surgeries: A Retrospective Analysis Study. Dig Dis 2020;38(6):449–57.
9. Chindamo MC, Marques MA. Bleeding risk assessment for venous thromboembolism prophylaxis J Vasc Bras, 20, 2021. p. e20200109.
10. Anderson DR, Morgano GP, Bennett C, et al. American Society of Hematology 2019 guidelines for management of venous thromboembolism: prevention of venous thromboembolism in surgical hospitalized patients. Blood Advances 2019;3(23):3898–944.
11. Edwards JZ, Pulido PA, Ezzet KA, et al. Portable Compression Device and Low-Molecular-Weight Heparin Compared With Low-Molecular-Weight Heparin for Thromboprophylaxis After Total Joint Arthroplasty. J Arthroplasty 2008;23(8):1122–7.
12. Spyropoulos AC, Hussein M, Lin J, et al. Rates of symptomatic venous thromboembolism in US surgical patients: a retrospective administrative database study. J Thromb Thrombolysis 2009;28(4):458–64.

13. Anderson DR, Dunbar M, Murnaghan J, et al. Aspirin or Rivaroxaban for VTE Prophylaxis after Hip or Knee Arthroplasty. N Engl J Med 2018;378(8):699–707.

14. Murphy PB, Vogt KN, Lau BD, et al. Venous Thromboembolism Prevention in Emergency General Surgery. JAMA Surgery 2018;153(5):479.

15. Cohen AT, Tapson VF, Bergmann JF, et al. Venous thromboembolism risk and prophylaxis in the acute hospital care setting (ENDORSE study): a multinational cross-sectional study. Lancet 2008;371(9610):387–94.

16. Kakkar VV, Balibrea JL, MARTÍNEZ-GONZÁLEZ J, et al. Extended prophylaxis with bemiparin for the prevention of venous thromboembolism after abdominal or pelvic surgery for cancer: the CANBESURE randomized study. J Thromb Haemostasis 2010;8(6):1223–9.

17. Eikelboom JW, Quinlan DJ, Douketis JD. Extended-duration prophylaxis against venous thromboembolism after total hip or knee replacement: a meta-analysis of the randomised trials. Lancet 2001;358(9275):9–15.

18. Sobieraj DM, Lee S, Coleman CI, et al. Prolonged Versus Standard-Duration Venous Thromboprophylaxis in Major Orthopedic Surgery. Ann Intern Med 2012;156(10):720.

19. Simon SJ, Patell R, Zwicker JI, et al. Venous thromboembolism in total hip and total knee arthroplasty. JAMA Netw Open 2023;6(12):e2345883.

20. CRISTAL Study Group. Effect of aspirin vs enoxaparin on symptomatic venous thromboembolism in patients undergoing hip or knee arthroplasty: The CRISTAL Randomized Trial. JAMA 2022;328(8):719–27.

21. Aspirin or Low-Molecular-Weight Heparin for Thromboprophylaxis after a Fracture. N Engl J Med 2023;388(3):203–13.

22. Presume J, Ferreira J, Ribeiras R, et al. Achieving higher efficacy without compromising safety with factor XI inhibitors versus low molecular weight heparin for the prevention of venous thromboembolism in major orthopedic surgery—Systematic review and meta-analysis. J Thromb Haemostasis 2022;20(12):2930–8.

23. Zee AA, van Lieshout K, van der Heide M, et al. Low molecular weight heparin for prevention of venous thromboembolism in patients with lower-limb immobilization. Cochrane Database Syst Rev 2014;(4):CD006681.

24. National Institute for Health Care and Clinical Excellence. Venous thromboembolism in over 16s: reducing the risk of hospital-acquired deep vein thrombosis or pulmonary embolism. NICE Guideline [NG89] 2019. Available at: https://www.nice.org.uk/guidance/ng89.

25. Bahl V, Hu HM, Henke PK, et al. A validation study of a retrospective venous thromboembolism risk scoring method. Ann Surg 2010;251(2):344–50.

26. Felder S, Rasmussen MS, King R, et al. Prolonged thromboprophylaxis with low molecular weight heparin for abdominal or pelvic surgery. Cochrane Database Syst Rev 2019;8(8):CD004318.

27. Key NS, Khorana AA, Kuderer NM, et al. Venous thromboembolism prophylaxis and treatment in patients with cancer: ASCO Guideline Update. J Clin Oncol 2023;41(16):3063–71.

28. Shargall Y, Wiercioch W, Brunelli A, et al. Joint 2022 European Society of Thoracic Surgeons and The American Association for Thoracic Surgery guidelines for the prevention of cancer-associated venous thromboembolism in thoracic surgery. J Thorac Cardiovasc Surg 2023;165(3):794–824.e6.

29. Bartlett MA, Mauck KF, Stephenson CR, et al. Perioperative venous thromboembolism prophylaxis. Mayo Clin Proc 2020;95(12):2775–98.

30. Mechanick JI, Apovian C, Brethauer S, et al. Clinical Practice Guidelines for the Perioperative Nutrition, Metabolic, and Nonsurgical Support of Patients

Undergoing Bariatric Procedures – 2019 Update: Cosponsored by American Association of Clinical Endocrinologists/American College of Endocrinology, The Obesity Society, American Society for Metabolic and Bariatric Surgery. Obesity Medicine Association, and American Society of Anesthesiologists. Obesity 2020;28(4).

31. Tikkinen KAO, Cartwright R, Gould MK, et al. EAU Guidelines on Thromboprophylaxis in Urological Surgery. Presented at the EAU Annual Congress Amsterdam; 2022. 978-94-92671-16-5.

32. American College of Obstetricians and Gynecologists' Committee on Practice Bulletins—Gynecology. Prevention of Venous Thromboembolism in Gynecologic Surgery: ACOG Practice Bulletin, Number 232. Obstet Gynecol 2021;138(1): e1–15.

33. Khan T, Vohra R S, Homer-Vanniasinkam S. Perioperative Thromboprophylaxis and Anticoagulation in Patients Undergoing Non-Cardiac Vascular Surgery. Curr Vasc Pharmacol 2011;9(1):48–53.

34. Ho KM, Bham E, Pavey W. Incidence of Venous Thromboembolism and Benefits and Risks of Thromboprophylaxis After Cardiac Surgery: A Systematic Review and Meta-Analysis. J Am Heart Assoc 2015;4(10).

35. Di Nisio M, Peinemann F, Porreca E, et al. Primary prophylaxis for venous thromboembolism in patients undergoing cardiac or thoracic surgery. Cochrane Database Syst Rev 2015.

36. Shargall Y, Brunelli A, Murthy S, et al. Venous thromboembolism prophylaxis in thoracic surgery patients: an international survey. Eur J Cardio Thorac Surg 2019;57(2):331–7.

37. Cramer JD, Shuman AG, Brenner M. Antithrombotic Therapy for Venous Thromboembolism and Prevention of Thrombosis in Otolaryngology–Head and Neck Surgery: State of the Art Review 2018;158(4):627–36.

38. Moubayed SP, Eskander A, Mourad MW, et al. Systematic review and meta-analysis of venous thromboembolism in otolaryngology-head and neck surgery. Head Neck 2017;39(6):1249–58.

39. Yorkgitis BK, Berndtson AE, Cross A, et al. American Association for the Surgery of Trauma/American College of Surgeons-Committee on Trauma Clinical Protocol for inpatient venous thromboembolism prophylaxis after trauma. J Trauma Acute Care Surg 2022;92(3):597–604.

40. Douketis JD, Spyropoulos AC, Murad MH, et al. Perioperative Management of Antithrombotic Therapy: An American College of Chest Physicians Clinical Practice Guideline. Chest 2022;162(5):e207–43. Epub 2022 Aug 11. Erratum in: Chest. 2023 Jul;164(1):267.

41. Colacci M, Tseng EK, Sacks CA, et al. Oral Anticoagulant Utilization in the United States and United Kingdom. J Gen Intern Med 2020;35(8):2505–7. Epub 2020 Jun 8.

42. Bonaca MP, Bauersachs RM, Anand SS, et al. Rivaroxaban in peripheral artery disease after revascularization. N Engl J Med 2020;382(21):1994–2004. Epub 2020 Mar 28.

43. Omling E, Jarnheimer A, Rose J, et al. Population-based incidence rate of inpatient and outpatient surgical procedures in a high-income country. Br J Surg 2018;105(1):86–95. Epub 2017 Nov 13.

44. Steinberg BA, Gao H, Shrader P, et al. International trends in clinical characteristics and oral anticoagulation treatment for patients with atrial fibrillation: Results from the GARFIELD-AF, ORBIT-AF I, and ORBIT-AF II registries. Am Heart J 2017;194:132–40. Epub 2017 Aug 24.

45. Spyropoulos AC, Brohi K, Caprini J, et al. SSC Subcommittee on Perioperative and Critical Care Thrombosis and Haemostasis of the International Society on Thrombosis and Haemostasis. Scientific and Standardization Committee Communication: Guidance document on the periprocedural management of patients on chronic oral anticoagulant therapy: Recommendations for standardized reporting of procedural/surgical bleed risk and patient-specific thromboembolic risk. J Thromb Haemostasis 2019;17(11):1966-72. Epub 2019 Aug 22.
46. Narouze S, Benzon HT, Provenzano D, et al. Interventional Spine and Pain Procedures in Patients on Antiplatelet and Anticoagulant Medications (Second Edition): Guidelines From the American Society of Regional Anesthesia and Pain Medicine, the European Society of Regional Anaesthesia and Pain Therapy, the American Academy of Pain Medicine, the International Neuromodulation Society, the North American Neuromodulation Society, and the World Institute of Pain. Reg Anesth Pain Med. 2018 Apr;43(3):225-262.
47. Birnie DH, Healey JS, Wells GA, et al, BRUISE CONTROL Investigators. Pacemaker or defibrillator surgery without interruption of anticoagulation. N Engl J Med 2013;368(22):2084-93. Epub 2013 May 9.
48. Steib A, Barre J, Mertes M, et al. Can oral vitamin K before elective surgery substitute for preoperative heparin bridging in patients on vitamin K antagonists? J Thromb Haemostasis 2010;8(3):499-503. Epub 2009 Nov 12.
49. White RH, McKittrick T, Hutchinson R, et al. Temporary discontinuation of warfarin therapy: changes in the international normalized ratio. Ann Intern Med 1995; 122(1):40-2.
50. Schulman S, Hwang HG, Eikelboom JW, et al. Loading dose vs. maintenance dose of warfarin for reinitiation after invasive procedures: a randomized trial. J Thromb Haemostasis 2014;12(8):1254-9. Epub 2014 Jun 25.
51. Baumgartner C, de Kouchkovsky I, Whitaker E, et al. Periprocedural Bridging in Patients with Venous Thromboembolism: A Systematic Review. Am J Med 2019; 132(6):722-32.e7. Epub 2019 Jan 16.
52. Barnes GD, Li Y, Gu X, et al. Periprocedural bridging anticoagulation in patients with venous thromboembolism: A registry-based cohort study. J Thromb Haemostasis 2020;18(8):2025-30. Epub 2020 Jun 25.
53. Douketis JD, Spyropoulos AC, Kaatz S, et al. Perioperative Bridging Anticoagulation in Patients with Atrial Fibrillation. N Engl J Med 2015;373(9):823-33. Epub 2015 Jun 22.
54. Kovacs MJ, Wells PS, Anderson DR, et al. PERIOP2 Investigators. operative low molecular weight heparin bridging treatment for patients at high risk of arterial thromboembolism (PERIOP2): double blind randomised controlled trial. BMJ 2021;373:n1205.
55. Otto CM, Nishimura RA, Bonow RO, et al. 2020 ACC/AHA Guideline for the Management of Patients With Valvular Heart Disease: A Report of the American College of Cardiology/American Heart Association Joint Committee on Clinical Practice Guidelines. Circulation 2021;143(5). e72-e227. Epub 2020 Dec 17. Erratum in: Circulation. 2021 Feb 2;143(5):e229. Erratum in: Circulation. 2023 Aug 22;148(8):e8. Erratum in: Circulation. 2023 Nov 14;148(20):e185.
56. Hylek EM, Regan S, Go As, et al. Clinical predictors of prolonged delay in return of the international normalized ratio to within the therapeutic range after excessive anticoagulation with warfarin. Ann Intern Med 2001;135(6):393-400.
57. Levy JH, Connors JM, Steiner ME, et al. Management of oral anticoagulants prior to emergency surgery or with major bleeding: A survey of perioperative practices in North America: Communication from the Scientific and Standardization

Committees on Perioperative and Critical Care Haemostasis and Thrombosis of the International Society on Thrombosis and Haemostasis. Res Pract Thromb Haemost 2020;4(4):562–8.

58. Hindley B, Lip GYH, McCloskey AP, et al. Pharmacokinetics and pharmacodynamics of direct oral anticoagulants. Expet Opin Drug Metab Toxicol 2023; 19(12):911–23.

59. Stangier J, Rathgen K, Stähle H, et al. Influence of renal impairment on the pharmacokinetics and pharmacodynamics of oral dabigatran etexilate: an open-label, parallel-group, single-centre study. Clin Pharmacokinet 2010;49(4):259–68.

60. Nazha B, Pandya B, Cohen J, et al. Periprocedural outcomes of direct oral anticoagulants versus warfarin in nonvalvular atrial fibrillation. Circulation 2018; 138(14):1402–11.

61. Pillarisetti J, Maybrook R, Parikh V, et al. Peri-procedural use of direct anticoagulation agents during cardiac device implantation: vitamin K antagonists vs direct oral anticoagulants. J Intervent Card Electrophysiol 2020;58(2):141–6.

62. Reynolds MR, Allison JS, Natale A, et al. A prospective randomized trial of apixaban dosing during atrial fibrillation ablation: the AEIOU trial. JACC Clin Electrophysiol 2018;4(5):580–8.

63. Nakamura K, Naito S, Sasaki T, et al. Uninterrupted vs. interrupted periprocedural direct oral anticoagulants for catheter ablation of atrial fibrillation: a prospective randomized single-centre study on post-ablation thrombo-embolic and haemorrhagic events. Europace 2019;21(2):259–67.

64. Yu HT, Shim J, Park J, et al. When is it appropriate to stop non-vitamin K antagonist oral anticoagulants before catheter ablation of atrial fibrillation? A multi-centre prospective randomized study. Eur Heart J 2019;40(19):1531–7.

65. Douketis JD, Spyropoulos AC, Duncan J, et al. Perioperative management of patients with atrial fibrillation receiving a direct oral anticoagulant. JAMA Intern Med 2019;179(11):1469–78.

66. Kaserer A, Kiavialaitis GE, Braun J, et al. Impact of rivaroxaban plasma concentration on perioperative red blood cell loss. Transfusion 2020;60(1):197–205.

67. Hofer H, Oberladstätter D, Schlimp CJ, et al. Role of DOAC plasma concentration on perioperative blood loss and transfusion requirements in patients with hip fractures. Eur J Trauma Emerg Surg 2023;49(1):165–72.

68. Pollack CV Jr, Reilly PA, van Ryn J, et al. Idarucizumab for dabigatran reversal - full cohort analysis. N Engl J Med 2017;377(5):431–41.

69. Connolly SJ, Crowther M, Eikelboom JW, et al, ANNEXA-4 Investigators. Full study report of andexanet alfa for bleeding associated with factor Xa inhibitors. N Engl J Med 2019;380(14):1326–35.

70. Cuker A, Burnett A, Triller D, et al. Reversal of direct oral anticoagulants: Guidance from the Anticoagulation Forum. Am J Hematol 2019;94(6):697–709.

71. Schwartz JB. Potential effect of substituting estimated glomerular filtration rate for estimated creatinine clearance for dosing of direct oral anticoagulants. J Am Geriatr Soc 2016;64(10):1996–2002.

72. Shaw JR, Kaplovitch E, Douketis J. Periprocedural management of oral anticoagulation. Med Clin North Am 2020;104(4):709–26.

Coronary Disease Risk Prediction, Risk Reduction, and Postoperative Myocardial Injury

Matthew A. Pappas, MD, MPH, FHM[a,b,c,*],
Leonard S. Feldman, MD[d], Andrew D. Auerbach, MD, MPH, MHM[e]

KEYWORDS

- Preoperative period • Perioperative care • Cardiovascular diagnostic techniques

KEY POINTS

- Patients with urgent medical conditions, including previously-undiagnosed or suboptimally-managed acute cardiac disease, should have those high-acuity conditions addressed before elective surgery.
- Workup and diagnosis of cardiac disease in previously-undiagnosed, asymptomatic persons will not reduce cardiac complications, but will act as a barrier to surgery and delay surgery when completed.
- Multiple tools exist to predict incident perioperative cardiac events, with different limitations.
- Assessing whether the expected benefit of surgery outweighs the expected harms remains a key role of preoperative assessment. When current risk assessment tools leave that decision unclear, biochemistries can refine risk predictions.
- With the possible exception of withholding angiotensin-converting enzyme inhibitors or angiotensin receptor blockers in the 24 hours before surgery, preoperative management changes that reduce the risk of cardiac complications have been elusive.

INTRODUCTION/BACKGROUND

Worldwide, more than 10 million adults each year have a cardiac complication within the 30 days after major noncardiac surgery.[1] Cardiac complications account for at least one-third of perioperative deaths, increase both costs of care and duration of post-surgical hospitalization, and worsen long-term patient outcomes.[2–5]

[a] Department of Hospital Medicine, Cleveland Clinic, Cleveland, OH, USA; [b] Center for Value-based Care Research, Cleveland Clinic, Cleveland, OH, USA; [c] Outcomes Research Consortium, Cleveland, OH, USA; [d] Departments of Medicine and Pediatrics, Division of Hospital Medicine, Johns Hopkins Hospital, Baltimore, MD, USA; [e] Department of Hospital Medicine, University of California, San Francisco, CA, USA
* Corresponding author. 9500 Euclid Avenue, Mail Stop G-10, Cleveland, OH 44195.
E-mail address: pappasm@ccf.org

Med Clin N Am 108 (2024) 1039–1051
https://doi.org/10.1016/j.mcna.2024.06.003 **medical.theclinics.com**
0025-7125/24/© 2024 Elsevier Inc. All rights are reserved, including those for text and data mining, AI training, and similar technologies.

For patients at risk of perioperative cardiac complications, the preoperative evaluation can serve multiple purposes. First, for patients with poorly treated medical conditions, it allows physicians to prioritize medical care that may be more urgent than elective surgery (such as evaluation of exertional angina or management of decompensated heart failure). Second, it allows a careful prediction of the risk of operative complications, to both ensure the expected benefit of a proposed surgery exceeds the expected harms and facilitate good patient decisions. Third, it allows physicians to make temporary changes to patient management to reduce operative risk, such as withholding anticoagulants or antiplatelet agents. These 3 important goals—diagnosis of existing medical conditions, prediction of surgical benefit and harm, and management of chronic conditions—require different bodies of evidence and require the preoperative physician to perform different tasks. The authors therefore discuss each of the 3 goals separately.

DISCUSSION
Diagnosis of Previously-Undiagnosed or Suboptimally-Managed Disease

For more than 45 years, it has been standard practice to delay all but the most urgent surgical procedures for patients with active coronary syndromes or decompensated heart failure.[6] Management of those syndromes is not unique to the preoperative setting, and should take precedence over preoperative testing in all but the most urgent surgical scenarios.[7–10] In general, postponing elective surgery is the core approach to reducing cardiac risk for patients with acute cardiac issues.[6]

Coronary artery disease (CAD) has well-known risk factors, develops over time, and is often asymptomatic. This has led to the observation that CAD is under-recognized in persons without recent testing, and the theory that diagnosing and treating CAD in asymptomatic persons could in turn reduce surgical risk. Observational studies in the 1980s suggested that coronary revascularization might be associated with lower morbidity and/or mortality in subsequent noncardiac surgery.[11] However, a large randomized trial of patients evaluated for vascular surgery, the Coronary Artery Revascularization Prophylaxis Trial, showed no difference in short-term or long-term mortality with coronary revascularization; this study remains the core counterargument to any approach which emphasizes diagnosis of CAD and revascularization before surgery.[12]

Medications have also been examined as a potential approach to reducing operative cardiac risk. Many medications have been studied, and some are promising (discussed in detail below). Still, none of those medications require a diagnosis of CAD for appropriate use. As such, we see no changes to preoperative management that would support pursuing a diagnosis of CAD in asymptomatic persons.[13]

In rare situations where physicians wanted to pursue a diagnosis of CAD, models to estimate the pretest probability of CAD from outpatient settings are likely reasonably representative (none have been specifically validated in a preoperative population). In contemporary outpatient settings, the best-performing model appears to be CAD2.[8,14] Previous work applied this model to a large single-center cohort of patients considering a wide range of noncardiac surgeries, finding a median pretest probability of CAD of 6.5% (interquartile range: 2.6% to 15.1%).[15,16] In this probability range, functional stress testing is likely not diagnostically helpful, and coronary computed tomography angiography (CTA) would generally be the preferred diagnostic modality if a diagnosis is pursued.[8,17,18] Diagnostic workup in an asymptomatic patient would also likely delay and deter surgery, without offering clear patient benefit.[19] Physicians pursuing such a workup must first have a clear rationale for how making a diagnosis of stable CAD will improve their patient's health. Otherwise, such workup likely contributes to over diagnosis, and should not be pursued.[20]

Predicting Risk of Perioperative Cardiac Complications

Current society guidelines suggest any of 3 tools for predicting incident cardiovascular events: the Revised Cardiac Risk Index (RCRI), the American College of Surgeons' National Surgical Quality Improvement Program (ACS-NSQIP), or the Myocardial Injury or Cardiac Arrest (MICA).[21–23] Other tools have been published as well, with the American University of Beirut HAS2 (AUB-HAS2) among the most promising.[24] Here, the authors focus on the 3 widely recommended tools.

The most-studied risk prediction tool, RCRI, was developed based on a cohort of 4315 patients at a single center between 1989 and 1994.[25] The cohort included 98 events in a composite endpoint that included myocardial infarction (MI), pulmonary edema, ventricular fibrillation, complete heart block, or cardiac arrest. Consenting patients had sampling of creatine kinase (CK) with reflex testing of creatine kinase myocardial band (CK-MB), with other follow-up data collected by manual chart review. This cohort predated the first universal definition of MI.[26]

The American College of Surgeons' National Surgical Quality Improvement Program (NSQIP) calculator predicts many different complications based on cases sampled from completed surgeries at participating hospitals. Compared to the cohort used to create RCRI, the dataset underlying ACS-NSQIP is substantially larger and potentially more representative of patients who complete surgery in the US hospitals. However, the calculator's design and implementation limit study in external datasets: its terms of use prohibit automated access, and model weights have never been published. Therefore, confidence in the model's performance rests on reported internal validation and limited external validations that have generally focused on specific procedures.[27,28] The most recent version of the calculator, which transitioned from a regression-based modeling approach to a machine learning-based approach, used approximately 5 million patient records from 2016 through 2020, with 10,676 cardiac events.[29]

The myocardial infarction or cardiac arrest (MICA) model used 2 years of the NSQIP dataset (2007 and 2008) to derive a logistic regression predictor of the same cardiac endpoint—MI or cardiac arrest.[30] Those 2 years of the NSQIP dataset included 468,795 cases, with 2772 outcome events. The authors' published model weights alongside the original derivation, which has allowed other authors to apply the model to other cohorts.[15,16] Owing to the smaller dataset, the authors grouped surgeries into 21 categories, rather than relying on individual current procedural terminology (CPT®) codes. Categorizing surgeries is a reasonable strategy to limit overfitting, but because different surgeries likely have different inherent cardiac risk, this may be a source of imprecision compared to ACS-NSQIP.[31] These years of the NSQIP cohort straddled the first and second universal definitions of MI.[32]

Most perioperative myocardial infarctions occur within 48 hours of surgery.[5] Perhaps because of analgesic use, many such patients do not report symptoms of ischemia.[33] Still more patients will have elevated cardiac biomarkers that do not meet the universal definition of MI, called "myocardial injury after noncardiac surgery (MINS)." As with MI, MINS is strongly associated with 30-day post-operative mortality.[1,34] Physicians tasked with estimating operative risk may therefore wish to estimate the risk of MINS as a surrogate endpoint, but preoperative tools to do so are limited. A state-of-the-art machine learning algorithm developed in the Vascular events In noncardiac Surgery patients cOhort evaluatioN (VISION) Study cohort has been published, but has not yet been validated in a different dataset and would require integration into an electronic health record (EHR).[35] For prediction of MINS, RCRI, whose development cohort included routine sampling of cardiac enzymes, has theoretic advantages over the prediction tools based on NSQIP data. Still, RCRI has not been specifically validated for this purpose, and other ready-to-use calculators are lacking. Validation of any prediction tool for this purpose would require a separate cohort with routine measurement of cardiac biomarkers. Without routine measurement of biomarkers, many MIs and most cases of MINS would be undetected.

Comparisons between RCRI and MICA have found substantial discordance in predicted rates of cardiac complications.[36] See **Table 1**. As described earlier, this discordance has many reasons, including patient populations in different eras of ambulatory surgery, different outcome definitions, differences in spectrum of risk factors (such as broader definitions of hypertension in more recent decades), and differences in specificity of risk factors (RCRI categorizes surgeries into 4 groups, MICA categorizes surgeries into 21 groups, and ACS-NSQIP uses CPT codes as an input).[25,27,30] Other issues likely amplify discordance in these prediction tools. First, many prediction models have poor external calibration that is, the difference between predicted from observed events.[37] Second, dichotomizing a continuous risk measure—the 2014 American College of Cardiology/American Heart Association (ACC/AHA) guidelines recommend a risk threshold of 1% when considering further testing—will ensure that very small differences in predicted risk around that threshold lead to different recommendations. In a large Canadian cohort, all patients—even those with an RCRI of 0—had a predicted cardiac complication rate above 1%.[22] A risk threshold may be justified for some preoperative decisions, but ideal risk thresholds should be based on the expected benefits and harms of the care options, not selected arbitrarily.

Many other measurement scales likely have prognostic value but are not designed to predict risk of cardiac complications. Most prominently, the American Society of Anesthesiologists' (ASA) physical status classification system is likely correlated with a patient's risk of a major adverse cardiac event.[38] (Indeed, as part of the development of RCRI, the authors compared their tool to ASA class, which predicted cardiac risk, albeit with lower discrimination than RCRI.[6]) The Duke Activity Status Index (DASI) has prognostic value, and frailty risk scores do as well.[39] However, type of surgery is an important predictor of surgical risk, and tools that assess only patient-level measures such as these are likely to be inferior tools that incorporate some information about the type of surgery. Many such tools also rely on subjective assessments, which could lead to suboptimal reliability. When a patient's predicted perioperative cardiac risk is germane, physicians should use a calculator designed for that purpose.

Some authors have proposed using measures like DASI to assess patient functional status in conjunction with a procedure-specific cardiac risk assessment.[39,40] Current ACC/AHA guidelines suggest a similar approach—estimating patient functional status for patients at elevated risk of an adverse cardiac event when considering cardiac testing.[21] However, there is little reason to think that pursuing a diagnosis of stable CAD would be more helpful in patients whose functional status is above or below some threshold. The authors' practice therefore differs from the 2014 guideline in that they consider a patient's current functional status (and any improvements to patient function that are hoped for with surgery) into a qualitative assessment of the expected benefit of surgical management.

Additional Prognostic Measures

Both preoperative B-type natriuretic peptide (BNP) and N-terminal pro B-type natriuretic peptide (NT-pro-BNP) likely have prognostic value when added to RCRI.[41–43] Current Canadian guidelines recommend measurement of NT-pro-BNP for patients

Table 1

Outcomes considered adverse cardiac events in the revised cardiac risk index and myocardial infarction or cardiac arrest prediction tools

	Revised Cardiac Risk Index	Gupta-Myocardial Infarction or Cardiac Arrest
Myocardial Infarction	• CK-MB >5% • CK-MB >3% & electrocardiogram changes	• ST elevation >1 mm in ≧2 contiguous leads • New LBBB • New Q wave in ≧2 contiguous leads • New troponin elevation >3x ULN + "suspected myocardial injury"
Cardiac arrest	"Ventricular fibrillation or primary cardiac arrest"	"Absence of cardiac rhythm or presence of chaotic cardiac rhythm that results in loss of consciousness requiring the initiation of any component of basic and/or advanced cardiac life support"
Pulmonary edema	"Radiologist reading consistent with pulmonary edema in a plausible clinical setting"	×
Complete heart block	✓	×

Abbreviations: CK-MB, creatine kinase myocardial band; LBBB, left bundle branch block; ULN, upper limit of normal.

65 years of age or older and for patients at least 45 years of age with cardiovascular disease or an RCRI of 1 or greater.[22] Multiple thresholds above which BNP or NT-pro-BNP can be considered "elevated" have been reported.[44] The relationship between preoperative natriuretic peptide levels and perioperative cardiac events is likely a continuous one, but prediction tools incorporating BNP or NT-pro-BNP as a continuous variable in addition to other patient-level and surgery-level predictors are lacking.[44]

Preoperative troponin also has incremental risk prediction when added to RCRI, with predictive ability similar to natriuretic peptides.[43,45,46] European guidelines emphasize troponin over natriuretic peptides for reasons of cost, availability, and the ability to compare postoperative measurements against the preoperative value.[23] As with natriuretic peptides, prediction models that incorporate troponin as a continuous variable in addition to other patient-level and surgery-specific predictors are lacking.

Other biochemical results could plausibly improve risk predictions as well. For example, a single-center cohort study found improved prediction of MI when preoperative hemoglobin was added to RCRI.[16] Hemoglobin has the advantage of being almost universally available and inexpensive, but external validation of a prediction tool that incorporates hemoglobin is lacking.

Cardiac test results other than biochemistries have been less successful at improving predictions. A prospective study found that coronary CTA results overestimated perioperative risk, which could lead to inappropriate decisions to delay or cancel surgeries.[47] Left ventricular ejection fraction from resting echocardiography also predicts perioperative cardiac events, but underperforms NT-pro-BNP.[48] And in the largest cohort study to date with detailed clinical data, stress test results did not improve predicted risk of MI when added to variables included in RCRI or MICA.[16] Because cardiac disease is a predictor of surgical risk, it remains possible that making a new diagnosis of CAD could modestly improve predictions. However, that would only refine 1 predictor in a multivariable model. A preponderance of evidence suggests that, when the decision to proceed to surgery requires a more refined estimate of perioperative cardiac risk, biochemical testing will be more useful than functional or anatomic cardiac testing.

For multiple reasons, future efforts would do well to incorporate modeling tools directly into the EHR. First, it is difficult to incorporate multiple predictors and complex relationships into readily memorized tools like RCRI. Adding predictors such as hemoglobin would be dramatically easier with a built-in prediction tool capable of interfacing with the patient record.[16] Second, the data entry currently required to use tools such as ACS-NSQIP or MICA is unnecessary and tedious, potentially limiting their use. Third, because different systems document and encode information differently, models derived at different systems could identify different predictors.[49] Fourth, even if they used the same predictors, many prediction models (including outpatient models of incident cardiac events) have poor external calibration.[37] Locally-informed models could be calibrated to local event rates. To the authors' knowledge, no such models are currently available for major EHR systems.

Management Changes to Reduce Operative Cardiac Risk

In general, patients with medical conditions that require immediate attention (and whose surgery can be delayed safely) should have their acute medical issue addressed before surgery. Postponing elective surgery until after treatment of acute decompensated heart failure or unstable angina has long been standard practice. Although outcomes research to demonstrate improved outcomes is lacking, most experts support delaying elective surgery and addressing other acute medical issues as well.

For patients without medical issues of greater urgency than the proposed surgery, physicians then must determine whether the expected benefits of surgery outweigh the expected harms. If the expected harms exceed the expected benefits, surgery should be canceled. Every surgery confers some irreducible risk, and canceling surgery will certainly reduce surgical mortality.

If surgery offers expected net benefit, the goal is to reduce the risk of surgery to the extent possible. Unfortunately, many interventions hypothesized to reduce surgical risk have proven disappointing. Most notably, coronary revascularization did not reduce mortality in an adequately-powered trial in a high-risk population.[12] A large randomized trial suggested that clonidine did not reduce MI or death compared to placebo; there is little reason to think other alpha-agonists would be more helpful.[50,51] The best-available evidence suggests that initiating a beta-blocker within 24 hours of surgery will reduce nonfatal MI but increase the risk of death, stroke, hypotension, and bradycardia.[52] Other data suggest that preoperative withdrawal of beta blockers is associated with increased postoperative mortality.[53,54] The authors here discuss changes in the near-term preoperative setting; patients with a clear long-term indication for beta blockade who have been suboptimally-managed are considered more fully in the above-mentioned text). Calcium channel blocker initiation has been tested in small trials, but the largest meta-analysis included only 5 MIs and this remains a hypothesis without high-quality evidence.[55] Statins are associated with lower perioperative risk, but this may be healthy user bias, and efforts to randomize patients to preoperative statin initiation have been limited by low enrollment.[56–60] Overall, little evidence supports initiating, withholding, or making dose changes for any of these medications.

One possible exception comes in the form of ACE-inhibitors and angiotensin receptor blockers (ARBs). Trials that compared withholding ACE-inhibitors or ARBs have not been powered to demonstrate differences in MI; however, withholding those agents appears to reduce the rate of intraoperative hypotension.[22] Because hypotension may be a key mediator of adverse events, there is reason to believe that withholding these agents before surgery may improve outcomes. Although the quality of evidence is low, at least 1 major guideline recommends withholding ACE-inhibitors and ARBs starting 24 hours before noncardiac surgery.[22]

Decisions regarding antiplatelet agents, including aspirin, are influenced by the estimated risk of perioperative bleeding and the risk of perioperative thrombotic events. Randomized trial data suggest that aspirin increases the risk of major bleeding without reducing the risk of MI or mortality.[61] There is little reason to start aspirin (or any other antiplatelet agent) based on operative cardiac risk. For patients already taking an antiplatelet agent, whether to continue that agent is controversial, and guidelines differ.[22,62] Eventually after percutaneous coronary intervention, the incremental risk of MI or in-stent thrombosis from stopping an antiplatelet agent would be less consequential than the incremental risk of bleeding with continuing that agent. However, as with other similar questions, an estimate of the optimal timing for that complex set of trade-offs would require simulation methods.[63] For the moment, whether aspirin can be safely withheld for a patient with an indwelling stent, and whether the harm of potential bleeding is sufficient to justify the incremental risk of MI, should remain based on the consensus of the treating physicians. Like other authors, we generally favor withholding aspirin before intracranial or spinal procedures owing to the severe consequences of bleeding at those surgical sites.[62] Based on very low certainty of evidence, current guidelines suggest that when antiplatelet agents are withheld, aspirin be withheld for 7 days or fewer, clopidogrel be withheld for 5 days, ticagrelor for 3 to 5 days, and prasugrel for 7 days.[62] The authors follow those ranges when withholding antiplatelet agents.

Future studies of interventions could plausibly use MINS as a biochemical intermediate endpoint. Although MINS would be a surrogate endpoint, it is clearly related to 30-day postoperative mortality and an order of magnitude more common than MI.[1,34] Many management changes that were hypothesized to improve perioperative outcomes have failed to do so in randomized trials. MINS offers a promising surrogate: in exchange for routine sampling of cardiac biomarkers in high-risk patients, researchers could more rapidly test whether management changes reduce the cardiac risk incurred by surgery. In the interim, for patients without acute medical conditions for whom the expected benefits of surgery outweigh the expected harms, precious few management changes will reduce perioperative cardiac risk. Moreover, there are no interventions that reduce mortality among patients who have MINS. Still, the AHA "encourage [s] serial [troponin] measurement in the 2 to 3 days after noncardiac inpatient surgery in selected at-risk patients."[44] The authors generally do not favor routine monitoring, but when patients are at elevated risk and better postoperative prognostic information could inform care, troponin measurements would be reasonable. See **Table 2**.

Table 2 Summary of recommendations	
When considering...	**The Authors Recommend...**
Whether a patient has undiagnosed obstructive coronary disease	Recognizing that workup and diagnosis of cardiac disease in previously-undiagnosed, asymptomatic persons will not reduce cardiac complications, will act as a barrier to surgery and delay surgery when completed, and will not improve patient outcomes In rare circumstances where a diagnosis of stable coronary disease might be useful, consider a patient's pretest probability using the CAD2 model before pursuing further workup
Whether a patient's expected benefit from surgery exceeds the expected harms	Estimating risk of an incident major perioperative cardiac event using the Myocardial Infarction or Cardiac Arrest (MICA) model
Whether to proceed with surgery when the expected benefits and expected harms are finely balanced, after use of a multivariable risk model to estimate surgical risk	Refining risk estimates with preoperative biochemical testing (either N-terminal pro B-type natriuretic peptide [NT-pro-BNP] or troponin)
Whether to make medication changes before noncardiac surgery	Withholding angiotensin-converting enzyme inhibitors or angiotensin receptor blockers in the 24 h before surgery Withholding antiplatelet agents before intracranial or spinal procedures (3–5 d for ticagrelor, 5 d for clopidogrel, 7 d for aspirin or prasugrel) unless a nonendothelialized coronary stent demands ongoing use
Patient prognosis after high-risk surgery	When patients are at elevated risk and postoperative prognosis is of interest, consider measuring daily troponin in the 48 or 72 h following surgery to screen for myocardial injury after noncardiac surgery

SUMMARY

Cardiac complications are the most common cause of perioperative mortality. Patients with symptoms from previously-undiagnosed or suboptimally-managed cardiac disease should, with exceptions for urgent surgery, have their procedures delayed to allow treatment of urgent cardiac conditions. Cardiac workup of asymptomatic persons with suspected CAD will, on average, reduce the rate of surgical completion and delay surgery for patients who ultimately have the operation, without improving cardiac outcomes. Multiple tools exist to predict risk of a perioperative cardiac complication, and biochemistries are likely the best way to refine a risk prediction when the benefits and harms of a proposed surgery are still finely balanced. Preoperative management changes that could reduce operative cardiac risk remain frustratingly elusive.

CLINICS CARE POINTS

- For all but the most urgent surgical procedures, patients with active coronary syndromes or decompensated heart failure should have surgery postponed.
- Workup and diagnosis of cardiac disease in previously-undiagnosed, asymptomatic persons will not reduce cardiac complications, will act as a barrier to surgery and delay surgery when completed, and will not improve patient outcomes.
- In rare circumstances where a diagnosis of stable coronary disease might be useful, consider a patient's pretest probability using the CAD2 model before pursuing further workup.
- For stable patients considering elective noncardiac surgery, prediction tools such as the Myocardial Infarction or Cardiac Arrest (MICA) calculator can estimate incident perioperative cardiac events, and biochemical testing can be used to further refine estimated incidence.

DISCLOSURES

Dr M.A. Pappas reports receiving funding from NIH, United States/NHLBI (K08HL141598), including salary support during the writing of this article. Dr A.D. Auerbach reports research funding from AHRQ, United States and NIH, royalties from UpToDate, Inc., and equity in a company (Kuretic), all unrelated to this work. Dr L.S. Feldman reports that he has no relevant relationships, activities, or interests.

REFERENCES

1. Botto F, Alonso-Coello P, Chan MTV, et al. Myocardial injury after noncardiac surgery: a large, international, prospective cohort study establishing diagnostic criteria, characteristics, predictors, and 30-day outcomes. Anesthesiology 2014; 120(3):564–78.
2. Udeh BL, Dalton JE, Hata JS, et al. Economic trends from 2003 to 2010 for perioperative myocardial infarction: a retrospective, cohort study. Anesthesiology 2014;121(1):36–45.
3. Van Waes JAR, Nathoe HM, De Graaff JC, et al. Myocardial injury after noncardiac surgery and its association with short-term mortality. Circulation 2013; 127(23):2264–71.
4. Van Waes JAR, Grobben RB, Nathoe HM, et al. One-year mortality, causes of death, and cardiac interventions in patients with postoperative myocardial injury. Anesth Analg 2016;123(1):29–37.

5. Devereaux PJ, Xavier D, Pogue J, et al. Characteristics and short-term prognosis of perioperative myocardial infarction in patients undergoing noncardiac surgery: a cohort study. Ann Intern Med 2011;154(8):523–8.

6. Goldman L, Caldera DL, Nussbaum SR, et al. Multifactorial index of cardiac risk in noncardiac surgical procedures. N Engl J Med 1977;297(16):845–50.

7. Cooper A, Calvert N, Skinner J, et al. Chest pain of recent onset: Assessment and diagnosis of recent onset chest pain or discomfort of suspected cardiac origin. National Institute for Health and Care Excellence. 2010. Available at: https://www.nice.org.uk/guidance/cg95/update/CG95/documents/chest-paindiscomfort-of-recent-onset-prepublication-check-full-guideline2. [Accessed 12 February 2021].

8. Genders TSS, Petersen SE, Pugliese F, et al. The optimal imaging strategy for patients with stable chest pain. Ann Intern Med 2015;162(7):474.

9. Fihn SD, Gardin JM, Abrams J, et al. 2012 ACCF/AHA/ACP/AATS/PCNA/SCAI/STS guideline for the diagnosis and management of patients with stable ischemic heart disease. Circulation 2012;126(25):3097–137.

10. Heidenreich PA, Bozkurt B, Aguilar D, et al. 2022 AHA/ACC/HFSA Guideline for the Management of Heart Failure: A Report of the American College of Cardiology/American Heart Association Joint Committee on Clinical Practice Guidelines. J Am Coll Cardiol 2022;79(17):e263–421.

11. Rihal CS, Eagle KA, Mickel MC, et al. Surgical therapy for coronary artery disease among patients with combined coronary artery and peripheral vascular disease. Circulation 1995;91(1):46–53.

12. McFalls EO, Ward HB, Moritz TE, et al. Coronary-artery revascularization before elective major vascular surgery. N Engl J Med 2004;351(27):2795–804.

13. Goff DC, Lloyd-Jones DM, Bennett G, et al. 2013 ACC/AHA guideline on the assessment of cardiovascular risk: A report of the American college of cardiology/American heart association task force on practice guidelines. Circulation 2014;129(25 SUPPL. 1):49–73.

14. Genders TSS, Steyerberg EW, Hunink MGM, et al. Prediction model to estimate presence of coronary artery disease: Retrospective pooled analysis of existing cohorts. BMJ 2012;344(7862).

15. Pappas MA, Sessler DI, Auerbach AD, et al. Variation in preoperative stress testing by patient, physician and surgical type: a cohort study. BMJ Open 2021;11(9):e048052.

16. Pappas MA, Auerbach AD, Kattan MW, et al. Diagnostic and prognostic value of cardiac stress testing before major noncardiac surgery. J Clin Anesth 2023. https://doi.org/10.1016/j.jclinane.2023.111193.

17. Pappas MA, Auerbach AD, Kattan MW, et al. Diagnostic and prognostic value of cardiac stress testing before major noncardiac surgery—A cohort study. J Clin Anesth 2023;90:111193.

18. Genders T, Meijboom W, Meijs M, et al. CT coronary angiography in patients suspected of having coronary artery disease: decision making from various perspectives in the face of uncertainty. Radiology 2009;253(3):734–44.

19. Pappas MA, Auerbach AD, Kattan MW, et al. Consequences of preoperative cardiac stress testing—A cohort study. J Clin Anesth 2023;90:111158.

20. Brodersen J, Schwartz LM, Heneghan C, et al. Overdiagnosis: what it is and what it isn't. BMJ Evidence-Based Med. 2018;23(1):1–3.

21. Fleisher LA, Fleischmann KE, Auerbach AD, et al. 2014 ACC/AHA guideline on perioperative cardiovascular evaluation and management of patients undergoing noncardiac surgery: executive summary: a report of the American College of

Cardiology/American Heart Association Task Force on Practice Guidelines. Circulation 2014;130(24):2215–45.

22. Duceppe E, Parlow J, MacDonald P, et al. Canadian Cardiovascular Society Guidelines on Perioperative Cardiac Risk Assessment and Management for Patients Who Undergo Noncardiac Surgery. Can J Cardiol 2017;33(1):17–32.

23. Halvorsen S, Mehilli J, Cassese S, et al. 2022 ESC Guidelines on cardiovascular assessment and management of patients undergoing non-cardiac surgeryDeveloped by the task force for cardiovascular assessment and management of patients undergoing non-cardiac surgery of the European Society of Cardiology (ESC) Endorsed by the European Society of Anaesthesiology and Intensive Care (ESAIC). Eur Heart J 2022;43(39):3826–924.

24. Dakik HA, Sbaity E, Msheik A, et al. AUB-HAS2 cardiovascular risk index: performance in surgical subpopulations and comparison to the revised cardiac risk index. J Am Heart Assoc 2020;9(10).

25. Lee TH, Marcantonio ER, Mangione CM, et al. Derivation and prospective validation of a simple index for prediction of cardiac risk of major noncardiac surgery. Circulation 1999;100(10):1043–9.

26. Antman E, Bassand JP, Klein W, et al. Myocardial infarction redefined - A consensus document of The Joint European Society of Cardiology/American College of Cardiology Committee f or the redefinition of myocardial infarction. J Am Coll Cardiol 2000;36(3):959–69.

27. Bilimoria K, Liu Y, Paruch J, et al. Development and evaluation of the universal ACS NSQIP surgical risk calculator: a decision aid and informed consent tool for patients and surgeons. J Am Coll Surg 2013;217(5).

28. Cohen ME, Liu Y, Ko CY, et al. An Examination of American College of Surgeons NSQIP Surgical Risk Calculator Accuracy. J Am Coll Surg 2017;224(5): 787–95.e1.

29. Liu Y, Ko CY, Hall BL, et al. American College of Surgeons NSQIP Risk Calculator Accuracy Using a Machine Learning Algorithm Compared with Regression. J Am Coll Surg 2023;236(5):1024–30.

30. Gupta PK, Gupta H, Sundaram A, et al. Development and validation of a risk calculator for prediction of cardiac risk after surgery. Circulation 2011;124(4): 381–7.

31. Liu JB, Liu Y, Cohen ME, et al. Defining the intrinsic cardiac risks of operations to improve preoperative cardiac risk assessments. Anesthesiology 2018;128(2): 283–92.

32. Thygesen K, Members TF, Alpert JS, et al. Universal definition of myocardial infarction: Kristian Thygesen, Joseph S. Alpert and Harvey D. White on behalf of the Joint ESC/ACCF/AHA/WHF Task Force for the Redefinition of Myocardial Infarction. Eur Heart J 2007;28(20):2525–38.

33. Devereaux PJ, Goldman L, Cook DJ, et al. Perioperative cardiac events in patients undergoing noncardiac surgery: a review of the magnitude of the problem, the pathophysiology of the events and methods to estimate and communicate risk. CMAJ (Can Med Assoc J) 2005;173(6):627–34.

34. Devereaux PJ, Biccard BM, Sigamani A, et al. Association of postoperative high-sensitivity troponin levels with myocardial injury and 30-day mortality among patients undergoing noncardiac surgery. JAMA 2017;317(16):1642–51.

35. Nolde JM, Schlaich MP, Sessler DI, et al. Machine learning to predict myocardial injury and death after non-cardiac surgery. Anaesthesia 2023;78(7):853–60.

36. Pappas MA, Sessler DI, Rothberg MB. Anticipated rates and costs of guideline-concordant preoperative stress testing. Anesth Analg 2019;128(2):241–6.

37. Sussman JB, Wiitala WL, Zawistowski M, et al. The veterans affairs cardiac risk score: recalibrating the atherosclerotic cardiovascular disease score for applied use. Med Care 2017;55(9):864–70.

38. Wolters U, Wolf T, Stützer H, et al. ASA classification and perioperative variables as predictors of postoperative outcome. BJA Br J Anaesth 1996;77(2):217–22.

39. Wijeysundera DN, Beattie WS, Hillis GS, et al. Integration of the Duke Activity Status Index into preoperative risk evaluation: a multicentre prospective cohort study. Br J Anaesth 2020;124(3):261–70.

40. Wijeysundera DN, Pearse RM, Shulman MA, et al. Assessment of functional capacity before major non-cardiac surgery: an international, prospective cohort study. Lancet 2018;391(10140):2631–40.

41. Karthikeyan G, Moncur RA, Levine O, et al. Is a pre-operative brain natriuretic peptide or N-terminal pro-B-type natriuretic peptide measurement an independent predictor of adverse cardiovascular outcomes within 30 days of noncardiac surgery? A systematic review and meta-analysis of observational studies. J Am Coll Cardiol 2009;54(17):1599–606.

42. Rodseth RN, Biccard BM, Le Manach Y, et al. The prognostic value of pre-operative and post-operative B-type natriuretic peptides in patients undergoing noncardiac surgery: B-type natriuretic peptide and N-terminal fragment of pro-B-type natriuretic peptide: a systematic review and individual patient data meta-analysis. J Am Coll Cardiol 2014;63(2):170–80.

43. Vernooij LM, van Klei WA, Moons KGM, et al. The comparative and added prognostic value of biomarkers to the Revised Cardiac Risk Index for preoperative prediction of major adverse cardiac events and all-cause mortality in patients who undergo noncardiac surgery. Cochrane Database Syst Rev 2021;12(12).

44. Ruetzler K, Smilowitz NR, Berger JS, et al. Diagnosis and management of patients with myocardial injury after noncardiac surgery: a scientific statement from the American Heart Association. Circulation 2021;144(19):E287–305.

45. Weber M, Luchner A, Manfred S, et al. Incremental value of high-sensitive troponin T in addition to the revised cardiac index for peri-operative risk stratification in non-cardiac surgery. Eur Heart J 2013;34(11):853–62.

46. Shen JT, Xu M, Wu Y, et al. Association of pre-operative troponin levels with major adverse cardiac events and mortality after noncardiac surgery: A systematic review and meta-analysis. Eur J Anaesthesiol 2018;35(11):815–24.

47. Sheth T, Chan M, Butler C, et al. Prognostic capabilities of coronary computed tomographic angiography before non-cardiac surgery: prospective cohort study. BMJ 2015;350.

48. Park SJ, Choi JH, Cho SJ, et al. Comparison of transthoracic echocardiography with N-terminal pro-brain natriuretic Peptide as a tool for risk stratification of patients undergoing major noncardiac surgery. Korean Circ J 2011;41(9):505–11.

49. Oh J, Makar M, Fusco C, et al. A generalizable, data-driven approach to predict daily risk of clostridium difficile infection at two large academic health centers. Infect Control Hosp Epidemiol 2018;39(4):425–33.

50. Devereaux PJ, Sessler DI, Leslie K, et al. Clonidine in patients undergoing noncardiac surgery. N Engl J Med 2014;370(16):1504–13.

51. Duncan D, Sankar A, Beattie WS, et al. Alpha-2 adrenergic agonists for the prevention of cardiac complications among adults undergoing surgery. Cochrane Database Syst Rev 2018;3(3).

52. Blessberger H, Kammler J, Domanovits H, et al. Perioperative beta-blockers for preventing surgery-related mortality and morbidity. Cochrane Database Syst Rev 2018;3(3).

53. Wallace AW, Au S, Cason BA. Association of the pattern of use of perioperative β-blockade and postoperative mortality. Anesthesiology 2010;113(4):794–805.
54. Kertai MD, Cooter M, Pollard RJ, et al. Is compliance with surgical care improvement project cardiac (SCIP-card-2) measures for perioperative β-blockers associated with reduced incidence of mortality and cardiovascular-related critical quality indicators after noncardiac surgery? Anesth Analg 2018;126(6):1829–38.
55. Wijeysundera DN, Beattie WS. Calcium channel blockers for reducing cardiac morbidity after noncardiac surgery: a meta-analysis. Anesth Analg 2003;97(3): 634–41.
56. Berwanger O, Manach Y Le, Suzumura EA, et al. Association between preoperative statin use and major cardiovascular complications among patients undergoing non-cardiac surgery: The VISION study. Eur Heart J 2016;37(2):177–85.
57. Putzu A, de Carvalho e Silva CMPD, de Almeida JP, et al. Perioperative statin therapy in cardiac and non-cardiac surgery: a systematic review and meta-analysis of randomized controlled trials. Ann Intensive Care 2018;8(1):95.
58. Berwanger O, de Barros e Silva PGM, Barbosa RR, et al. Atorvastatin for high-risk statin-naïve patients undergoing noncardiac surgery: The Lowering the Risk of Operative Complications Using Atorvastatin Loading Dose (LOAD) randomized trial. Am Heart J 2017;184:88–96.
59. Bass AR, Szymonifka JD, Rondina MT, et al. Postoperative myocardial injury and inflammation is not blunted by a trial of atorvastatin in orthopedic surgery patients. HSS J 2018;14(1):67–76.
60. Marcucci M, Duceppe E, Le Manach Y, et al. Tranexamic acid and rosuvastatin in patients at risk of cardiovascular events after noncardiac surgery: a pilot of the POISE-3 randomized controlled trial. Pilot feasibility Stud 2020;6(1).
61. Devereaux PJ, Mrkobrada M, Sessler DI, et al. Aspirin in patients undergoing noncardiac surgery. N Engl J Med 2014;370(16):1494–503.
62. Douketis JD, Spyropoulos AC, Murad MH, et al. Perioperative management of antithrombotic therapy: an American College of Chest Physicians Clinical Practice Guideline. Chest 2022;162(5):e207–43.
63. Pappas MA, Evans N, Rizk MK, et al. Resuming anticoagulation following upper gastrointestinal bleeding among patients with nonvalvular atrial fibrillation-a microsimulation analysis. J Hosp Med 2019;14(7).

Perioperative Care of Heart Failure, Arrhythmias, and Valvular Heart Disease

Avital Y. O'Glasser, MD, SFHM, DFPM[a,b,*], Efrén C. Manjarrez, MD, SFHM[c]

KEYWORDS

- Heart failure • Arrhythmia • Atrial fibrillation • Anticoagulation
- Valvular heart disease • Aortic stenosis • Mitral regurgitation • MACE

KEY POINTS

- Heart failure is a risk factor for postoperative adverse events independent of ischemic heart disease.
- The associated perioperative risk of heart failure stratifies by type of heart failure and presence of heart failure symptoms.
- Arrhythmia management, especially when incidentally or newly detected in the preoperative period, remains a clinical challenge.
- New postoperative atrial fibrillation increases the risk of adverse events including stroke risk.
- Valvular heart disease remains a risk factor for adverse events, and the timing of (re) assessment of murmurs/valvular disease may be a clinical challenge.

INTRODUCTION

Far from providing "clearance", a dedicated preoperative assessment must be a holistic review of a patient's known chronic medical conditions as well as an exploration for as yet undiagnosed risk factors or risk factors that might have progressed in severity. "*Is this patient cleared for surgery*" is often code word for "*does this patient have cardiac clearance*"—and even more specifically, is often the code word for "*does this patient need a stress test?*" As this review article will explore, an appropriately

[a] Department of Medicine, Division of Hospital Medicine, Oregon Health and Science University, 3485 Southwest Bond Avenue, CHH2 8008, Portland, OR 97239, USA; [b] Department of Anesthesiology and Perioperative Medicine, Oregon Health and Science University, 3485 Southwest Bond Avenue, CHH2 8008, Portland, OR 97239, USA; [c] Department of Medicine, Division of Hospital Medicine, University of Miami Miller School of Medicine, Miami, FL, USA
* Corresponding author.
E-mail address: oglassea@ohsu.edu
Twitter: @aoglasser (A.Y.O.)

Med Clin N Am 108 (2024) 1053–1064
https://doi.org/10.1016/j.mcna.2024.05.001
medical.theclinics.com

robust preoperative cardiac assessment includes not only an ischemic risk evaluation but evaluation for non-ischemic cardiac conditions. Patients with cardiac conditions outside of coronary artery disease—namely heart failure, arrhythmias, and valvular disease—need patient-centered, evidenced based perioperative management strategies to mitigate risk across the spectrum of care and improve patient both outcomes and experiences.

Heart Failure

An estimated more than 64 million people have heart failure,[1] and many of these patients require non cardiac surgery annually given the approximately 300 million major surgeries performed annually worldwide.[2] However, practice guidelines have a paucity of content to guide office-based internal medicine physicians and hospitalists on perioperative heart failure management. The European Society of Cardiology (ESC) 2022 guidelines, the most recent society guidelines to guide care, have 2 pages.[2] Much of the focus on perioperative cardiac care has historically focused on perioperative coronary artery disease (CAD) both known and occult, despite heart failure related complications being a bigger driver of postoperative complications than ischemic heart disease.[3]

Much data regarding the associated risk of perioperative heart failure have emerged since the last iteration of the American College of Cardiology (ACC)/American Heart Association (AHA) perioperative guidelines.[4] This includes nuances regarding risk based on systolic versus diastolic heart failure, degree of left ventricle (LV) dysfunction, right heart failure, and patient symptomatology. In a large retrospective cohort of over 600,000 veterans, 8% of whom had heart failure, mortality for heart failure patients was 5.49% with an adjusted odds ratio (aOR) = 1.67.[5] Mortality increased with decreasing ejection fraction (EF) from 4.88% for EF greater than 50% to 8.34% with EF less than 30%, aORs from 1.51 to 2.35; mortality in symptomatic heart failure had an aOR of 9.07 versus 4.1 for asymptomatic heart failure.[4]

Perioperative diastolic dysfunction is itself a risk factor for 30 days adverse outcomes in noncardiac surgery. In one meta-analysis of 13 studies and almost 4000 patients, diastolic dysfunction was associated with an increased risk of perioperative heart failure exacerbation (OR = 3.90), myocardial infarction (OR = 1.74), and major adverse cardiac events (OR = 2.03); mortality was not found to be statistically significant.[6] The authors postulate that diastolic filling is worsened during the stress of the perioperative period in patients with suspected nonobstructive coronary disease and diastolic dysfunction.

In addition to preoperative concerns, clinicians must be astute to the potential for acute, decompensated heart failure postoperatively. In a prospective study of 9000 patients, the incidence of acute postoperative heart failure was 2.5%.[7] About half was new onset heart failure versus exacerbation of known heart failure; 10% of patients with known chronic heart failure developed postoperative exacerbations. Additionally, new onset heart failure postoperatively was most likely diastolic heart failure.[7] See **Fig. 1**.

Perioperative major adverse cardiac events (MACE) is increased with any heart failure diagnosis. However, certain surgery types are associated with higher risk of heart failure-related complications. In a large database review of 22 million patients over 3 years, the aOR of inpatient mortality for any heart failure diagnosis was 2.15.[8] The aOR ranged from 1.53 in vascular surgery to 7.05 in orthopedics. In this study, heart failure was also associated with the risk of acute ischemic stroke, acute pulmonary embolism, and cardiac arrest. See **Fig. 2**.

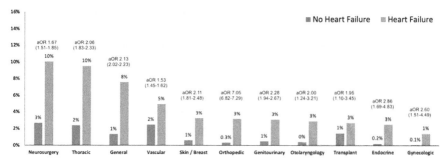

Fig. 1. In-hospital mortality by non-cardiac surgical subtype in patients with and without a diagnosis of heart. (Nathaniel R Smilowitz, Darcy Banco, Stuart D Katz, Joshua A Beckman, Jeffery S Berger, Association between heart failure and perioperative outcomes in patients undergoing non-cardiac surgery, European Heart Journal - Quality of Care and Clinical Outcomes, Volume 7, Issue 1, January 2021, Pages 68–75, https://doi.org/10.1093/ehjqcco/qcz066.)

PREOPERATIVE RISK ASSESSMENT

The most recent iteration of the ACC/AHA guidelines recommends patients with symptomatic heart failure be treated according to ACC clinical practice guidelines.[4] They furthermore suggest use of a validated risk prediction tool for MACE (Class IIA recommendation). The guidelines suggest 3 risk predictors: The Revised Cardiac Risk Index (C Statistical 0.76–0.80), the American College of Surgeons National Surgical Quality Improvement Program (NSQIP) Myocardial Infarction and Cardiac Arrest, and American College of Surgeons NSQIP Surgical Risk Calculator (C Statistical 0.81–0.94).[4]

The 2014 ACC/AHA guidelines also indicate (Class IIA) that it is reasonable for patients with dyspnea of unknown origin or heart failure with worsening dyspnea or other interval change in clinical status to undergo preoperative evaluation of LV function with

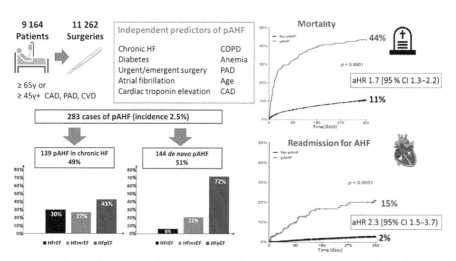

Fig. 2. Incidence, phenotypes, determinants, and outcomes of acute heart failure after non-cardiac surgery (pAHF). (*From* Gualandro DM, Puelacher C, Chew MS, et al. Acute heart failure after non-cardiac surgery: incidence, phenotypes, determinants, and outcomes. Eur J Heart Fail. 2023 Mar;25(3):347–357. https://doi.org/10.1002/ejhf.2773. Epub 2023 Feb 7. PMID: 36644890.)

a 2-D echocardiogram (ECHO) (Class IIA).[4] Reassessment of LV function in clinically stable patients may be considered especially if has been at least a year since last ECHO assessment (Class IIB). Routine preoperative evaluation of LV function is not recommended for patients without signs or symptoms concerning for undiagnosed heart failure (Class III). The European Cardiology Society (ECS) guidelines do recommend a preoperative ECHO in patients with pre-test suspicious of underlying disease[2]; the Canadian Cardiovascular Society preoperative guidelines recommend against ECHO in the preoperative setting.[9]

The 2014 ACC/AHA guidelines did not give clear recommendations regarding the use of biomarkers for preoperative cardiac risk assessment and evaluation.[4] However, more recent literature and other society guidelines have made recommendations. The VISION group found that patients with preoperative nt-pro-BNP levels greater than 200 pg/mL had a greater than 20% risk of myocardial injury after noncardiac surgery (MINS) and vascular death.[10] The outcomes were driven by MINS more than mortality.[10] The Canadian Cardiovascular Society preoperative guidelines suggest ordering a preoperative nt-pro-BNP in patients of age more than 65, age 45 to 64 with significant known coronary/cardiovascular disease, or have an revised cardiac risk index (RCRI) greater than or equal to 1.9. The recent ESC guidelines do not give clear recommendations on nt-pro-BNP other than to suggest an ECHO in patients with elevated values.[2]

The ACC/AHA,4 ESC,2 and Canadian[9] guidelines all recommend perioperative guideline directed management treatment (GDMT). All 3 guidelines recommend against initiation of beta blockers preoperatively unless multiple cardiac risk factors are present. However, there is a Class I recommendation to continue them in patients chronically taking them for CAD, heart failure, arrhythmias, or hypertension. Regarding renin-angiotensin-aldosterone system inhibitors, data and guidance are significantly mixed in the perioperative literature and clinical practices including in the 3 society guidelines.[2,4,9] Neither the ACC/AHA nor Canadian guidelines provide guidance on diuretics.[4,9] The ESC guidelines discuss caution in taking oral diuretics in the morning of surgery given the risk of electrolyte disturbances, namely hypokalemia and the risk of arrhythmia.[2] The newest GDMT agents for heart failure are the SGLT-2-inhibitors, which are recommended regardless of the presence of coexisting diabetes mellitus. Multiple societies including the ESC recommend holding SGLT-2-inhibitors for 3 to 4 days preoperatively because of the risk of euglycemic diabetic ketoacidosis.[2]

Office-based internists and hospitalists have 5 major management goals to optimize heart failure patients for surgery: preoperative risk assessment, goals of care discussions with patients regarding perioperative risks associated with heart failure, achieve euvolemia, symptom reduction preoperatively, and optimize guideline directed medical therapy. Furthermore, decisions need to be made on ambulatory versus inpatient surgery in a multi-disciplinary manner with surgery, cardiology, and our anesthesiology colleagues.

ADDITIONAL ETIOLOGIES OF HEART FAILURE

Patients with hypertrophic obstructive cardiomyopathy are at added risk based on left ventricular outflow tract obstruction and the associated pathophysiology of the condition. They will require an echo and specialty consult with cardiology and anesthesiology, with attention to preload based on volume status and heart rate control.[11]

Congenital heart disease includes a very broad set of abnormalities, and it may lead to chronic heart failure. It is impossible to merge all types of congenital heart disease into a single preoperative assessment requirement, and we advise being aware of and referencing separate guidelines.[12,13]

Arrhythmias

As written in the 2007 ACC/AHA perioperative guidelines, "significant arrhythmias" require further evaluation and management before non-emergency, non-cardiac surgery.[14] Patients with stable arrhythmias also require appropriate consideration and management before surgeries.[4] This includes assessment of associated etiology and concurrent comorbid conditions, availability of appropriate cardiac tests (eg, ECHO to exclude structural heart disease), rate and/or rhythm control medication management, and anticoagulation decisions.[4] Some patients with arrhythmias may have an associated cardiac implanted electrical device (CIED) that requires additional perioperative considerations. Symptomatology, including palpitations and other cardiopulmonary symptoms, should be explored as part of the preoperative risk assessment. We recommend including the following information in the preoperative consult: device type, date and clinical indication for implantation, whether the patient is pacemaker dependent, any recent therapies given by the device, the effect of magnet placement perioperatively, and battery life.

In addition to preoperative assessment of known or suspected arrhythmias, patients may develop arrhythmias intraoperatively or postoperatively. New onset perioperative arrhythmias may require immediate rate and rhythm control strategies, especially in a patient experiencing hemodynamic instability or other new cardiac events (eg, postoperative myocardial infarction/MINS or decompensated heart failure). New postoperative arrhythmias cannot be assumed to be transiently restricted to be perioperative, necessitating transitions of care back to primary care and/or new cardiology outpatient referrals.

ATRIAL FIBRILLATION

As the most common arrhythmia, atrial fibrillation is frequently encountered in the preoperative setting; atrial flutter management parallels atrial fibrillation management in this setting.[4,15,16]

Stable patients with a preoperative history of atrial fibrillation "generally do not require modification of medication management or special evaluation in the perioperative period, other than adjustment of anticoagulation."[4] In the clinical setting, this entails reviewing patient symptoms (**Box 1**), medication regimen, and prior cardiac

---

Box 1
Patient-centered evaluation of arrhythmias preop (ROS)

- Specific arrhythmia details
- Associated comorbid conditions (heart failure, CAD, structural heart disease including congenital heart disease, thyroid disease, alcohol intake, OSA)
- Patient-specific associated symptoms
- Patient-specific precipitants/exacerbating factors
- Frequency of symptoms or time in the arrhythmia
- Rate control medications
- Rhythm control medications
- Anticoagulation, if indicated
- Past cardiac testing (ECHO, stress, extended monitoring)
- Presence of CIED (pacemaker, ICD, loop recorder)

testing. Attention should be paid to symptoms and signs of other cardiac pathologies, especially those that might be destabilized by the presence of atrial fibrillation such as heart failure or ischemic heart disease. Chronic rate control therapy, including beta-blockers, as well as rhythm control/anti-arrhythmic medications, should be continued preoperatively including on the day of surgery.[4,15] These medications should also be continued postoperatively, though clinicians should monitor hemodynamic parameters to determine if beta-blockers need dose adjustments.[4]

Whether or not incidentally discovered atrial fibrillation in the preoperative setting requires delay or cancellation of surgery is a clinical challenge. Limited guidance given a paucity of studies, and risk/benefit discussions should be held about the potential harm of delaying noncardiac surgery, especially for asymptomatic patients and those who have baseline rate control. Incidental atrial fibrillation should likely have the same preliminary evaluation that non-preoperative atrial fibrillation requires, including alcohol intake, thyroid function, electrolytes, obstructive sleep apnea screening, and assessment for underlying structural heart disease.[17,18] Any preoperative considerations of cardioversion must consider that patients need uninterrupted anticoagulation for several weeks after cardioversion given the increased stroke risk.[19]

New onset of intraoperative atrial fibrillation, with or without a rapid ventricular response, is a clinical challenge anesthesiologists might encounter. Surgery and patient-related risk factors may or may not be reversible, especially in the intraoperative setting. This includes but is not limited to catecholamine surge, hypervolemic and hypovolemic, anemia, hypoxia, hypotension, sepsis, hypokalemia, and hypomagnesemia.[15,20–22] Intraoperative rate control agents can be administered, while intraoperative cardioversion for unstable patients might be necessary.[15]

Clinicians might also diagnose and manage new postoperative atrial fibrillation. New onset atrial fibrillation is the most common postoperative arrhythmia, reported in appropriately 2% of noncardiac surgeries.[16] The HART score (hypertension, age, surgical risk, and thyroid dysfunction) is validated to predict the risk of postoperative atrial fibrillation; 6 or more points predicts postoperative atrial fibrillation with 70% sensitivity and 72% specificity (**Table 1**).[16] A differential for new onset atrial fibrillation or new onset rapid ventricular response (RVR) should be explored, with reversible triggers addressed. Rate control should be pursued, with cardioversion considered for unstable patients.

Mounting evidence demonstrates that postoperative atrial fibrillation does not exist in the vacuum of the immediate postoperative setting. Multiple studies demonstrate the risk associated with atrial fibrillation after noncardiac surgery including recurrent atrial fibrillation,[23,24] stroke/TIA,[25–32] myocardial infarction,[28,29] heart failure,[31,33] and mortality[27–29,31]

Table 1	
The HART score risk for postoperative atrial fibrillation	
Variable	**Points**
Hypertension	1
< 65 yo	0
65–74 yo	1
75+ yo	2
Low risk surgery	0
Intermediate risk surgery	3
High risk surgery	3
Thyroid dysfunction	1

The risks of postoperative recurrent atrial fibrillation and increased stroke risk make immediate postoperative anticoagulation decisions challenging; long term anticoagulation should be considered in patients at risk for stroke utilizing shared decision making.[18] Timely outpatient follow-up via primary care and/or cardiology, with clear communications surrounding transitions of care, is vital to continue medication management and arrange any recommended outpatient testing such as ECHOs.[17,18]

In addition to rate/rhythm control management, preoperative atrial fibrillation also requires management of anticoagulant therapy. In the last decade, both updated bridging guidelines and the increasingly prevalent use of the direct oral anticoagulant (DOACs) have revolutionized perioperative management of anticoagulation.[34] Low and very low risk bleeding procedures may not need procedural interruption of anticoagulation.[34] If anticoagulation needs to be interrupted, data now support that most patients with atrial fibrillation do not need bridging of warfarin with heparin or low molecular weight heparin as bridging is not associated with a reduction in thromboembolic events but is associated with increased harm including bleeding risk.[35] The guidelines now recommend bridging in patients with a high CHA2DS2-VA2Sc greater than 7 and recent (<3 months) ischemic stroke, TIA or systemic embolism. In these patients with an INR in the therapeutic range, warfarin can be stopped for 5 days before surgery.[34] The DOACs, with their shorter half-life, can be held before high bleeding risk surgery for 2 calendar days—the safety of this protocol is confirmed by the PAUSE study.[36] This window should be adjusted based on creatinine clearance and for lower bleeding risk procedures; the American Society of Regional Anesthesia (ASRA) guidelines also advise a longer hold before neuraxial anesthesia.[37] The DOACs do not require bridging.[34,36]

Postoperatively, in stable patients, warfarin can be resumed as early as postoperative night 0.[34] Given its much shorter half-life, the timing of initiating postoperative bridging with heparin or low molecular weight heparin must take into the account bleeding risk of the procedure. DOACs can be resumed between 24 and 72 hours post procedure depending on the bleeding risk.[34]

OTHER ARRHYTHMIAS

Patients may present with an established history of bradyarrhythmias or tachyarrhythmias or with symptoms concerning for an undiagnosed arrhythmia warranting evaluation.[4] Sinus bradycardia can be normal in many patients, and a preoperative history should explore etiologies for such including regular physical activity. Symptomatic or inappropriate bradycardia should explore etiology, including symptomatic hypothyroidism and medication effect. Bradycardia may also be caused by certain types of heart block, which warrant appropriate evaluation and management preoperatively for types associated with overall worse outcomes—namely 2nd degree type 2 and 3rd degree/complete heart block. Akin to atrial fibrillation, patients prescribed rate or rhythm control agents for tachyarrhythmias should continue their medications preoperatively including day of surgery; postoperative adjustments might be needed based on hemodynamic trends.[4] New onset postoperative arrhythmias should be evaluated and managed akin to the nonsurgical setting.

PALPITATIONS

Palpitations may be a non-specific symptom, with a range of benign and pathologic etiologies. The differential includes anxiety, stress, caffeine intake, thyroid disease, arrhythmia, and structural heart disease. Patients may have associated electrocardiogram (EKG) findings, such as premature atrial contractions, premature ventricular contractions, or other findings such as sustained arrhythmias. Premature ventricular contractions or non-sustained ventricular tachycardia identified perioperatively warrant consideration of the risk of underlying ischemic, structural, or conduction system heart disease, but in general do not inherently expose patients to an increased risk of major adverse cardiac events.[4]

Valvular Heart Disease

As written in the 2007 ACC/AHA perioperative guidelines, severe aortic stenosis disease needs to be evaluated and treated before non-emergency non-cardiac surgery.[4] Based on interval publications and recognizing the limited ability of physical examination to accurately grade murmur severity, the 2014 ACC/AHA guidelines extended criteria for patients needing preoperative assessment via echocardiography before surgery to patients with suspected moderate to severe valve disease as well as both regurgitant and stenotic lesions.[4]

The assessment of known valvular disease should include documentation of type of lesion (valve, regurgitant vs stenotic), severity, associated cardiac conditions, anticoagulation needs, and any indications for endocarditis prophylaxis. Symptomatic versus asymptomatic severe valve disease is an important medical decision-making branch point; it is crucial to assess cardiopulmonary symptoms, baseline functional capacity, and volume status.

The preoperative management of a patient with a new or previously unassessed murmur is a frequent source of consternation in the perioperative setting, including when to obtain echocardiography especially if surgery must be postponed/canceled to facilitate testing. Physical examination should aim to ascertain as many features of aortic or mitral valve murmurs as possible. The classic severe valve disease symptoms of dyspnea or volume overload may be absent. Rather, practitioners should have a high index of suspicion for nonspecific symptoms, such as fatigue, presyncope, and decline in functional capacity.

Aortic valve disease, the most prevalent valve disorder with aging, especially aortic stenosis, has long been associated with perioperative risk.[38] Newer research has shown improved—but still elevated—risk factor profiles perioperatively.[39,40] Severe aortic stenosis is associated with significant hemodynamic changes at baseline, putting patients at increased risk of perioperative myocardial infarction, death, and stroke.[41,42] Severe mitral regurgitation is also associated with increased perioperative risk of mortality, myocardial infarction, stroke, and heart failure.[43,44]

According to the 2014 ACC/AHA guidelines (Class 1), a preoperative ECHO should be obtained when moderate or severe stenotic or regurgitant mitral or aortic valve disease is suspected when there has been no ECHO in the preceding year or the patient has a change in clinical status.[4]

Symptomatic patients with severe stenotic or regurgitant valve disease should proceed with repair/replacement before non-cardiac surgery.[2,4,45] Different from the 2007 guidelines, the 2014 guideline outlines that non-cardiac surgery might be able to proceed if the patient is asymptomatic and with appropriate monitoring. Given the potential for patients with severe valve disease to have non-specific or vague symptoms, as well as the challenges in determining symptomatology in a patient with a low functional capacity for any reason, perioperative clinicians must be very cautious when labeling a patient truly asymptomatic from their severe valvular disease. Any patient proceeding to elective or non-elective surgery with concurrent severe valve disease requires careful interdisciplinary discussions and planning, including intraoperative invasive monitoring, postoperative admission location (ICU or ward), venue (hospital vs ambulatory), as well as risk/benefit counseling.

Valve Replacement Recipients

There are limited data to guide the preoperative assessment of patients with prior surgical valve replacements, especially the timing of follow-up ECHOs.[46] History and examination, looking for signs/symptoms of valve prosthesis compromise, is prudent, and ECHO should be considered in patients with concerning changes.[2,45]

Patients with prior mechanical valve replacements need anticoagulation management. If anticoagulation needs to be held, most but not all patients will meet criteria for bridging off warfarin. This includes patients at moderate or high risk for thromboembolic events; highest risk patients include those with any mitral valve prosthesis, caged-ball or tilting disc aortic valve prostheses, or stroke or TIA within the last 6 months.[47] Lowest risk patients include those with bileaflet aortic valve prostheses without atrial fibrillation or other stroke risk factors.[47] American College of Chest Physicians (ACCP) guidelines recommend that these lowest risk patients receive no bridging whereas higher risk patients do receive bridging.[45] Recent data from the PERIOP-2 trial indicate it might be necessary less frequently than current practice.[48] See Steven J. Wilson and colleagues' article, "Medical Clinics of North America – Periprocedural Anti-thrombotics: Prophylaxis and Interruption," in this issue outlines anticoagulation strategies for these patients.

In the past decade, use of transcatheter aortic valve replacements (TAVR) has expanded dramatically; balloon valvuloplasty has fallen out of favor. Emerging data help add to discussions about how long non-cardiac surgery must be delayed to permit intervention for severe aortic stenosis as open surgical aortic valve replacement may have a long recovery period—and if TAVR is an appropriate treatment modality for severe aortic stenosis when a patient has indications for non-cardiac surgery.[42] TAVR recipients appear to not have increased surgical risk with subsequent noncardiac surgery, as long as there are no valve prosthesis-related complications such as moderate or severe prosthesis-patient mismatch or paravalvular regurgitation.[42,49]

SUMMARY

As demonstrated in this review, cardiac conditions beyond coronary artery disease are major, and often the most significant, drivers of more challenging intraoperative management and postoperative adverse outcomes. Heart failure, valvular pathologies, and arrhythmias—both prior, chronic, or occult—need to be appropriately assessed in accordance with the available society guidelines. Multiple opportunities exist internal medicine physicians, both outpatient and inpatient focused, to augment and dynamically risk reduce the perioperative complications for these patient populations.

DISCLOSURE

The authors have nothing to disclose.

REFERENCES

1. Savarese G, Becher PM, Lund LH, et al. Global burden of heart failure: a comprehensive and updated review of epidemiology. Cardiovasc Res 2023;118(17): 3272–87.
2. Halvorsen S, Mehilli J, Cassese S, et al. 2022 ESC Guidelines on cardiovascular assessment and management of patients undergoing non-cardiac surgery. Eur Heart J 2022;43(39):3826–924.

3. van Diepen S, Bakal JA, McAlister FA, et al. Mortality and readmission of patients with heart failure, atrial fibrillation, or coronary artery disease undergoing noncardiac surgery: an analysis of 38 047 patients. Circulation 2011;124(3):289–96.

4. Fleisher LA, Fleischmann KE, Auerbach AD, et al. ACC/AHA guideline on perioperative cardiovascular evaluation and management of patients undergoing noncardiac surgery: a report of the American College of Cardiology/American Heart Association Task Force on practice guidelines. J Am Coll Cardiol 2014; 64(22):e77–137.

5. Lerman BJ, Popat RA, Assimes TL, et al. Association of left ventricular ejection fraction and symptoms with mortality after elective noncardiac surgery among patients with heart failure. JAMA 2019;321(6):572–9.

6. Fayad A, Ansari MT, Yang H, et al. Perioperative diastolic dysfunction in patients undergoing noncardiac surgery is an independent risk factor for cardiovascular events: a systematic review and meta-analysis. Anesthesiology 2016;125(1): 72–91.

7. Gualandro DM, Puelacher C, Chew MS, et al. Acute heart failure after noncardiac surgery: incidence, phenotypes, determinants and outcomes. Eur J Heart Fail 2023;25(3):347–57.

8. Smilowitz NR, Banco D, Katz SD, et al. Association between heart failure and perioperative outcomes in patients undergoing non-cardiac surgery. Eur Heart J Qual Care Clin Outcomes 2021;7(1):68–75.

9. Duceppe E, Parlow J, MacDonald P, et al. Canadian cardiovascular society guidelines on perioperative cardiac risk assessment and management for patients who undergo noncardiac surgery. Can J Cardiol 2017;33(1):17–32.

10. Duceppe E, Heels-Ansdell D, Devereaux PJ. Preoperative N-Terminal Pro-B-Type natriuretic peptide and cardiovascular events after noncardiac surgery. Ann Intern Med 2020;172(12):843.

11. Hensley N, Dietrich J, Nyhan D, et al. Hypertrophic cardiomyopathy: a review. Anesth Analg 2015;120(3):554–69.

12. Warnes CA, Williams RG, Bashore TM, et al. ACC/AHA 2008 Guidelines for the Management of Adults with Congenital Heart Disease: a report of the American College of Cardiology/American Heart Association Task Force on Practice Guidelines (writing committee to develop guidelines on the management of adults with congenital heart disease). Circulation 2008;118(23):e714–833.

13. Howard-Quijano K, Schwarzenberger JC. Acute care medicine: perioperative management of adult congenital heart disease. Am J Ther 2014;21(4):288–95.

14. Fleisher LA, Beckman JA, Brown KA, et al. ACC/AHA 2007 guidelines on perioperative cardiovascular evaluation and care for noncardiac surgery. J Am Coll Cardiol 2007;50(17):e159–241.

15. Karamchandani K, Khanna AK, Bose S, et al. Atrial fibrillation: current evidence and management strategies during the perioperative period. Anesth Analg 2020;130(1):2–13.

16. Stronati G, Mondelli C, Urbinati A, et al. Derivation and validation of a clinical score for predicting postoperative atrial fibrillation in noncardiac elective surgery (the HART Score). Am J Cardiol 2022;170:56–62.

17. January CT, Wann LS, Alpert JS, et al. 2014 AHA/ACC/HRS guideline for the management of patients with atrial fibrillation: executive summary: a report of the American College of Cardiology/American Heart Association Task Force on practice guidelines and the Heart Rhythm Society. Circulation 2014;130(23): 2071–104.

18. Hindricks G, Potpara T, Dagres N, et al. 2020 ESC Guidelines for the diagnosis and management of atrial fibrillation developed in collaboration with the European Association for Cardio-Thoracic Surgery (EACTS): The Task Force for the diagnosis and management of atrial fibrillation of the European Society of Cardiology (ESC) Developed with the special contribution of the European Heart Rhythm Association (EHRA) of the ESC. Eur Heart J 2021;42(5):373–498.

19. Forslund T, Braunschweig F, Holzmann MJ, et al. Early risk of stroke in patients undergoing acute versus elective cardioversion for atrial fibrillation. J Am Heart Assoc 2021;10(16):e021716.

20. Khan AM, Lubitz SA, Sullivan LM, et al. Low serum magnesium and the development of atrial fibrillation in the community: the Framingham Heart Study. Circulation 2013;127(1):33–8.

21. Krijthe BP, Heeringa J, Kors JA, et al. Serum potassium levels and the risk of atrial fibrillation: the Rotterdam Study. Int J Cardiol 2013;168(6):5411–5.

22. Farah R, Nassar M, Aboraya B, et al. Low serum potassium levels are associated with the risk of atrial fibrillation. Acta Cardiol 2021;76(8):887–90.

23. Lowres N, Hillis GS, Gladman MA, et al. Self-monitoring for recurrence of secondary atrial fibrillation following non-cardiac surgery or acute illness: A pilot study. Int J Cardiol Heart Vasc 2020;29:100566.

24. McIntyre WF, Vadakken ME, Connolly SJ, et al. Atrial fibrillation recurrence in patients with transient new-onset atrial fibrillation detected during hospitalization for noncardiac surgery or medical illness: a matched cohort study. Ann Intern Med 2023;176(10):1299–307.

25. Gialdini G, Nearing K, Bhave PD, et al. Perioperative atrial fibrillation and the long-term risk of ischemic stroke. JAMA 2014;312(6):616–22.

26. Butt JH, Olesen JB, Havers-Borgersen E, et al. Risk of thromboembolism associated with atrial fibrillation following noncardiac surgery. J Am Coll Cardiol 2018; 72(17):2027–36.

27. Lin MH, Kamel H, Singer DE, et al. Perioperative/postoperative atrial fibrillation and risk of subsequent stroke and/or mortality. Stroke 2019;50(6):1364–71.

28. AlTurki A, Marafi M, Proietti R, et al. Major adverse cardiovascular events associated with postoperative atrial fibrillation after noncardiac surgery: a systematic review and meta-analysis. Circ Arrhythm Electrophysiol 2020;13(1):e007437.

29. Conen D, Alonso-Coello P, Douketis J, et al. Risk of stroke and other adverse outcomes in patients with perioperative atrial fibrillation 1 year after non-cardiac surgery. Eur Heart J 2020;41(5):645–51.

30. Siontis KC, Gersh BJ, Weston SA, et al. Association of new-onset atrial fibrillation after noncardiac surgery with subsequent stroke and transient ischemic attack. JAMA 2020;324(9):871–8.

31. Prasada S, Desai MY, Saad M, et al. Preoperative atrial fibrillation and cardiovascular outcomes after noncardiac surgery. J Am Coll Cardiol 2022;79(25): 2471–85.

32. Siontis KC, Gersh BJ, Weston SA, et al. Associations of atrial fibrillation after noncardiac surgery with stroke, subsequent arrhythmia, and death: a cohort study. Ann Intern Med 2022;175(8):1065–72.

33. Goyal P, Kim M, Krishnan U, et al. Post-operative atrial fibrillation and risk of heart failure hospitalization. Eur Heart J 2022;43(31):2971–80.

34. Doherty JU, Gluckman TJ, Hucker WJ, et al. 2017 ACC Expert Consensus Decision Pathway for Periprocedural Management of Anticoagulation in Patients With Nonvalvular Atrial Fibrillation: A Report of the American College of Cardiology

Clinical Expert Consensus Document Task Force. J Am Coll Cardiol 2017;69(7): 871–98.

35. Douketis JD, Spyropoulos AC, Kaatz S, et al. Perioperative bridging anticoagulation in patients with atrial fibrillation. N Engl J Med 2015;373(9):823–33.

36. Douketis JD, Spyropoulos AC, Duncan J, et al. Perioperative management of patients with atrial fibrillation receiving a direct oral anticoagulant. JAMA Intern Med 2019;179(11):1469–78.

37. Horlocker TT, Vandermeulen E, Kopp SL, et al. Regional anesthesia in the patient receiving antithrombotic or thrombolytic therapy: american society of regional anesthesia and pain medicine evidence-based guidelines (Fourth Edition). Reg Anesth Pain Med 2018;43(3):263–309.

38. Meers JB, Townsley MM. Aortic stenosis and noncardiac surgery in the era of transcatheter aortic valve replacement. J Cardiothorac Vasc Anesth 2020;34(8): 2234–44.

39. Agarwal S, Rajamanickam A, Bajaj NS, et al. Impact of aortic stenosis on postoperative outcomes after noncardiac surgeries. Circ Cardiovasc Qual Outcomes 2013;6(2):193–200.

40. Samarendra P, Mangione MP. Aortic stenosis and perioperative risk with noncardiac surgery. J Am Coll Cardiol 2015;65(3):295–302.

41. Tai YH, Chang CC, Yeh CC, et al. Adverse outcomes after noncardiac surgery in patients with aortic stenosis. Sci Rep 2021;11(1):19517.

42. Okuno T, Demirel C, Tomii D, et al. Risk and timing of noncardiac surgery after transcatheter aortic valve implantation. JAMA Netw Open 2022;5(7):e2220689.

43. Bajaj NS, Agarwal S, Rajamanickam A, et al. Impact of severe mitral regurgitation on postoperative outcomes after noncardiac surgery. Am J Med 2013;126(6): 529–35.

44. Richter EW, Shehata IM, Elsayed-Awad HM, et al. Mitral Regurgitation in Patients Undergoing Noncardiac Surgery. Semin CardioThorac Vasc Anesth 2022;26(1): 54–67.

45. Otto CM, Nishimura RA, Bonow RO, et al. 2020 ACC/AHA Guideline for the Management of Patients With Valvular Heart Disease: A Report of the American College of Cardiology/American Heart Association Joint Committee on Clinical Practice Guidelines. Circulation 2021;143(5):e72–227.

46. Luis SA, Dohaei A, Chandrashekar P, et al. Impact of aortic valve replacement for severe aortic stenosis on perioperative outcomes following major noncardiac surgery. Mayo Clin Proc 2020;95(4):727–37.

47. Douketis JD, Spyropoulos AC, Spencer FA, et al. Perioperative management of antithrombotic therapy: Antithrombotic Therapy and Prevention of Thrombosis, 9th ed: American College of Chest Physicians Evidence-Based Clinical Practice Guidelines. Chest 2012;141(2 Suppl):e326S–50S.

48. Kovacs MJ, Wells PS, Anderson DR, et al. Postoperative low molecular weight heparin bridging treatment for patients at high risk of arterial thromboembolism (PERIOP2): double blind randomised controlled trial. BMJ 2021;373:n1205.

49. Kai T, Izumo M, Okuno T, et al. Prevalence and clinical outcomes of noncardiac surgery after transcatheter aortic valve replacement. Am J Cardiol 2024;210: 259–65.

Anemia and Transfusion Medicine

Smita K. Kalra, MD[a],*, Moises Auron, MD[b]

KEYWORDS

- Perioperative anemia • Transfusion medicine • Pre-operative anemia
- Anemia and surgery

KEY POINTS

- Peri-operative anemia is highly prevalent and remains an independent predictor for post-operative mortality and morbidity.
- Pre-operative evaluation should focus on identifying the cause of anemia and optimization strategies should focus on increasing red cell mass and correcting any nutritional deficiencies.
- Intravenous iron is safe and can be used for correcting pre-operative and post-operative anemia, especially when iron deficiency anemia is present.
- International normalized ratio should not be used as the sole measure of coagulopathy when considering reversal strategies as it may not accurately reflect thrombin generation and actual hemostasis.

EPIDEMIOLOGY AND MORBIDITY OF PERIOPERATIVE ANEMIA

Anemia is a condition where the number of red blood cells (RBCs) or the hemoglobin (Hgb) concentration within them is lower than normal. World Health Organization (WHO) defines anemia as Hgb as less than 12 g/dL in non-pregnant women, less than 11 g/dL in pregnant women and less than 13 g/dL in men.[1] Globally, there were 1.76 billion prevalent cases of anemia in 2019.[2]

Peri-operative anemia is a common condition encountered in adult surgical patients. It is increasingly recognized as a predictor of post-operative morbidity and mortality. Additionally, patients with perioperative anemia have increased risk of infection and length of stay (LOS) leading to increased resource utilization.[3,4] Pre-operative anemia is the number one predictor for the need for perioperative RBC transfusion. RBC transfusion, in turn, can have many downstream complications including risks

[a] UCI Hospitalist Program, Department of Medicine, University of California Irvine Medical Center, Orange, CA, USA; [b] Department of Hospital Medicine, Cleveland Clinic, 9500 Euclid Avenue, Cleveland, OH 44195, USA
* Corresponding author. UCI Hospitalist Program, 333 City Boulevard West, Suite 500, Orange, CA 92868.
E-mail address: skkalra@hs.uci.edu

Med Clin N Am 108 (2024) 1065–1085
https://doi.org/10.1016/j.mcna.2024.04.002   medical.theclinics.com

from ABO incompatibility, transfusion reactions, infections, circulatory overload, and acute lung injury. The estimates of pre-operative anemia are highly variable based on the literature with a range from 5% to 75%.[5] In post-operative patients, this number can be as high as 90%.[5] Women tend to have higher risk of post-operative anemia as they have low circulating blood volume compared with men, so the same amount of blood loss leads to a more significant effect on the loss of blood volume that may lead to higher transfusion rates in women.[6] Therefore, in perioperative settings, a target Hgb of greater than 13 g/dL should be considered irrespective of sexes.[7,8]

With an aging surgical population, the prevalence of anemia in elderly patients is of considerable importance. A retrospective study of 310,311 elderly veterans with pre-operative anemia demonstrated that every percentage-point decrease in pre-operative hematocrit value below 39% was associated with a 1.6% increased 30-day postoperative mortality.[9] Another study of elderly patients (age >65 years) using prospective American College of Surgeons National Surgical Quality Improvement Program database of 31,857 patients undergoing elective vascular surgery found that 47% of the study population was anemic.[10] Patients with anemia had significantly higher rates of cardiac events and post-operative mortality leading authors to conclude that identification and treatment of anemia should be important components of pre-operative care for patients undergoing vascular operations.[10]

A retrospective study of 7759 non-cardiac surgery patients showed about 40% prevalence of preoperative anemia, which was in turn associated with a nearly 5-fold increase in the odds of post-operative mortality.[11] A systematic review of ortho-pedic hip and knee surgeries showed that perioperative anemia was associated with a blood transfusion rate of 45 ± 25% and 44 ± 15%, post-operative infections, poorer physical functioning and recovery, and increased LOS and mortality.[12] Sequeira and colleagues conducted a study of iron deficiency anemia (IDA) using national insurance database of patients who underwent Total Hip Arthroplasty (THA) between 2005 and 2014 evaluating rates of post-operative medical complications, surgery-related complications, hospital readmission, emergency department visits, and mortality.[13] Additionally, 90-day and day of surgery cost and LOS were calculated.[13] In total, 98,681 patients with a pre-operative diagnosis of IDA who underwent THA were identified and compared with 386,724 controls. Not only was IDA associated with increased risk of 30-day emergency department visits and 30-day readmission but also IDA was also associated with an increased 90-day medical complication rate, 1-year peri-prosthetic joint infection, revision, dislocation, and fracture. Patients with IDA accrued higher hospital charges ($27,658.27 vs $16,709.18, $P<.001$) and lower hospital reim-bursement ($5509.90 vs $3605.59, $P<.001$) while evaluating the economic impact.[13] One may conclude that severe anemia is responsible for adverse post-operative out-comes, but in a retrospective study of 227,425 non-cardiac surgery patients, even mild anemia (hematocrit between 38%–28% in men and 35%–28% in women) was independently associated with increased 30-day morbidity and mortality.[14]

An important goal of pre-operative anemia optimization is to increase hemoglobin levels enough to avoid blood transfusion. Another outcome that must be prevented is the development of myocardial ischemia. Recently in the non-cardiac surgery pop-ulation, peri-operative anemia correlates with an increased risk of myocardial ischemia in non-cardiac surgery (MINS). A retrospective cohort analysis of 6141 pa-tients, from which 4480 were evaluated, demonstrated MINS in 155 patients (inci-dence of 3.5%) in the overall cohort; the incidence was 0% among patients whose postoperative hemoglobin was greater than 13 g/dL and it rose up to 8.5% among pa-tients whose minimum post-operative hemoglobin was less than 8 g/dL. The risk for developing MINS was 1.29 [HR 1.29, 95% CI 1.16–1.42; $P<.001$] for every 1 g/dL decrease in post-operative hemoglobin in both time-varying covariate analysis and sensitivity analyses.[15] Another single center retrospective study of 35,170 patients comparing 22,062 (62.7%) patients with normal hemoglobin versus 13,108 (37.3%) with post-operative anemia in whom 11,919 sets of patients were analyzed with propensity score matching, demonstrated a higher incidence of MINS among patients with anemia [14.5 versus 21.0%, (OR) 1.57, 95% CI 1.47–1.68; $P<.001$]. The estimated threshold for pre-operative hemoglobin associated with MINS was 12.2 g/dL (AUC 0.622).[16]

EVALUATION OF PERIOPERATIVE ANEMIA

Anemia is a single marker for adverse peri-operative outcomes, especially in elderly patients.[14,17–20] Therefore, once identified, an appropriate evaluation for the etiology of anemia pre-operatively must be pursued, to optimize Hgb values with non-transfusion interventions, which subsequently decreases the risk of adverse outcomes and receiving allogeneic blood product transfusions in the peri-operative period.

Peri-operative blood management and optimization include correction of coagulopathy, source control of hemorrhage, enhancement of patient's tolerance to anemia, as well as improving the hemoglobin and hematocrit.[21] However, the modifiable risk factors that can be corrected without transfusion of blood products are often nutritional (hematinic) deficiencies, which include mostly iron, cyanocobalamin (vitamin B12), and folic acid. Zinc and copper deficiencies can also cause refractory anemia and must be considered.[22,23] Also, hematinic deficiency even in patients without anemia are associated with adverse outcomes. Among patients undergoing cardiac surgery, even those who are not anemic, the presence of iron deficiency was correlated with adverse outcomes, and therefore, its pre-operative optimization enhances overall prognosis.[24]

There are multiple algorithms designed to evaluate anemia. The authors propose a simplified, yet comprehensive algorithm that allows one to evaluate anemia (Hb < 13 g/dL irrespective of gender) pre-operatively (**Fig. 1**). A detailed history is fundamental. It should include: history or symptoms of anemia, transfusion history, history of

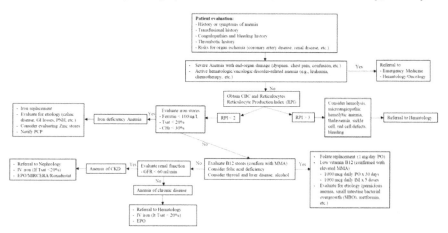

Fig. 1. Algorithm for evaluation and optimization of pre-operative anemia (Hb < 13 g/dL). (*Adapted from* Warner MA, Shore-Lesserson L, Shander A, Patel SY, Perelman SI, Guinn NR. Perioperative Anemia: Prevention, Diagnosis, and Management Throughout the Spectrum of Perioperative Care. Anesth Analg. 2020 May;130(5):1364-1380. https://doi.org/10.1213/ANE.0000000000004727. PMID: 32167979.)

coagulopathies, and bleeding, as well as thrombosis, in addition to the risk factors for end organ ischemia (coronary artery disease, renal disease, and so forth.).[25,26] The pre-operative optimization will focus mostly on stable patients in whom there is opportunity to optimize the anemia. Patients with severe anemia with end-organ damage (dyspnea, chest pain, confusion, and so forth.), as well as with active hematologic-oncologic disorder-related anemia (eg, leukemia, chemotherapy, and so forth.) should be referred to a hematologist.[26]

The reticulocyte production index (RPI) allows differentiation of hypoproliferative from hyperproliferative conditions. Elevated RPI (>3) points most commonly to underlying hemolysis, and therefore, formal Hematology referral is warranted.[5,25,26]

In the preoperative realm, it is hypoproliferative anemia (RPI < 2) that the authors focus most given that its etiology is often secondary to nutritional deficiencies and therefore, can be corrected with supplementation. Since the most common nutritional deficiency associated with anemia is iron deficiency,[27] the algorithm starts with formal assessment of iron stores. This includes measurement of transferrin saturation, ferritin levels, and reticulocyte hemoglobin content (CHr). Iron deficiency is defined by ferritin less than 100 µg/L, transferrin saturation less than 20%, or CHr less than 30%.[26] Less common nutritional deficiency causes of anemia include copper and zinc deficiency, the latter being more common; in our practice, formal evaluation for zinc deficiency is done, especially among patients with low alkaline phosphatase, and if identified, replacement is recommended.[28]

If the iron stores are normal, then the focus of evaluation shifts toward identifying cyanocobalamin deficiency, confirming it with elevated methylmalonic acid. Folic acid deficiency must also be considered; however, its evaluation is considered not essential as it can be easily supplemented both enterally and parenterally with rapid correction of stores.[29] As with other hematinic deficiencies, formal identification of underlying etiology is warranted for long-term optimization.

In patients in whom no significant hematinic levels deficiencies are found, then consider identifying anemia of chronic inflammation and anemia of chronic renal disease.

OPTIMIZATION OF ANEMIA

Anemia is often a sign of underlying disease. Therefore, the first step in anemia optimization is to identify and treat the disease that is causing anemia, as discussed previously. Once the etiology of anemia has been identified and treated, best practice is to try to optimize anemia before any major surgery.

Optimizing Iron Deficiency Anemia

Given that IDA is the most common etiology of anemia in surgical patients, there have been multiple studies assessing outcomes of treatment of IDA before surgery. These studies have looked at both oral and intravenous (IV) iron use and their role in reducing blood transfusions or other post-operative complications.

Oral iron: Oral iron replacement is cheap and easily available, but the effectiveness is reduced by poor absorption and gastrointestinal side effects like constipation, diarrhea, abdominal discomfort, and metallic taste. Multiple formulations are available (**Table 1**); the authors suggest ferrous sulfate given its broader availability and cost. Non-adherence to daily iron has been estimated to range from 10% to 32%.[30] Intestinal bacterial overgrowth in metabolic syndrome, uremia and chronic use of antacids, calcium supplements and, prior gastric bypass surgery have all been shown to reduce absorption of key nutrients in the intestine, including iron.[31] Furthermore, it can take 3–6 months to completely replenish iron stores depending on the severity of IDA.

Table 1 Oral iron formulations	
Formulation	**Elemental Iron Content/Tab**
Ferric citrate	210 mg/g
Ferric maltol	30 mg/30 mg
Ferrous fumarate	106 mg/324 mg
Ferrous gluconate	27 mg/240 mg; 38 mg/324 mg
Ferrous sulfate	65 mg/325 mg
Ferric pyrophosphate	120 mg/g
Polysaccharide iron complex	Variable over the counter-eg, 50 mg/50 mg
Carbonyl iron	1000 mg/g

Although it may be reasonable to delay some elective surgeries, like THA, to allow complete replenishment of iron stores; other time sensitive surgeries, like those for cancer, cannot be delayed. If oral iron is used for repletion, the recommended dose is 60 mg to 120 mg of elemental iron per day. Of this dose, there is wide variation in the percentage absorbed ranging from 2% to 30% depending on food intake or not. It is recommended to periodically check Hgb during this time to assess response. Recent data provide evidence that higher daily dosages of iron can increase hepcidin activity that will in turn decrease enteral iron absorption through its effect on the ferroportin pathway.[32] A randomized trial to study alternate day dosing versus daily dosing found that providing iron supplements on alternate days and in single doses optimizes iron absorption and might be a preferable dosing regimen.[33,34] In another randomized study of 200 adults with IDA comparing alternate day single 120 mg dose iron sulfate to daily single 60 mg dose found no significant difference in Hgb improvement at 8 weeks.[30] A guide to commonly available oral iron formulations is shown in **Table 1**. If Hgb checked 4 weeks before surgery shows no response to oral iron despite compliance, then IV iron should be recommended.

Parenteral iron: Parenteral or IV iron has traditionally been reserved as a last resort because of its cost and associated risk of adverse reactions. However, the newer formulations have much improved safety profile and, with increased awareness, it is being widely accepted as a superior treatment option when compared with oral iron. IV iron has a superior bioavailability compared with oral iron. The currently available IV iron formulations and their recommended dosages are shown in **Table 2**. IV iron is especially useful in patients with functional iron deficiency where chronic inflammation often leads to poor enteral absorption of oral iron. IV iron also allows for a faster response as seen with Hgb improvement as early as 5 days to at most 3 weeks after infusion.[35] This can be a crucial factor in decision making when surgery cannot be significantly delayed.

The evidence on the benefit of IV iron on reduction of blood utilization and other post-operative complications has, so far, been mixed. In a randomized controlled trial of patients undergoing major abdominal surgery, 72 patients with IDA were enrolled and given either IV iron or placebo.[36] A 60% reduction in allogeneic blood transfusion and shorter LOS was observed in IV iron group. There was no difference in morbidity, mortality, or quality of life between IV iron and placebo.[36] But another well-conducted randomized trial evaluating IV iron infusion versus placebo before major abdominal surgery did not reveal a benefit towards transfusion reduction or mortality.[37] The pre-operative IV iron to treat anemia before major abdominal surgery trial, which was a double-blind randomized controlled trial in 487 adult patients with pre-operative anemia undergoing elective major open abdominal surgery who were randomized to

Table 2
Different intravenous iron formulations currently approved for use in the United States[45]

Generic Name	US Brand Name	Plasma Half Life (hr)	Need for Test Dose	Single Total Dose Infusion	Suggested Dosage and Frequency (for 1000 mg Deficit)
Iron Dextran	Infed	20	Yes	Yes	25 mg test dose followed by 1000 mg single dose.
Sodium Ferric Gluconate	Ferrlecit	1	No	No	125 mg IV daily up to 8 doses.
Iron Sucrose	Venofer	6	No	No	200 mg daily up to 5 doses.
Ferumoxytol	Feraheme	15	No	No	510 mg every 3–8 d for 2 doses.
Ferric Carboxymaltose	Injectafer	16	No	No	15 mg/kg every 7 d for 2 doses.
Ferric Derisomaltose (Iron isomaltoside)	Monoferric	20	No	Yes	1000 mg single dose.

Adapted from Kalra SK TB, Khambaty M, Manjarrez E. Post-operative Anemia After Major Surgery: a Brief Review. Current Emergency and Hospital Medicine Reports. 16 June 2021 2021;9: 89–95.

receive IV iron (244) or placebo (243) 10 days to 42 days before surgery. End points were risk of the composite outcome of blood transfusion or death and number of blood transfusions from randomization to 30 days post-operatively. There was no superiority of IV iron versus placebo to decrease the need for blood transfusion (RR 0.98, 95% CI 0.68–1.43; $P=.93$).[37] There was a significant trend for reduced readmissions in this trial raising the possibility of benefit of IV iron in post-operative recovery. Nonetheless, the results from this study reinforced the findings from a 2019 Cochrane review of 6 randomized controlled trials of 372 anemic patients, which did not reveal a benefit in reducing red cell transfusions in patients who were treated with pre-operative oral, or IV iron supplementation compared with no treatment, placebo, or usual care.[38] On the other hand, a recent meta-analysis of randomized trials using preoperative IV iron compared with oral iron or placebo in colorectal surgery patients showed that use of IV iron reduced the risk of blood transfusion compared with oral iron or placebo. There was no mortality difference between the groups.[39]

Studies have also evaluated the benefit of erythrocyte stimulating agents (ESAs) and IV iron used concurrently. In patients with anemia and iron deficiency, preoperative treatment with a single dose of IV ferric derisomaltose and darbepoetin decreased the proportion of participants who received a peri-operative blood transfusion compared with treatment with oral ferrous sulphate.[40] In a prospective randomized trial of 1006 patients undergoing cardiac surgery, an ultra-short-term combination treatment with IV iron, subcutaneous erythropoietin alpha, vitamin B12, and oral folic acid reduced RBC and total allogeneic blood product transfusions in patients with pre-operative anemia or isolated iron deficiency.[41] IV iron has also been studied in non-anemic iron deficient patients. In a randomized trial of 60 non-anemic cardiac surgery patients, a single peri-operative 1000 mg dose of IV iron isomaltoside significantly increased the Hgb level and prevented anemia 4 weeks after surgery, with a short-term safety profile like placebo.[42]

As noticeable, most of the studies have been in pre-operative setting and there is limited evidence of use of IV iron in post-operative period. A consensus guideline published in 2017 recommended use of IV iron for post-operative anemia.[43] It was postulated that post-surgical inflammation is likely to render oral iron ineffective because of increased levels of hepcidin and IV iron can bypass this risk.[43]

Adverse events: Clinicians are often hesitant to use IV iron because of fear of infusion reactions and anaphylaxis. The concern for infusion reactions was evaluated recently in which overall risk for anaphylaxis and other infusion reactions with IV iron formulations was low, especially with newer formulations.[44] In this multicenter cohort, 35,737 IV iron infusions were administered to 12,237 patients, the incidence of infusion reactions was 3.9%, with only 2 total documented epinephrine administrations. Surprisingly, the incidence of adverse events among those who received premedication was 23-fold higher compared with those who did not. However, many patients who received premedication had a prior history of reactions to IV iron.[44]

Despite a lack of level one evidence for the benefit of IV iron, it is still a best practice to replenish iron stores before major surgery, especially those associated with significant blood loss (>300 mL), and the cost of IV iron can potentially be offset by cost saving from reduced transfusion. In summary, the authors recommend an individualized approach with careful consideration of potential risks and benefits before recommending either oral or IV iron therapy.

Optimizing Anemia of Chronic Disease

Anemia of chronic disease is also commonly encountered preoperatively, where patients may have anemia from chronic kidney disease (CKD) or chronic inflammation from an underlying condition. In these conditions, the iron metabolism is also impaired because of ineffective erythropoiesis. Therefore, it is important to assess for concomitant iron deficiency in these patients and to optimize both conditions.

Erythrocyte Stimulating Agents (ESAs): There is insufficient erythropoietin production in patients with CKD that commonly leads to anemia. ESAs have been extensively studied and used in CKD, especially those on dialysis. The 2012 KDIGO (Kidney Disease: Improving Global Outcomes) Clinical Practice Guideline for anemia in CKD suggests initiating ESAs to maintain Hgb of 9.0 g/dL to 10.0 g/dL, with the goal of preventing the Hgb from being less than 9 g/dL. However, individualization of therapy is reasonable as some patients may benefit from initiation of ESAs at a Hgb more than 10 g/dL. For all patients, ESAs should be discontinued if the Hgb exceeds 13 g/dL, and for most patients, ESAs should be stopped when the Hgb is more than 11.5 g/dL.[46] ESAs are currently approved by Food and Drug Administration (FDA) for use in surgical patients to reduce the transfusions in certain major surgery patients. It is beneficial even in non-CKD patients who are anemic and are at risk for significant blood loss during surgery. Studies on use of ESAs have consistently shown a reduction in blood transfusions.[47–50] Of these studies, those in orthopedic surgeries, have shown to have consistent improvement in Hgb with use of ESA along with decreased transfusions. The use of ESAs must be balanced against potential risk of increased thromboembolism risk, and there is FDA advisory to bear caution in patients with heart disease, stroke, and uncontrolled hypertension. Additionally, there is a risk for cancer progression. The 2019 update from American Society of Hematology and Clinical Oncology on the use of ESAs suggested that ESAs can be used in patients with cancer with chemotherapy-induced anemia and low risk of myelodysplastic syndromes.[51] Expert opinion and guidance recommend use in patients who are on chemotherapy with a palliative intent.[51] When ESAs are used pre-operatively, the authors recommend concomitant use of IV iron to prevent patients from developing a functional iron deficiency.

A novel product for anemia optimization in end stage renal disease is Roxadustat, an oral hypoxia-inducible factor prolyl hydroxylase inhibitor that stimulates erythropoiesis and regulates iron metabolism.[52] In renal transplant patients, there is evidence that Roxadustat effectively optimizes anemia and may have renoprotective effects.[53]

Optimizing Other Nutritional Deficiencies

Although IDA is the most common cause of anemia from nutritional deficiencies, there are other vitamins and minerals that are also vital for production of RBC and Hgb. The most important of these include vitamin B12, folic acid, zinc, and copper. Vitamin B12 deficiency takes months to years to develop and manifests with macrocytic and megaloblastic morphology of RBC. Likewise, folate deficiency (although uncommon in US due to fortification of food with folic acid) can lead to macrocytic anemia. In patients with malnutrition, more than one vitamin and mineral deficiency may be present, and the patient may have a normocytic anemia with concomitant deficiency of iron, b12 and folate. B12 deficiency is easily corrected with high dose oral B12, but a careful history should be obtained to rule out malabsorption as the cause of B12 deficiency. In the absence of intrinsic factor, oral B12 is unlikely to be absorbed and injectable form of B12 will be required. Additionally, patients with severe symptomatic anemia from B12 deficiency should also be treated with injectable B12. The authors recommend a weekly 1000 µg intramuscular injection until levels normalize, followed by monthly or every other month maintenance dose administration. When treated appropriately, vitamin B12 deficiency can be corrected within a month. Routine testing of folate levels in patients with anemia has been called into question because of issues around the assays and their reliability.[29] It may be reasonable to treat with folic acid at a dose of 400 µg - 1000 µg when there is a high suspicion for deficiency followed by testing Hgb in 1 week to 2 weeks to measure for an increase in Hgb levels.[29] As discussed earlier, a pragmatic approach of treatment for as little as 1 day before surgery using IV iron, subcutaneous erythropoietin alpha, vitamin B12, and oral folic acid has been shown to be effective in reducing RBC transfusion in cardiac surgery patients with pre-operative anemia.[41]

Copper associated anemia is uncommon as most adults get enough copper through their usual diet. Copper deficiency can manifest in times of either increased demand like pregnancy and lactation or low intake as seen with anorexia and malnutrition. Copper is mainly absorbed in stomach and proximal duodenum so malabsorption (inflammatory bowel disease, celiac disease, gastrectomy, bowel resection, and post bariatric surgery) or increased losses (protein losing enteropathy, prolonged diarrhea, and tropical sprue) can also lead to deficiency. Zinc is a competitive inhibitor of oral copper absorption, and excessive zinc consumption can lead to copper deficiency. Iatrogenic deficiency can manifest when parenteral nutrition or enteric nutrition is not supplemented with copper. Copper deficiency affects normal hematopoiesis resulting in anemia and leukopenia. Although the exact mechanism of anemia in copper deficiency is unclear, copper is an important regulator of iron homeostasis. Copper is a vital component in the ferroxidase enzymes, hephaestin and ceruloplasmin. Hephaestus is located in the duodenal mucosa and helps in the oxidation of ferrous iron. Ceruloplasmin is essential for iron transfer from monocyte-macrophage to plasma.[23] Treatment includes oral or IV copper replacement in the form of copper gluconate, copper sulfate, or copper chloride. If concomitant zinc deficiency is present, copper should be repleted first before initiating treatment with zinc.

TRANSFUSION APPROACH TO ANEMIA

There has been a perception that patients may be arbitrarily transfused with hemoglobin thresholds higher than required. Acute normovolemic hemodilution studies allowed to recognize in different patient populations, including elderly and stable cardiac patients, tolerance to progressively lower hemoglobin targets without significant adverse outcomes and demonstrating normal cardiovascular response.[54] Subsequently, to evaluate this response in real clinical scenarios, landmark studies were done, demonstrating the tolerance to lower hemoglobin thresholds for transfusion, with similar or even better outcomes when compared with patients transfused at higher hemoglobin thresholds (**Table 3**).

The recommendations for anemia optimization with transfusion of allogeneic blood were recently updated by the Association for the Advancement of Blood & Biotherapies (AABB) and the recommendations are for restrictive transfusion thresholds as below.[70]

- Hemoglobin 7 g/dL
- Hospitalized adult patients who are hemodynamically stable.
- Hospitalized adult patients with hematologic and oncologic disorders.
- Hemoglobin 7.5 g/dL - patients undergoing cardiac surgery.
- Hemoglobin 8 g/dL – patients undergoing orthopedic surgery or those with pre-existing cardiovascular disease.

The guidelines did not provide specific recommendations regarding patients with acute coronary syndromes. However, the Myocardial Ischemia and Transfusion (MINT) trial has since been published.[68] This randomized controlled study evaluated 3504 patients, comparing a restrictive transfusion threshold (Hgb 7 or 8 g/dL) with a liberal transfusion threshold (Hgb < 10 g/dL), with the primary outcome being a composite of myocardial infarction or death at 30 days. The primary outcome occurred in 16.9% versus 14.5% (liberal vs restrictive) (RR 1.15; 95% CI, 0.99–1.34; P=.07). Death occurred in 9.9% versus 8.3% (liberal vs restrictive) (RR 1.19; 95% CI, 0.96–1.47) and myocardial infarction occurred in 8.5% versus 7.2% (liberal vs restrictive) (RR 1.19; 95% CI, 0.94–1.49). The authors concluded that although the liberal transfusion strategy did not significantly reduce the outcomes, they could not exclude potential harms of restrictive strategies.[68]

SPECIAL CONSIDERATIONS
Sickle Cell Disease

Patients with sickle cell disease (SCD) undergoing surgery have a higher risk of morbidity and mortality compared with the general population because of risk of sickle cell crisis and chronic organ damage from prior crisis episodes.[71–73] Risks are greater for patients homozygous for hemoglobin S (SCD-SS) or with both sickle and β-zero-thalassemia mutations (SCD-S β0-thalassemia) compared with those with trait or heterozygous mutation. Several studies have evaluated the best management strategies for SCD patients undergoing surgical procedures. One of the recommendations is to correct anemia by giving RBC transfusion or exchange transfusion before surgery. One study evaluated liberal strategy, where patients were transfused to maintain HbS concentration less than 30% compared with a conservative approach for transfusion in which Hgb is maintained at 10 g/dL, and authors found no difference in complication rates between the 2 strategies.[74] One of the oldest studies in this area is The Cooperative Study of Sickle Cell Disease that observed 3765 patients between 1978 and 1988 with a mean follow-up of 5.3 plus minus 2.0 years.[75] This study showed that peri-operative transfusions in SCD patients reduced the risk of sickle cell related complications. The Transfusion Alternatives Preoperatively in Sickle cell disease study (TAPS Study) was a randomized trial of 70 patients with SCD-SS or SCD-S

Table 3
Landmark randomized clinical trials evaluating Hgb threshold for transfusion

Authors/Trial	Hgb Threshold in G/dL (Conservative Group)	Hgb Threshold in G/dL (Liberal Group)	Patient Population/Setting	Number of Patients	Primary Outcome	Outcome Liberal vs Restrictive
Hebert et al,[55] 1999 TRICC	7	10	MICU	838	30-d mortality	Unchanged
Lacroix et al,[56] 2007 TRIPICU	7	9.5	PICU	637	28-d mortality or multiorgan dysfunction	Unchanged
Hajjar et al,[57] 2010 TRACS	8	10	Cardiac surgery	502	30-d mortality and severe morbidity	Unchanged
Carson et al,[58] 2011 FOCUS	8	10	Elderly hip fracture	2016	60-d mortality or inability to walk 10 ft	Unchanged
Villanueva et al,[59] 2013	7	9	Severe GI Bleeding	921	45 d rate of death	Worse in Liberal
Holst et al,[60] 2014	7	9	Septic shock	1005	90 d mortality	Unchanged
Robertson et al,[61] 2014	7	10	Traumatic Brain Injury	200	Neurologic recovery at 6 mo	Increased adverse events in liberal group
Jairath et al,[62] 2015 TRIGGER	8	10	GI bleeding	936	28-d mortality or further bleeding	Unchanged
Murphy et al,[63] 2015 Titer2	7.5	9	Cardiac surgery	2007	Ischemia or infection within 3 mo	Unchanged
Mazer et al,[64] 2017; Mazer et al,[65] 2018 TRICS III	7.5	9.5	Cardiac surgery	5243	28 d and 6-mo composite mortality, MI, stroke, or new renal failure needing dialysis	Unchanged

Study						
Garg et al,[66] 2019 TRICS III AKI Substudy	7.5	9.5	Cardiac surgery	4531	Perioperative AKI within 7 d of surgery	Unchanged
Ducrocq et al,[67] 2021 REALITY	8	10	Acute MI with anemia	668	Major adverse cardiovascular outcome	Unchanged
Carson et al,[68] 2023 MINT	7/8	10	Acute MI and anemia	3504	30-d Recurrent MI or death	Liberal transfusion did not significantly reduce outcomes.
Mullis et al,[69] 2024	5.5	7	Asymptomatic musculoskeletal injured trauma patients (age 18–50) who are no longer in the initial resuscitative period.	65	Postoperative infection, other post-operative complications, and Musculoskeletal Functional Assessment scores	Lower infection rate. Similar functional outcomes at 6 mo or 1 y.

β0-thalassemia evaluating preoperative transfusion strategy for low or medium risk surgeries and found a reduced risk of post-operative complications in persons with SCD-SS undergoing medium risk surgery when their preoperative hemoglobin level was increased to 10 g/dL.[76] Additionally, without pre-operative transfusion, the need for peri-operative transfusion was increased in patients with SCD.[76]

The risks of transfusion in SCD include hyper viscosity and increased sickling from over-transfusion, hemolytic and non-hemolytic transfusion reactions, and transmission of infection. An updated Cochrane review in 2020 concluded that there is insufficient evidence from randomized trials to determine whether conservative pre-operative RBC transfusion is as effective as aggressive pre-operative RBC transfusion in preventing disease or surgery related complications in people with SCD.[77] Current consensus in both US[78] and United Kingdome[79] supports pre-operative RBC transfusion in patients with SCD who are undergoing elective surgeries. The American College of Hematology recommends that the decision-making should be individualized based on genotype, the risk level of surgery, baseline total Hgb, complications with prior transfusions, and disease severity. The task force favors pre-operative transfusion in surgeries requiring general anesthesia and lasting more than 1 hour and a goal Hgb of greater than 9 g/dL is favored.[78] The British Society of Hematology task force also recommends pre-operative transfusion in SCD patients undergoing medium- to high-risk surgeries for a goal Hgb of 10 g/dL.[79]

The authors recommend ensuring that the patients are normothermic, euvolemic, have normal oxygenation, and appropriate pain control. Also, folic acid replacement must be continued peri-operatively. As in other clinical contexts, optimization of hematinic substrates is appropriate with caution to avoid development of secondary hemosiderosis. Patients undergoing medium- to high-risk surgery should have pre-operative hemoglobin optimized to 10 g/dL and a multidisciplinary approach between hematology, blood bank, anesthesia, primary care physician, hospitalist, and surgeon is recommended.

Jehovah Witness and Patients in Whom Blood Is Not an Option

A very challenging situation in the peri-operative setting is the care of patients who refuse blood products transfusion for personal or religious beliefs, of which Jehovah's Witnesses are the most commonly encountered patient examples. There are over 8 million Jehovah's witnesses worldwide and their belief command its followers to abstain from blood transfusions or accepting other blood products even if there is a threat to their life. This can provide both ethical and clinical challenges in peri-operative care and, therefore, pre-operative optimization of anemia and coagulation status, as well as minimizing blood loss is of utmost importance. Although Jehovah's Witnesses do not accept autologous blood donation, they will accept blood if it is retained within a closed circuit, such as through cell salvage, acute normovolemic hemodilution, cardiopulmonary bypass, dialysis, and plasmapheresis. The authors recommend a clear discussion with patients and documentation about what they would accept.[80]

The optimization of anemia requires an appropriate evaluation of the hematologic disorders, with a focus on the immediately treatable conditions and may require multiple substrate supplementations (iron, folate, zinc, etc.) in addition to erythropoietic agents. Although, the optimization process should begin at least 6 weeks before surgery,[80] short-term optimization is possible as demonstrated in a randomized controlled trial in cardiac surgery, with simultaneous administration of IV iron, (20 mg/kg ferric carboxymaltose), erythropoietin (40,000 U subcutaneous erythropoietin alpha), parenteral cyanocobalamin (1 mg subcutaneous), and folic acid (5 mg p.o.) and consequent decreased post-operative transfusion requirements.[41] An important consideration in Jehovah witness patients is that erythropoietic agents should not contain human albumin; the agents darbepoetin alfa and epoetin alfa-epx are appropriate in this population.

There are multiple therapeutics approved to treat coagulopathy including antifibrinolytics (eg, tranexamic acid), recombinant factor VIIa, 4 factor prothrombin complex concentrates (4PCC), fibrinogen concentrates, and thrombopoietin receptor agonists.[81]

Post-operatively, minimizing laboratory tests, and using smaller (pediatric size) tubes for collection is recommended.[45,80,82]

INTRAVENOUS IRON IN PATIENT WITH INFECTIONS

The use of IV iron has been associated with increased risk for infections. However, iron deficiency and anemia are also associated with increased infection risk.[83] Limitations of the evidence include heterogeneity in clinical practice, as well as variability in reporting of infections as adverse clinical outcomes.[84]

Iron is a strong substrate for multiple bacteria, including *Escherichia coli, Klebsiella, Pseudomonas, Salmonella, Yersinia, Listeria, Staphylococcus,* and *Haemophilus influenzae.* The evidence of correlation between increased bacterial growth proportional and transferrin saturation comes from in vitro studies.[85]

A recent large systematic review and meta-analysis of 154 randomized controlled trials with 32,920 patients, aimed to examine the risk of infection associated with IV iron when compared with enteral iron or no iron. Intravenous iron was associated with a 17% increased risk of infections when compared to oral iron or no iron. IV iron was associated with increase in hemoglobin with a mean difference of 0.57 g/dL, and the risk of allogenic RBC transfusion was decreased by 7%. There was no meaningful effect of IV iron on mortality or LOS.[84]

Therefore, caution should be exercised when considering the use of IV iron in patients with severe infections, balancing the associated risk with allogeneic RBC transfusions. In the authors' practice, if source control has been established, the patient has been receiving appropriate antimicrobial therapy with demonstration of improvement in clinical features (eg, fever and hemodynamic status) and acute phase reactants (eg, C reactive protein, procalcitonin, etc.) then IV iron can be administered, especially for patients who refuse RBC transfusions.

PLASMA TRANSFUSION

Plasma is the component of whole blood that consists of protein C, protein S, antithrombin, albumin, tissue factor pathway inhibitor and the coagulation factors.[86]

Although plasma is overused as a blood product worldwide, being transfused in up to 1% of all hospitalized patients, the evidence supporting its appropriate use is insufficient. In the US, the overuse of plasma includes its transfusion for International normalized ratio (INR) less than 1.8, with up to 22.5% of patients receiving it for INR less than 1.6. Of note, the appropriate dosing for plasma is based on body weight and is 10 mL/kg to 20 mL/kg; this dose augments the concentration of coagulation factors by 20%; therefore, subtherapeutic doses are clinically ineffective, yet carry the risk associated with transfusion like transfusion associated circulatory overload.[87]

In the periprocedural setting, its most common utilization is for treatment of coagulopathy in actively bleeding patients, as well as for pre-operative optimization. Its most appropriate use is in the setting of active bleeding to treat significant deficiency of multiple coagulation factors. Warfarin reversal is a common scenario where plasma has been routinely used. However, currently there is preference for the use of vitamin K and 4PCC. In patients with bleeding because of vitamin K antagonists (warfarin) or vitamin K deficiency, plasma can be used when vitamin K or 4PCC are not immediately available.[87]

Other clinical scenarios where plasma is used include massive transfusion protocol and liver disease. Massive transfusion protocol (MTP) must be considered in patients undergoing surgeries with high bleeding risk. In MTP, a combination of plasma, red blood cells, and plasma is transfused at a ratio of 1:1:1 ratio. Nonetheless, increased volume of plasma as compared with RBCs can cause decrease in hematocrit levels, as well as dilution of fibrinogen.[87]

Plasma transfusion when INR is less than or equal to 2 is not supported by evidence because of lack of improvement of outcomes or laboratories values. In addition, there should be awareness that the Prothrombin time (PT) or INR levels below 2.0 correlate with normal concentration (>30%) of most clotting factors, hence making plasma transfusions unnecessary.[88] In addition, the PT/INR value is not the sole indicator of the status of hemostasis or thrombosis in some populations, as can be demonstrated in patients with chronic liver disease, who have a balanced coagulation profile with a prothrombotic risk associated with plasma use.[89] Also, in the patients with liver disease, fresh frozen plasma (FFP) can cause volume expansion with consequent increase in portal pressure increasing the risk of variceal bleeding.[90]

The Society for Interventional Radiology guidelines has very conservative recommendations: for patients undergoing a low bleeding risk procedure (eg, central venous access, paracentesis, thoracentesis, etc.), is recommended INR less than or equal to a range of 2.0 to 3.0; the only indication for plasma use in these patients is if femoral arterial access is needed; in patients undergoing a high bleeding risk procedure (deep organ biopsy) the society recommends that the INR be less than 1.5 to 1.8.[91]

Caution must be held with the sole use of INR to assess coagulopathy, as it may not accurately reflect the current rate of thrombin generation and actual hemostasis.[92,93] Therefore, in addition to the INR, clinicians must have awareness of other tests to assess coagulopathy, especially, the viscoelastic tests, which include Thromboelastogram (TEG) and rotatory thromboelastometry (ROTEM), which have decreased inappropriate blood products transfused without adverse clinical outcomes.[94,95]

Recent strategies to allow for safer and easy to use plasma products, especially in environments with limited resources, has allowed to develop a newer plasma product – the lyophilized plasma (LyP) which has the benefit of room temperature storage, pathogen-reduction, and rapid reconstitution, with similar clinical effectiveness to FFP. It can also be partially reconstituted to 50% of the volume, conferring a similar hemostatic benefit with decreased transfused volume, although with obvious higher colloid osmotic pressure than FFP.[87]

PLATELET TRANSFUSION

An important element to consider before invasive procedures is the platelet count. However, clinicians must appraise certain aspects involving the assessment of periprocedural thrombocytopenia, as well as the challenges associated with platelet transfusion; platelets are expensive and often are not readily available; have a short half-life (must be used within 5 days); they are stored at room temperature, which increases the risk of bacterial contamination; they carry a high risk of transfusion reactions and alloimmunization; and clinician compliance with recommended transfusion thresholds is often not optimal.[96–98]

A unit of platelet (either as a pool of 5 concentrates from different donors with same ABO group and Rhesus factor diluted in plasma or obtained directly from apheresis)

Table 4
Current platelet thresholds recommended for transfusion by the Association for the Advancement of Blood & Biotherapies,[98] the British Committee for Standards in Haematology[102] and the Society for Interventional Radiology[91]

Society	Platelet Threshold	Indications
AABB/BSH	$\leq 10 \times 10^9$/L	Decrease spontaneous bleeding.
AABB/BSH	$< 20 \times 10^9$/L	Central venous catheter
AABB	$< 50 \times 10^9$/L	Lumbar puncture (AABB)
BSH	$< 40 \times 10^9$/L	Lumbar puncture (BSH)
AABB/BSH	$< 50 \times 10^9$/L	Major elective surgery
AABB/BSH	$< 100 \times 10^9$/L	Neurosurgery and ophthalmology
SIR	$< 20 \times 10^9$/L	Percutaneous procedures with low risk of bleeding: lumbar puncture, chest tube, central venous catheter, paracentesis/thoracentesis, etc.
SIR	$< 50 \times 10^9$/L	Percutaneous procedures with high bleeding risk: arterial access from femoral artery, deep organ biopsy, deep organ abscess drain, etc.

increase the circulating platelet number by 20 cells/μL to 30,000 cells/μL.[99] Platelets in the United States (US) are treated with a photochemical process with ultraviolet light that inactivates pathogens, as well as residual leukocytes, decreasing the risk of graft-vs-host disease and increase its storage life from 5 days to 7 days. However, this process significantly raises the cost associated with platelet transfusion.[100]

Clinicians must have awareness of 3 main conditions that can be associated with periprocedural thrombocytopenia. Pseudothrombocytopenia occurs when platelets aggregate in ethylenediamine tetraacetic acid-anticoagulated blood, and this can be assessed with direct microscopy of a RBC smear, or with measurement of platelet count with a citrate-anticoagulated blood. Hemodilution from the use of crystalloids and plasma can also decrease the circulating number of platelets. A third cause is consumption of platelets, in the setting of activation of coagulation cascade secondary to bleeding, inflammation, sepsis, and so forth.[101] Another condition that can occur is the development of heparin induced thrombocytopenia. The autoimmune conditions associated with thrombocytopenia often present as already identified underlying comorbid conditions, rather than a newly developed condition.

The current thresholds for platelet transfusion recommended by the AABB,[98] the British Committee for Standards in Haematology (BSH)[102] guidelines, and the Society

Table 5
Elements that contribute to coagulation effectiveness and thrombopoiesis

Mechanism	Recommendation
Improve endothelial function	Treat sepsis
Enhance platelet adhesion	Use desmopressin to increase circulating levels of von Willebrand factor
Optimization of coagulation factors	Use of recombinant factor VIIa Fibrinogen
Prevent fibrin degradation	Use of antifibrinolytics (tranexamic acid and aminocaproic acid)
Enhance thrombopoiesis	Use thrombopoietin receptor agonists (romiplostim, eltrombopag, avatrombopag, etc.)

for Interventional Radiology (SIR)[91] can be seen in **Table 4**. The recommendation is transfusing single apheresis unit or equivalent.

An important consideration in the periprocedural setting is when platelets are not available, or when patients refuse platelet transfusion. In this context, the optimization of all elements of coagulation, as well as of thrombopoiesis are paramount (**Table 5**).

In addition to platelet count, especially in the setting of active bleeding and concerns for coagulopathy, viscoelastic testing also offers an accurate perspective to guide optimization of coagulation function.[94,95]

SUMMARY

Peri-operative anemia is highly prevalent and remains an independent predictor for post-operative mortality and morbidity. Pre-operative evaluation should focus on identifying the cause of anemia and optimization strategies should focus on increasing red cell mass and correcting any nutritional deficiencies. IV iron is safe and can be used for correcting pre-operative and post-operative anemia, especially when IDA is present. Benefit of IV iron in reducing transfusion or mortality remains controversial. Multiple randomized trials have shown non-inferiority of restrictive strategies for RBC transfusion in surgical patients, and the authors support this approach. Indiscriminate use of plasma or FFP is not supported by current evidence and care should be taken to avoid volume overload when using plasma. INR should not be used as the sole measure of coagulopathy when considering reversal strategies as it may not accurately reflect thrombin generation and actual hemostasis.

DISCLOSURE

None.

REFERENCES

1. Haemoglobin concentrations for the diagnosis of anaemia and assessment of severity. WHO. Available at: https://www.who.int/publications-detail-redirect/WHO-NMH-NHD-MNM-11.1.
2. Global Health Metrics. Anemia-Level 1 impairment. Lancet 2019;393.
3. Dunne JR, Malone D, Tracy JK, et al. Perioperative anemia: an independent risk factor for infection, mortality, and resource utilization in surgery. J Surg Res 2002;102(2):237–44.
4. Gomez-Ramirez S, Jerico C, Munoz M. Perioperative anemia: Prevalence, consequences and pathophysiology. Transfus Apher Sci 2019;58(4):369–74.
5. Shander A, Knight K, Thurer R, et al. Prevalence and outcomes of anemia in surgery: a systematic review of the literature. Am J Med 2004;116(Suppl 7A): 58S–69S.
6. Gombotz H, Rehak PH, Shander A, et al. Blood use in elective surgery: the Austrian benchmark study. Transfusion 2007;47(8):1468–80.
7. Munoz M, Acheson AG, Auerbach M, et al. International consensus statement on the peri-operative management of anaemia and iron deficiency. Anaesthesia 2017;72(2):233–47.
8. Shander A, Corwin HL, Meier J, et al. Recommendations From the International Consensus Conference on Anemia Management in Surgical Patients (ICCAMS). Ann Surg 2023;277(4):581–90.

9. Wu WC, Schifftner TL, Henderson WG, et al. Preoperative hematocrit levels and postoperative outcomes in older patients undergoing noncardiac surgery. JAMA 2007;297(22):2481–8.

10. Gupta PK, Sundaram A, Mactaggart JN, et al. Preoperative anemia is an independent predictor of postoperative mortality and adverse cardiac events in elderly patients undergoing elective vascular operations. Ann Surg 2013; 258(6):1096–102.

11. Beattie WS, Karkouti K, Wijeysundera DN, et al. Risk associated with preoperative anemia in noncardiac surgery: a single-center cohort study. Anesthesiology 2009;110(3):574–81.

12. Spahn DR. Anemia and patient blood management in hip and knee surgery: a systematic review of the literature. Anesthesiology 2010;113(2):482–95.

13. Sequeira SB, Quinlan ND, Althoff AD, et al. Iron deficiency anemia is associated with increased early postoperative surgical and medical complications following total hip arthroplasty. J Arthroplasty 2021;36(3):1023–8.

14. Musallam KM, Tamim HM, Richards T, et al. Preoperative anaemia and postoperative outcomes in non-cardiac surgery: a retrospective cohort study. Lancet 2011;378(9800):1396–407.

15. Turan A, Cohen B, Rivas E, et al. Association between postoperative haemoglobin and myocardial injury after noncardiac surgery: a retrospective cohort analysis. Br J Anaesth 2021;126(1):94–101.

16. Kwon JH, Park J, Lee SH, et al. Pre-operative anaemia and myocardial injury after noncardiac surgery: A retrospective study. Eur J Anaesthesiol 2021;38(6): 582–90.

17. Baron DM, Hochrieser H, Posch M, et al. Preoperative anaemia is associated with poor clinical outcome in non-cardiac surgery patients. Br J Anaesth 2014;113(3):416–23.

18. Sim YE, Abdullah HR. Implications of anemia in the elderly undergoing surgery. Clin Geriatr Med 2019;35(3):391–405.

19. Sim YE, Wee HE, Ang AL, et al. Prevalence of preoperative anemia, abnormal mean corpuscular volume and red cell distribution width among surgical patients in Singapore, and their influence on one year mortality. PLoS One 2017; 12(8):e0182543.

20. Auron M, DCM MY. Preoperative anemia optimization: role of iron supplementation. J Xiangya Med 2018;3(37).

21. Desai N, Schofield N, Richards T. Perioperative patient blood management to improve outcomes. Anesth Analg 2018;127(5):1211–20.

22. Jeng SS, Chen YH. Association of Zinc with Anemia. Nutrients 2022;14(22).

23. Myint ZW, Oo TH, Thein KZ, et al. Copper deficiency anemia: review article. Ann Hematol 2018;97(9):1527–34.

24. Rossler J, Schoenrath F, Seifert B, et al. Iron deficiency is associated with higher mortality in patients undergoing cardiac surgery: a prospective study. Br J Anaesth 2020;124(1):25–34.

25. Piva E, Brugnara C, Chiandetti L, et al. Automated reticulocyte counting: state of the art and clinical applications in the evaluation of erythropoiesis. Clin Chem Lab Med 2010;48(10):1369–80.

26. Warner MA, Shore-Lesserson L, Shander A, et al. Perioperative anemia: prevention, diagnosis, and management throughout the spectrum of perioperative care. Anesth Analg 2020;130(5):1364–80.

27. Lin Y. Preoperative anemia-screening clinics. Hematology Am Soc Hematol Educ Program 2019;2019(1):570–6.

28. Ray CSSB, Jena I, Behera S, et al. Low Alkaline Phosphatase (ALP) In Adult Population an Indicator of Zinc (Zn) and Magnesium (Mg) Deficiency. Curr Res Nutr Food Sci 2017;5(3).

29. Breu AC, Theisen-Toupal J, Feldman LS. Serum and red blood cell folate testing on hospitalized patients. J Hosp Med 2015;10(11):753–5.

30. Pasupathy E, Kandasamy R, Thomas K, et al. Alternate day versus daily oral iron for treatment of iron deficiency anemia: a randomized controlled trial. Sci Rep 2023;13(1):1818.

31. Goddard AF, James MW, McIntyre AS, et al. Guidelines for the management of iron deficiency anaemia. Gut 2011;60(10):1309–16.

32. Moretti D, Goede JS, Zeder C, et al. Oral iron supplements increase hepcidin and decrease iron absorption from daily or twice-daily doses in iron-depleted young women. Blood 2015;126(17):1981–9.

33. Stoffel NU, Cercamondi CI, Brittenham G, et al. Iron absorption from oral iron supplements given on consecutive versus alternate days and as single morning doses versus twice-daily split dosing in iron-depleted women: two open-label, randomised controlled trials. Lancet Haematol 2017;4(11):e524–33.

34. Stoffel NU, Zeder C, Brittenham GM, et al. Iron absorption from supplements is greater with alternate day than with consecutive day dosing in iron-deficient anemic women. Haematologica 2020;105(5):1232–9.

35. Goodnough LT, Skikne B, Brugnara C. Erythropoietin, iron, and erythropoiesis. Blood 2000;96(3):823–33.

36. Froessler B, Palm P, Weber I, et al. The Important Role for Intravenous Iron in Perioperative Patient Blood Management in Major Abdominal Surgery: A Randomized Controlled Trial. Ann Surg 2016;264(1):41–6.

37. Richards T, Baikady RR, Clevenger B, et al. Preoperative intravenous iron to treat anaemia before major abdominal surgery (PREVENTT): a randomised, double-blind, controlled trial. Lancet 2020;396(10259):1353–61.

38. Ng O, Keeler BD, Mishra A, et al. Iron therapy for preoperative anaemia. Cochrane Database Syst Rev 2019;12(12):CD011588.

39. Lederhuber H, Massey LH, Abeysiri S, et al. Preoperative intravenous iron and the risk of blood transfusion in colorectal cancer surgery: meta-analysis of randomized clinical trials. Br J Surg 2024;(1):111.

40. Kong R, Hutchinson N, Hill A, et al. Randomised open-label trial comparing intravenous iron and an erythropoiesis-stimulating agent versus oral iron to treat preoperative anaemia in cardiac surgery (INITIATE trial). Br J Anaesth 2022; 128(5):796–805.

41. Spahn DR, Schoenrath F, Spahn GH, et al. Effect of ultra-short-term treatment of patients with iron deficiency or anaemia undergoing cardiac surgery: a prospective randomised trial. Lancet 2019;393(10187):2201–12.

42. Johansson PI, Rasmussen AS, Thomsen LL. Intravenous iron isomaltoside 1000 (Monofer(R)) reduces postoperative anaemia in preoperatively non-anaemic patients undergoing elective or subacute coronary artery bypass graft, valve replacement or a combination thereof: a randomized double-blind placebo-controlled clinical trial (the PROTECT trial). Vox Sang 2015;109(3):257–66.

43. Munoz M, Acheson AG, Bisbe E, et al. An international consensus statement on the management of postoperative anaemia after major surgical procedures. Anaesthesia 2018;73(11):1418–31.

44. Arastu AH, Elstrott BK, Martens KL, et al. Analysis of adverse events and intravenous iron infusion formulations in adults with and without prior infusion reactions. JAMA Netw Open 2022;5(3):e224488.

45. Kalra SKTB, Khambaty M, Manjarrez E. Post-operative anemia after major surgery: a brief review. Current Emergency and Hospital Medicine Reports 2021;9:89–95.
46. KDIGO clinical practice guideline for anemia in chronic kidney disease. Kidney Int 2012;2(4) (Suppl).
47. Bezwada HP, Nazarian DG, Henry DH, et al. Preoperative use of recombinant human erythropoietin before total joint arthroplasty. J Bone Joint Surg Am 2003;85(9):1795–800.
48. Bedair H, Yang J, Dwyer MK, et al. Preoperative erythropoietin alpha reduces postoperative transfusions in THA and TKA but may not be cost-effective. Clin Orthop Relat Res 2015;473(2):590–6.
49. Christodoulakis M, Tsiftsis DD, Hellenic Surgical Oncology Perioperative EPOSG. Preoperative epoetin alfa in colorectal surgery: a randomized, controlled study. Ann Surg Oncol 2005;12(9):718–25.
50. Weltert L, D'Alessandro S, Nardella S, et al. Preoperative very short-term, high-dose erythropoietin administration diminishes blood transfusion rate in off-pump coronary artery bypass: a randomized blind controlled study. J Thorac Cardiovasc Surg 2010;139(3):621–6 [discussion 626-7].
51. Bohlius J, Bohlke K, Castelli R, et al. Management of cancer-associated anemia with erythropoiesis-stimulating agents: ASCO/ASH clinical practice guideline update. J Clin Oncol 2019;37(15):1336–51.
52. Chen N, Hao C, Liu BC, et al. Roxadustat treatment for anemia in patients undergoing long-term dialysis. N Engl J Med 2019;381(11):1011–22.
53. Tang X, Liu F, Li Q, et al. Roxadustat for patients with posttransplant anemia: a narrative review. Kidney Dis 2024;10(1):32–8.
54. Auron M, Duran Castillo MY, Kumar A. Parsimonious blood use and lower transfusion triggers: What is the evidence? Cleve Clin J Med 2017;84(1):43–51.
55. Hebert PC, Wells G, Blajchman MA, et al. A multicenter, randomized, controlled clinical trial of transfusion requirements in critical care. Transfusion Requirements in Critical Care Investigators, Canadian Critical Care Trials Group. N Engl J Med 1999;340(6):409–17.
56. Lacroix J, Hebert PC, Hutchison JS, et al. Transfusion strategies for patients in pediatric intensive care units. N Engl J Med 2007;356(16):1609–19.
57. Hajjar LA, Vincent JL, Galas FR, et al. Transfusion requirements after cardiac surgery: the TRACS randomized controlled trial. JAMA 2010;304(14):1559–67.
58. Carson JL, Terrin ML, Noveck H, et al. Liberal or restrictive transfusion in high-risk patients after hip surgery. N Engl J Med 2011;365(26):2453–62.
59. Villanueva C, Colomo A, Bosch A, et al. Transfusion strategies for acute upper gastrointestinal bleeding. N Engl J Med 2013;368(1):11–21.
60. Holst LB, Haase N, Wetterslev J, et al. Lower versus higher hemoglobin threshold for transfusion in septic shock. N Engl J Med 2014;371(15):1381–91.
61. Robertson CS, Hannay HJ, Yamal JM, et al. Effect of erythropoietin and transfusion threshold on neurological recovery after traumatic brain injury: a randomized clinical trial. JAMA 2014;312(1):36–47.
62. Jairath V, Kahan BC, Gray A, et al. Restrictive versus liberal blood transfusion for acute upper gastrointestinal bleeding (TRIGGER): a pragmatic, open-label, cluster randomised feasibility trial. Lancet 2015;386(9989):137–44.
63. Murphy GJ, Pike K, Rogers CA, et al. Liberal or restrictive transfusion after cardiac surgery. N Engl J Med 2015;372(11):997–1008.
64. Mazer CD, Whitlock RP, Fergusson DA, et al. Six-month outcomes after restrictive or liberal transfusion for cardiac surgery. N Engl J Med 2018;379(13):1224–33.

65. Mazer CD, Whitlock RP, Fergusson DA, et al. Restrictive or liberal red-cell transfusion for cardiac surgery. N Engl J Med 2017;377(22):2133–44.

66. Garg AX, Badner N, Bagshaw SM, et al. Safety of a restrictive versus liberal approach to red blood cell transfusion on the outcome of AKI in patients undergoing cardiac surgery: a randomized clinical trial. J Am Soc Nephrol 2019; 30(7):1294–304.

67. Ducrocq G, Gonzalez-Juanatey JR, Puymirat E, et al. Effect of a restrictive vs liberal blood transfusion strategy on major cardiovascular events among patients with acute myocardial infarction and anemia: The REALITY randomized clinical trial. JAMA 2021;325(6):552–60.

68. Carson JL, Brooks MM, Hebert PC, et al. Restrictive or liberal transfusion strategy in myocardial infarction and anemia. N Engl J Med 2023;389(26):2446–56.

69. Mullis BH, Mullis LS, Kempton LB, et al. Orthopaedic Trauma and Anemia: Conservative versus Liberal Transfusion Strategy: A Prospective Randomized Study. J Orthop Trauma 2024;38(1):18–24.

70. Carson JL, Stanworth SJ, Guyatt G, et al. Red blood cell transfusion: 2023 AABB International Guidelines. JAMA 2023;330(19):1892–902.

71. Rutledge R, Croom RD 3rd, Davis JW Jr, et al. Cholelithiasis in sickle cell anemia: surgical considerations. South Med J 1986;79(1):28–30.

72. Esseltine DW, Baxter MR, Bevan JC. Sickle cell states and the anaesthetist. Can J Anaesth 1988;35(4):385–403.

73. Vichinsky EP, Neumayr LD, Haberkern C, et al. The perioperative complication rate of orthopedic surgery in sickle cell disease: report of the National Sickle Cell Surgery Study Group. Am J Hematol 1999;62(3):129–38.

74. Vichinsky EP, Haberkern CM, Neumayr L, et al. A comparison of conservative and aggressive transfusion regimens in the perioperative management of sickle cell disease. The Preoperative Transfusion in Sickle Cell Disease Study Group. N Engl J Med 1995;333(4):206–13.

75. Koshy M, Weiner SJ, Miller ST, et al. Surgery and anesthesia in sickle cell disease. Cooperative Study of Sickle Cell Diseases. Blood 1995;86(10):3676–84.

76. Howard J, Malfroy M, Llewelyn C, et al. The transfusion alternatives preoperatively in sickle cell disease (TAPS) study: a randomised, controlled, multicentre clinical trial. Lancet 2013;381(9870):930–8.

77. Estcourt LJ, Kimber C, Trivella M, et al. Preoperative blood transfusions for sickle cell disease. Cochrane Database Syst Rev 2020;7(7):CD003149.

78. Chou ST, Alsawas M, Fasano RM, et al. American Society of Hematology 2020 guidelines for sickle cell disease: transfusion support. Blood Adv 2020;4(2): 327–55.

79. Davis BA, Allard S, Qureshi A, et al. Guidelines on red cell transfusion in sickle cell disease Part II: indications for transfusion. Br J Haematol 2017;176(2): 192–209.

80. Klein AA, Bailey CR, Charlton A, et al. Association of Anaesthetists: anaesthesia and peri-operative care for Jehovah's Witnesses and patients who refuse blood. Anaesthesia 2019;74(1):74–82.

81. DeLoughery TG. Transfusion replacement strategies in Jehovah's Witnesses and others who decline blood products. Clin Adv Hematol Oncol 2020;18(12): 826–36.

82. Guinn NR, Resar LMS, Frank SM. Perioperative management of patients for whom transfusion is not an option. Anesthesiology 2021;134(6):939–48.

83. Abuga KM, Nairz M, MacLennan CA, et al. Severe anaemia, iron deficiency, and susceptibility to invasive bacterial infections. Wellcome Open Res 2023;8:48.

84. Shah AA, Donovan K, Seeley C, et al. Risk of infection associated with administration of intravenous iron: a systematic review and meta-analysis. JAMA Netw Open 2021;4(11):e2133935.
85. Daoud E, Nakhla E, Sharma R. Q: Is iron therapy for anemia harmful in the setting of infection? Cleve Clin J Med 2011;78(3):168–70.
86. Kor DJ, Stubbs JR, Gajic O. Perioperative coagulation management–fresh frozen plasma. Best Pract Res Clin Anaesthesiol 2010;24(1):51–64.
87. Benson MA, Tolich D, Callum JL, et al. Plasma: indications, controversies, and opportunities. Postgrad Med 2024.
88. Callum JDW, Mintz PDE. The use of blood components prior to invasive bedside procedures: a critical appraisal. In: Mintz PD, editor. Transfusion therapy: clinical principles and practice. 3rd edition. Chicago: AABB Press; 2010. p. 1–36.
89. O'Shea RS, Davitkov P, Ko CW, et al. AGA clinical practice guideline on the management of coagulation disorders in patients with cirrhosis. Gastroenterology 2021;161(5):1615–1627 e1.
90. de Franchis R, Bosch J, Garcia-Tsao G, et al. Baveno VII - Renewing consensus in portal hypertension. J Hepatol 2022;76(4):959–74.
91. Patel IJ, Rahim S, Davidson JC, et al. Society of Interventional Radiology Consensus Guidelines for the Periprocedural Management of Thrombotic and Bleeding Risk in Patients Undergoing Percutaneous Image-Guided Interventions-Part II: Recommendations: Endorsed by the Canadian Association for Interventional Radiology and the Cardiovascular and Interventional Radiological Society of Europe. J Vasc Intervent Radiol 2019;30(8):1168–1184 e1.
92. Tripodi A, Chantarangkul V, Primignani M, et al. Thrombin generation in plasma from patients with cirrhosis supplemented with normal plasma: considerations on the efficacy of treatment with fresh-frozen plasma. Intern Emerg Med 2012; 7(2):139–44.
93. Muller MC, Straat M, Meijers JC, et al. Fresh frozen plasma transfusion fails to influence the hemostatic balance in critically ill patients with a coagulopathy. J Thromb Haemostasis 2015;13(6):989–97.
94. Brill JB, Brenner M, Duchesne J, et al. The Role of TEG and ROTEM in damage control resuscitation. Shock 2021;56(1S):52–61.
95. Shenoy A, Louissaint J, Shannon C, et al. Viscoelastic testing prior to non-surgical procedures reduces blood product use without increasing bleeding risk in cirrhosis. Dig Dis Sci 2022;67(11):5290–9.
96. Marwaha N, Sharma RR. Consensus and controversies in platelet transfusion. Transfus Apher Sci 2009;41(2):127–33.
97. Sedhom R, Willett L. Do physicians adhere to platelet transfusion guidelines? Am J Med Qual 2016;31(4):383.
98. Kaufman RM, Djulbegovic B, Gernsheimer T, et al. Platelet transfusion: a clinical practice guideline from the AABB. Ann Intern Med 2015;162(3):205–13.
99. Hess AS, Ramamoorthy J, Hess JR. Perioperative platelet transfusions. Anesthesiology 2021;134(3):471–9.
100. Kacker S, Bloch EM, Ness PM, et al. Financial impact of alternative approaches to reduce bacterial contamination of platelet transfusions. Transfusion 2019; 59(4):1291–9.
101. Thiele T, Greinacher A. Platelet transfusion in perioperative medicine. Semin Thromb Hemost 2020;46(1):50–61.
102. Estcourt LJ, Birchall J, Allard S, et al. Guidelines for the use of platelet transfusions. Br J Haematol 2017;176(3):365–94.

Evaluation and Management of Perioperative Pulmonary Complications

Babar Junaidi, MD[a], Andrew Hawrylak, MD[b], Roop Kaw, MD[c,d,*]

KEYWORDS

- Perioperative • Postoperative pulmonary complications • Non-cardiac surgery
- Postoperative respiratory failure

KEY POINTS

- Pulmonary complications are common after noncardiac surgery especially among elderly patients with chronic cardiopulmonary diseases and can include respiratory failure and death.
- Patients at highest risk for pulmonary complications should be managed with regional/neuraxial anesthesia, protective ventilation, and monitored for reversal of neuromuscular blockade
- Patients with obesity should be screened and appropriately managed for obstructive sleep apnea (OSA) and/or obesity hypoventilation syndrome to avoid postoperative cardiac and pulmonary complications

INTRODUCTION

Pulmonary complications are the most common perioperative complication second to wound infection, occurring in up to 6.8% of patients in the postoperative period.[1,2] While a lot of focus is placed on the evaluation of cardiac risk in the perioperative setting, postoperative pulmonary complications (PPCs) pose an equal risk of morbidity and mortality.[1,3–5] Additionally, they can lead to increased length of stay (LOS), greater likelihood of intensive care unit (ICU) admission, and need for invasive or noninvasive ventilation.[4] Postoperative respiratory failure (PORF) has been reported

Funding source: None.

[a] Division of Hospital Medicine, Department of Medicine, Emory University Hospital, 310 Findley Way, Johns Creek, GA 30097, USA; [b] Baylor Scott & White Health, Baylor College of Medicine, 2401 South 31st Street, MS 01-410, Temple, TX 76052, USA; [c] Department of Hospital Medicine; [d] Outcomes Research Consortium, Department of Anesthesiology, Cleveland Clinic, 9500 Euclid Avenue, Suite M2-113, Cleveland, OH 44195, USA

* Corresponding author. Department of Hospital Medicine, Outcomes Research Consortium, 9500 Euclid Avenue, Suite M2-113, Cleveland, OH 44195.

E-mail address: kawr@ccf.org

Med Clin N Am 108 (2024) 1087–1100

https://doi.org/10.1016/j.mcna.2024.04.003
medical.theclinics.com

to have a 30 day mortality of 10% to 27%.[6–9] Studies have also shown that PPCs are better predictors of long-term mortality than postoperative cardiac events.[4,10]

RISK FACTORS

The risk factors for POCs can broadly be divided into patient-related risk factors and procedure-related risk factors.

Patient-Related Risk Factors

Patient-related risk factors are outlined in **Table 1**.

Procedure-Related Risk Factors

Procedure-related risk factors are of greater significance in the development of PPCs (**Table 2**).[1]

PREOPERATIVE EVALUATION OF RISK
History and Physical Examination

The evaluation of postoperative pulmonary risk starts with a thorough history and physical examination. This should focus on chronic conditions like COPD, asthma, and heart failure with close attention to documenting the severity and frequency of

Table 1
Patient-related risk factors for the postoperative pulmonary complications

Risk Factors[a]	Details
ADL/Functional dependence	The following increase risk of PPCs • Bedbound status • Use of assist devices • Requiring help for activities of daily living (ADLs)
Age	Age >65 y[1,4,5]
Chronic heart failure	Bigger predictor of PPCs than COPD[1]
OSA	
COPD	Sixth leading cause of death in the United States in 2021[11] despite decreasing prevalence[12] PPCs associated with COPD: • Increased length of stay (4 d vs 1 d) • Increased 30 d mortality (6.7% vs 1.4%) • Increased 30 d morbidity (25.8% vs 10.2%) • Pneumonia, respiratory failure • Prolonged ventilator support, increased risk of reintubation[13]
ASA Class	ASA Class 3–5[1,4]
Smoking tobacco products[1]	
Pulmonary Hypertension	
Respiratory Infection within 1 month	
COVID-19	Data from COVIDSurg collaborative reveal that 39.5% patients with COVID-19 7 days before or 30 d after surgery experience PPCs. The risk tends to persist for 7 wk[14] Risk is likely lower in the postvaccine era and with newer variants.[15]

[a] Prioritized by odds ratios.

Table 2
Procedure-related risk factors for postoperative pulmonary complications[1,4,5]

Risk Factors	Details
Site of surgery	In order of highest risk • Aortic[16] • Esophageal, intrathoracic, and upper abdominal[4] • Brain • Lower abdominal • ENT
Prolonged surgery	Duration >2 h (1,3)[1,4]
Emergency surgery[1,4]	
General anesthesia	Higher risk than neuraxial, other regional & local anesthesia[1,4]
Long-acting neuromuscular blockade[17]	Can cause PPCs including aspiration, airway obstruction, hypoxia and inability to extubate

symptoms, the need for rescue medication, recent respiratory infection, and hospitalizations. Social history detailing tobacco use and functional status should also be obtained. On physical examination emphasis should be placed on jugular venous pressure, large V waves, S3/4 gallop, rales or wheeze, hepatomegaly, ascites, and pedal edema. It is important diagnose incident heart failure, right ventricular (RV) dysfunction, and early RV failure during a preoperative examination. Preoperative evaluation (and management) of pulmonary hypertension is outside the scope of this study.

Chest Radiograph

Chest radiograph can be ordered for evaluation of an underlying condition. However, routine preoperative chest radiograph does not add to the preoperative management.

Pulmonary Functions Testing

Pulmonary function testing (PFT) does not need be performed on a routine basis. However, PFTs may be obtained if they aid in the classification and control and management of COPD or asthma. Patient's going for lung resection should have predictive postoperative forced expiratory volume in one second and the diffusing capacity for carbon monoxide calculated. Both values greater than 60% are associated with low risk of anatomic lung resection but any of the values less than 60% need to be complemented by a screening exercise test.[18]

Laboratory Tests

Albumin level of less than 3.5 g/dL and BUN greater than 21 mg/dL are associated with PPCs[1]

QUANTIFICATION OF POSTOPERATIVE PULMONARY RISK

ARISCAT score is a risk prediction model developed to help quantify the risk of PPCs using data from a large, multicenter prospective randomized study carried out in Europe.[5] The risk score designed was based on 7 objective measures outlined in **Table 3**. The ARISCAT index has been further validated by subsequent studies but may be cumbersome for some busy clinicians to use.

Several other risk calculators have been in use to estimate the incidence of PORF. The Gupta calculator,[8] which was created from the multivariate analysis of the

Table 3
ARISCAT index and Periscope score

Patient Health-Related Factors		ARISCAT Score	Periscope Risk Score
Patient related			
Age (years)	51–80	3	
	> 80	16	
Preoperative SpO$_2$	≥96%		
	91%–95%	8	7
	<90%	24	10
Respiratory infection within 1 month of surgery		17	
Preoperative hemoglobin	>10 g/dL	11	
Respiratory symptoms (at least 1)			10
History of chronic heart failure	No		
	NYHA class I		3
	NYHA class ≥II		8
History of Chronic Liver Disease			7
Procedure related			
Emergency Surgery		8	12
Duration of Surgery	≤2		
	2–3 h	16	5
	>3 h	23	10
Surgical Incision	Peripheral		
	Closed intrathoracic/ closed upper abdominal		3
	Open upper abdominal	15	7
	Open intrathoracic	24	12

Risk Stratification	Score	Incidence of PPC	Score	Incidence of PRF
Low	< 26	1.6%–3.4%	< 12	1.1%
Intermediate	26–44	13%–13.3%	12–22	4.6%
High	≥ 45	38%–42.1%	≥ 23	18.8%

Abbreviations: NYHA, New York Heart Association; PPC, postoperative pulmonary complications; PRF, postoperative respiratory failure; SpO$_2$, oxygen saturation.

American College of Surgeons 2007 and the 2008 National Surgical Quality Improvement dataset, estimated PORF at 3.1% with a 25.62% 30 day mortality. The same dataset was also used to create the Gupta calculator for likelihood of developing postoperative pneumonia.[19]

The PERISCOPE group[7] (see **Table 3**) also carried out a large, multicenter, prospective observational trial in Europe that included 5384 participants to develop a score to predict PORF. PORF was defined as the development of hypoxia measured by Pao$_2$ of less than 60 mm Hg or SpO$_2$ of less than 90% while breathing ambient air that required supplemental oxygen therapy or noninvasive or invasive ventilation within 5 days after surgery. The risk predictors identified were low preoperative oxygen saturation, respiratory symptoms a month before surgery, chronic liver disease, chronic heart failure, open intrathoracic or upper abdominal surgery, surgery lasting longer than 2 hours, and emergency surgery. The procedure-related factors seem to dominate the patient-related factors (odds ratio >2.7) and therefore intraoperative variables like tidal volume (V$_T$), intraoperative colloid, packed red blood cell and vasopressor use have been explored in recent literature.[20,21] A more recent predictive model can directly use data from the electronic health record, including intraoperative predictors for early identification of PORF and incorporate into clinical decision support systems.[22]

STRATEGIES TO REDUCE THE RISK OF POSTOPERATIVE PULMONARY COMPLICATIONS

Different measures can be taken in the preoperative, intraoperative, and postoperative periods to mitigate the development of PPCs.

Preoperative Measures

Optimization of chronic lung disease

Patients with COPD should be evaluated for symptoms and severity and classified according to the GOLD classification system. They should be treated accordingly with bronchodilators and glucocorticoids to achieve the best possible symptom control. It is best to delay surgery until appropriate symptom control is achieved in order to reduce to the risk of PPCs. Well-controlled asthma is not a risk factor for PPCs but poorly controlled asthma is, patients should be assessed for severity and treated accordingly prior to elective surgery.[23]

Smoking cessation

Smoking cessation more than 8 weeks prior to elective surgery helps reduce the development of PPCs. Multiple studies reveal that quitting smoking closer than that to the date of surgery is not protective.[24]

Pulmonary pre-habilitation

Use of preoperative inspiratory muscle training and cardiopulmonary physiotherapy 1 to 2 weeks before cardiac and major abdominal surgery has been shown to reduce the risk of PPCs.[25] Boden and colleagues showed number needed to treat (NNT) to be 4.[26]

Triage

Patients deemed high risk for PORF should not be scheduled for ambulatory surgery, irrespective of the choice of anesthesia but particularly if general anesthesia cannot be avoided.

Intraoperative Measures

Protective ventilation

Protective ventilation (recommended V_T <6–8 mL/Kg and high PEEP >6 cmH$_2$O) has been shown to decrease PPCs, death, and LOS (by 2 days) after abdominal surgery.[27] This was further confirmed by a meta-analysis of 34 high-quality studies showing that use of low V_T and moderate-to-high PEEP with or without recruitment maneuvers was associated with a lower incidence of the primary outcome of PPCs, secondary outcome of atelectasis and pneumonia.[28] No difference, however, was reported in acute respiratory distress syndrome or short-term mortality.

Avoidance of long-acting neuromuscular blockade

If neuromuscular blockade has not recovered spontaneously at the end of the surgery, reversal with sugammadex should be preferred over neostigmine at deep, moderate, and shallow depths, to avoid residual blockade.[29]

Use of neuraxial anesthesia

General anesthesia is associated with a higher risk of PPCs.[20,21] Neuraxial anesthesia has been shown to decrease PPCs in patients from a matched NSQIP database[30] and those undergoing lower extremity revascularization, major truncal, and lower limb surgery.[31]

Postoperative Measures

Postoperative triage
High risk patients should be triaged to a longer hold in post anesthesia care unit (PACU) or surgical ICU before they are sent to the floor.

Postoperative respiratory monitoring
While some authorities have advocated for, it remains unclear whether patients should be continuously monitored for postoperative respiratory events on medical–surgical floors after discharge from the PACU. More than 90% of episodes of prolonged oxygen desaturation in surgical patients can be missed[32] and with continuous pulse oximetry the odds of recognizing desaturation ($SpO_2<90$) within 1 hour can be 12 times higher when compared to standard monitoring.[33] However, no difference was reported for ICU transfer, reintubation, noninvasive ventilation, and LOS. Opioid-induced respiratory depression (OIRD) when measured using continuous oximetry and capnography, has been reported to occur in nearly half of the surgical and medical patients on hospital floors. The PRODIGY risk prediction tool identified increasing age, male sex, opioid naïve status, chronic heart failure, and sleep apnea were independently associated with postoperative respiratory depression. This screening tool correctly identified respiratory depression events 74% of the time, and the patients in the highest risk group were greater than 6 times more likely to develop OIRD.[34]

Lung expansion maneuvers
Incentive spirometry and lung expansion maneuvers like intermittent positive pressure breathing and positive airway pressure (PAP) have been shown to reduce the risk of PPCs[1] but this was not confirmed in a Cochrane review[35] probably because of low rate of PPCs in a lower risk patient population. Among patients undergoing abdominal surgery continuous PAP showed definite benefit.[36]

Early mobilization
Patients should be mobilized as soon as possible after surgery and several times a day if their situation allows. This helps with lung expansion.

Pain management
Epidural analgesia and intravenous (IV) patient-controlled analgesia-based opioid analgesia has shown better pulmonary outcomes compared to intermittent IV dosing.[37]

PERIOPERATIVE EVALUATION AND MANAGEMENT OF OBSTRUCTIVE SLEEP APNEA
OSA Increases Risk of Perioperative Complications

Pulmonary complications
Patients with a known diagnosis of OSA have been shown to be at an increased risk of postoperative hypoxemia, pneumonia, acute respiratory distress syndrome, unexpected perioperative intubation or mechanical ventilation, and unexpected ICU admission or readmission.[38,39] This risk seems to be independent of the type of surgery the patients are undergoing.[40,41] The increased risk for unexpected mechanical ventilation or noninvasive ventilation was further increased when OSA was comorbid with COPD or obesity hypoventilation syndrome (OHS).[42,43] Matched cohort studies[39] and meta-analyses[44,45] have demonstrated that the increased risk for postoperative respiratory complications occurs with patients with both known prior diagnosis of OSA and with patients diagnosed by both polysomnography and home apnea testing

immediately prior to surgery. The increased risk of respiratory complications has also been demonstrated in patients who screened positive for OSA of all levels of severity.[46]

Cardiac complications

OSA has also been shown to significantly increase the risk of perioperative cardiac complications after noncardiac surgery, such as new-onset and/or symptomatic atrial fibrillation, myocardial injury, acute congestive heart failure, and even cardiac death, with most cardiac complications associated with either severe or untreated OSA.[39,46] It is worth noting that among those with myocardial injury, only 5.5% met the criteria for myocardial infarction.[46] Although it is a common complication of cardiac surgery, symptomatic atrial fibrillation is significantly more common after cardiac surgery among patients with OSA.[47] These events are predicted by the severity of OSA in an exposure–response relationship.[48]

There is some evidence that OSA is associated with non-cardiopulmonary postoperative complications including delirium, acute kidney injury, and surgical-site infections; however, these findings are inconsistent across the medical literature.[42,46,49]

PREOPERATIVE SCREENING/EVALUATION FOR OSA

OSA is becoming increasingly prevalent, and has been rising since at least 1998.[38,42] Old estimates were that OSA affects 1 in 20 adults, with many of them being unrecognized and undiagnosed.[50] As the population ages but prevalence of obesity and severe obesity remain relatively static, the incidence of OSA is likely to continue to rise.[51,52] More modern estimates, primarily from Europe and North America, suggest that the prevalence of OSA in the general adult population ranges from 9% to 38% with risk factors including age, male sex, and higher body mass index.[53] Furthermore, OSA may be more common in patients with pre-existing COPD, with certain populations having been found to have as high as 65% comorbidity of the two conditions.[54] Just as in the general population, OSA remains mostly undiagnosed in the perioperative environment, therefore all patients at risk for OSA should be identified by screening before surgery.[55] A review of screening tools for surgical patients is provided in **Table 4**.

One of the many screening tools used to identify patients who would benefit from further diagnostic testing for OSA is the STOP-Bang Questionnaire.[56] This tool uses only 8 pieces of data, making it easy to use in the clinical setting, and higher scores are associated with increased rates of confirmed OSA diagnoses in both sleep clinic patients and surgical patients.[57] A later meta-analysis[58] specifically reviewed studies screening surgical patients for OSA, and found that STOP-Bang score of 3 or higher had high sensitivity and negative predictive value, making it a good tool to exclude OSA. Notably, STOP-Bang score was a poor predictor of postoperative cardiac complications and mortality, so its use should be limited to evaluating patients for the risk of OSA.[59]

Despite being able to rule out OSA with reasonable accuracy, STOP-Bang scores of 3 or higher only have 50% specificity for diagnosis of OSA.[58] More specific methods such as preoperative nocturnal pulse oximetry monitoring have been shown to predict postoperative cardiovascular events, and therefore may be useful as a screening tool.[48] Current evidence does not support canceling or delaying elective surgery while awaiting further evaluation for OSA with polysomnography except in patients with resting hypoxia, OHS, or severe pulmonary hypertension.[60] In a severely obese patient with severe OSA, a serum bicarbonate less than 27mEq/L helps to rule out OHS. Arterial blood gas should be obtained preoperatively if serum bicarbonate is greater than

Table 4
Comparison of OSA screening tools in surgical patients

	STOP-Bang Questionnaire (n,177)[116]	Berlin Questionnaire[62] (n,177)	ASA Checklist[62] (n = 177)	P-SAP Score[142] (n = 511)
Sensitivity	83.6 (75.8–89.7)	68.9 (59.8–76.9)	72.1 (63.3–79.9)	93.9 (91.8–96.6)
Specificity	56.3 (42.3–69.6)	56.4 (42.3–69.7)	38.2 (25.4–52.3)	32.3 (23.2–46.7)
PPV[a]	81.0 (73.0–87.4)	77.9 (68.8–85.2)	72.1 (63.3–79.9)	10.0 (9.0–24.0)
NPV[a]	60.7 (46.1–74.1)	44.9 (32.9–57.4)	38.2 (25.4–52.3)	99.0 (98.0–99.0)
LR+	1.9 (1.40–2.61)	1.57 (1.17–2.36)	1.16 (0.94–1.51)	1.38 (1.37–1.39)
LR–	0.29 (0.18–0.46)	0.55 (0.39–0.79)	0.73 (0.47–1.13)	0.18 (0.1 and –0.21)
DOR	6.58 (3.03–14.36)	2.85 (1.48–5.50)	1.59 (0.81–3.13)	7.40 (6.43–8.45)
ROC	0.80	0.69	0.78	0.82

Abbreviations: ASA, American Society of Anesthesiologists; DOR, diagnostic odds ratio; LR+, positive likelihood ratio; LR–, negative likelihood ratio; NPV, negative predictive value; OSA, obstructive sleep apnea; PPV, positive predictive value; ROC, area under receiver operative characteristic curve.
[a] Predictive values are highly dependent on the prevalence of OSA, which was 69% in the evaluation of STOP-Bang, Berlin, and ASA checklist, and 7.1% for the P-SAP score.

From Chung F, Memtsoudis SG, Ramachandran SK, Nagappa M, Opperer M, Cozowicz C, Patrawala S, Lam D, Kumar A, Joshi GP, Fleetham J, Ayas N, Collop N, Doufas AG, Eikermann M, Englesakis M, Gali B, Gay P, Hernandez AV, Kaw R, Kezirian EJ, Malhotra A, Mokhlesi B, Parthasarathy S, Stierer T, Wappler F, Hillman DR, Auckley D. Society of Anesthesia and Sleep Medicine Guidelines on Preoperative Screening and Assessment of Adult Patients With Obstructive Sleep Apnea. Anesth Analg. 2016 Aug;123(2):452-73. https://doi.org/10.1213/ANE.0000000000001416. PMID: 27442772; PMCID: PMC4956681.

27mEq/L.[61] Such evaluations may be routine in patients undergoing bariatric surgery or upper airway surgery.[60]

INTRAOPERATIVE MANAGEMENT OF OSA

There is mixed evidence that regional anesthesia should be preferred over general anesthesia in patients with OSA, with the most meta-analyses and guideline statements recommending regional anesthesia when possible.[62–64] However, patients requiring procedural sedation with propofol, especially deep sedation, are at risk for respiratory compromise and require heightened vigilance.[64] Opioids have respiratory depressant effects and IV benzodiazepines can induce upper airway collapse, and therefore should be used with caution in patients with OSA.[65] Intraoperative tidal volume should be set to 6 to 8 mL/kg based on ideal body weight rather than measured body weight and high levels of PEEP (12 cm H_2O) do not reduce PPCs.[66]

POSTOPERATIVE MANAGEMENT OF OSA

In general, patients who are being treated for OSA prior to elective surgery have better clinical outcomes than those who are undiagnosed or noncompliant with PAP at the time of surgery.[67–70] Therefore, patients should be encouraged to bring their own PAP device and resume PAP at home settings perioperatively. The use of PAP in the perioperative period on previously PAP-naive patients has been shown to reduce the rate of hypoxemia events, apnea–hypopnea index, and the need for reintubation after noncardiac surgery, although the evidence is largely low quality[36,71] and inadequate, patient compliance with PAP therapy in the postoperative period can make these benefits difficult to measure.[72] Among patients undergoing elective noncardiac surgery, consistent PAP adherence has been found to be as low as 50%, despite the noted benefits of patients compliant with PAP treatment.[73] Patients who undergo cardiac surgery also benefit from PAP, as they have been shown to have decreased risk of postoperative atrial fibrillation when patients have been known to be compliant with PAP before surgery.[69] Among patients undergoing bariatric surgery, PAP treatment for 1 h in the postanesthesia care unit also reduced OIRD.[74] The timing of perioperative PAP administration is heterogenous in the medical literature, with many trials evaluating only preoperative or postoperative use but usually not both, which might explain some of the lack of benefit of PAP therapy in some trials and even meta-analyses.[75] Use of PAP therapy in patients previously undiagnosed with suspected OSA lacks evidence from randomized controlled trial (RCTs) and should be considered only on a case-by-case basis, preferably under the guidance of a Sleep Medicine specialist.[55]

SUMMARY

Postoperative pulmonary complications are quite common especially in the elderly after upper abdominal, thoracic, and prolonged surgery. PORF is often underdiagnosed and misattributed as complication of other morbidities but has lately been recognized as a patient safety indicator amenable to prevention in the hospital. Protective ventilation, monitoring for neuromuscular blockade, and postoperative respiratory monitoring are evolving fields of study to make better outcomes possible in future. Patients with obesity need to effectively screened for OSA and evaluated before elective surgery if OHS or pulmonary hypertension is suspected.

DISCLOSURES

R. Kaw serves as consultant for Medtronic.

REFERENCES

1. Smetana GW, Lawrence VA, Cornell JE, et al. Preoperative pulmonary risk stratification for noncardiothoracic surgery: systematic review for the American College of Physicians. Ann Intern Med 2006;144(8):581–95.
2. Khuri SF, Henderson WG, DePalma RG, et al. Determinants of long-term survival after major surgery and the adverse effect of postoperative complications. Ann Surg 2005;242(3):326–41 [discussion 341-3].
3. Miskovic A, Lumb AB. Postoperative pulmonary complications. Br J Anaesth 2017;118(3):317–34.
4. Fernandez-Bustamante A, Frendl G, Sprung J, et al. Postoperative pulmonary complications, early mortality, and hospital stay following noncardiothoracic surgery: a multicenter study by the perioperative research network investigators. JAMA Surg 2017;152(2):157–66.
5. Canet J, Gallart L, Gomar C, et al. Prediction of postoperative pulmonary complications in a population-based surgical cohort. Anesthesiology 2010;113(6):1338–50.
6. Arozullah AM, Daley J, Henderson WG, et al. Multifactorial risk index for predicting postoperative respiratory failure in men after major noncardiac surgery. The National Veterans Administration Surgical Quality Improvement Program. Ann Surg 2000;232(2):242–53.
7. Canet J, Sabate S, Mazo V, et al. Development and validation of a score to predict postoperative respiratory failure in a multicentre European cohort: A prospective, observational study. Eur J Anaesthesiol 2015;32(7):458–70.
8. Gupta H, Gupta PK, Fang X, et al. Development and validation of a risk calculator predicting postoperative respiratory failure. Chest 2011;140(5):1207–15.
9. Johnson RG, Arozullah AM, Neumayer L, et al. Multivariable predictors of postoperative respiratory failure after general and vascular surgery: results from the patient safety in surgery study. J Am Coll Surg 2007;204(6):1188–98.
10. Manku K, Bacchetti P, Leung JM. Prognostic significance of postoperative in-hospital complications in elderly patients. I. Long-term survival. Anesth Analg 2003;96(2):583–9, table of contents.
11. Xu J, Murphy SL, Kochanek KD, et al. Mortality in the United States, 2021. NCHS Data Brief 2022;456:1–8. Available at: https://www.ncbi.nlm.nih.gov/pubmed/36598387.
12. Liu Y, Carlson SA, Watson KB, et al. Trends in the prevalence of chronic obstructive pulmonary disease among adults aged >/=18 years - United States, 2011-2021. MMWR Morb Mortal Wkly Rep 2023;72(46):1250–6.
13. Gupta H, Ramanan B, Gupta PK, et al. Impact of COPD on postoperative outcomes: results from a national database. Chest 2013;143(6):1599–606.
14. Collaborative CO. Outcomes and their state-level variation in patients undergoing surgery with perioperative SARS-CoV-2 Infection in the USA: A Prospective Multicenter Study. Ann Surg 2022;275(2):247–51.
15. McInerney CD, Kotze A, Bacon S, et al. Postoperative mortality and complications in patients with and without pre-operative SARS-CoV-2 infection: a service evaluation of 24 million linked records using OpenSAFELY. Anaesthesia 2023;78(6):692–700.
16. Arozullah AM, Khuri SF, Henderson WG, et al, Participants in the National Veterans Affairs Surgical Quality Improvement P. Development and validation of a multifactorial risk index for predicting postoperative pneumonia after major noncardiac surgery. Ann Intern Med 2001;135(10):847–57.

17. Murphy GS, Szokol JW, Marymont JH, et al. Residual neuromuscular blockade and critical respiratory events in the postanesthesia care unit. Anesth Analg 2008;107(1):130–7.

18. Brunelli A, Kim AW, Berger KI, et al. Physiologic evaluation of the patient with lung cancer being considered for resectional surgery: Diagnosis and management of lung cancer, 3rd ed: American College of Chest Physicians evidence-based clinical practice guidelines. Chest 2013;143(5 Suppl):e166S–90S.

19. Gupta H, Gupta PK, Schuller D, et al. Development and validation of a risk calculator for predicting postoperative pneumonia. Mayo Clin Proc 2013;88(11): 1241–9.

20. Lukannek C, Shaefi S, Platzbecker K, et al. The development and validation of the Score for the Prediction of Postoperative Respiratory Complications (SPORC-2) to predict the requirement for early postoperative tracheal re-intubation: a hospital registry study. Anaesthesia 2019;74(9):1165–74.

21. Neto AS, da Costa LGV, Hemmes SNT, et al. The LAS VEGAS risk score for prediction of postoperative pulmonary complications: An observational study. Eur J Anaesthesiol 2018;35(9):691–701.

22. Stocking JC, Drake C, Aldrich JM, et al. Outcomes and risk factors for delayed-onset postoperative respiratory failure: a multi-center case-control study by the University of California Critical Care Research Collaborative (UC(3)RC). BMC Anesthesiol 2022;22(1):146.

23. Woods BD, Sladen RN. Perioperative considerations for the patient with asthma and bronchospasm. Br J Anaesth 2009;103(Suppl 1):i57–65.

24. Mills E, Eyawo O, Lockhart I, et al. Smoking cessation reduces postoperative complications: a systematic review and meta-analysis. Am J Med 2011;124(2): 144–154 e8.

25. Katsura M, Kuriyama A, Takeshima T, et al. Preoperative inspiratory muscle training for postoperative pulmonary complications in adults undergoing cardiac and major abdominal surgery. Cochrane Database Syst Rev 2015;2015(10): CD010356.

26. Boden I, Skinner EH, Browning L, et al. Preoperative physiotherapy for the prevention of respiratory complications after upper abdominal surgery: pragmatic, double blinded, multicentre randomised controlled trial. BMJ 2018;360:j5916.

27. Futier E, Constantin JM, Paugam-Burtz C, et al. A trial of intraoperative low-tidal-volume ventilation in abdominal surgery. N Engl J Med 2013;369(5):428–37.

28. Deng QW, Tan WC, Zhao BC, et al. Intraoperative ventilation strategies to prevent postoperative pulmonary complications: a network meta-analysis of randomised controlled trials. Br J Anaesth 2020;124(3):324–35.

29. Thilen SR, Weigel WA, Todd MM, et al. American Society of Anesthesiologists Practice Guidelines for Monitoring and Antagonism of Neuromuscular Blockade: A Report by the American Society of Anesthesiologists Task Force on Neuromuscular Blockade. Anesthesiology 2023;138(1):13–41.

30. Saied NN, Helwani MA, Weavind LM, et al. Effect of anaesthesia type on postoperative mortality and morbidities: a matched analysis of the NSQIP database. Br J Anaesth 2017;118(1):105–11.

31. Smith LM, Cozowicz C, Uda Y, et al. Neuraxial and combined neuraxial/general anesthesia compared to general anesthesia for major truncal and lower limb surgery: a systematic review and meta-analysis. Anesth Analg 2017;125(6): 1931–45.

32. Sun Z, Sessler DI, Dalton JE, et al. Postoperative hypoxemia is common and persistent: a prospective blinded observational study. Anesth Analg 2015; 121(3):709–15.

33. Khanna AK, Banga A, Rigdon J, et al. Role of continuous pulse oximetry and capnography monitoring in the prevention of postoperative respiratory failure, postoperative opioid-induced respiratory depression and adverse outcomes on hospital wards: A systematic review and meta-analysis. J Clin Anesth 2024;94: 111374.

34. Khanna AK, Bergese SD, Jungquist CR, et al. Prediction of opioid-induced respiratory depression on inpatient wards using continuous capnography and oximetry: an international prospective, observational trial. Anesth Analg 2020;131(4): 1012–24.

35. do Nascimento Junior P, Módolo NS, Andrade S, et al. Incentive spirometry for prevention of postoperative pulmonary complications in upper abdominal surgery. Cochrane Database Syst Rev 2014;2014(2):Cd006058 (In eng).

36. Ireland CJ, Chapman TM, Mathew SF, et al. Continuous positive airway pressure (CPAP) during the postoperative period for prevention of postoperative morbidity and mortality following major abdominal surgery. Cochrane Database Syst Rev 2014;2014(8):CD008930.

37. Nishimori M, Low JH, Zheng H, et al. Epidural pain relief versus systemic opioid-based pain relief for abdominal aortic surgery. Cochrane Database Syst Rev 2012;(7):CD005059.

38. Memtsoudis S, Liu SS, Ma Y, et al. Perioperative pulmonary outcomes in patients with sleep apnea after noncardiac surgery. Anesth Analg 2011;112(1):113–21.

39. Mutter TC, Chateau D, Moffatt M, et al. A matched cohort study of postoperative outcomes in obstructive sleep apnea: could preoperative diagnosis and treatment prevent complications? Anesthesiology 2014;121(4):707–18.

40. Kaw R, Pasupuleti V, Walker E, et al. Postoperative complications in patients with obstructive sleep apnea. Chest 2012;141(2):436–41.

41. Mokhlesi B, Hovda MD, Vekhter B, et al. Sleep-disordered breathing and postoperative outcomes after elective surgery: analysis of the nationwide inpatient sample. Chest 2013;144(3):903–14.

42. Memtsoudis SG, Stundner O, Rasul R, et al. The impact of sleep apnea on postoperative utilization of resources and adverse outcomes. Anesth Analg 2014; 118(2):407–18.

43. Kaw R, Bhateja P, Paz YMH, et al. Postoperative complications in patients with unrecognized obesity hypoventilation syndrome undergoing elective noncardiac surgery. Chest 2016;149(1):84–91.

44. Pivetta B, Sun Y, Nagappa M, et al. Postoperative outcomes in surgical patients with obstructive sleep apnoea diagnosed by sleep studies: a meta-analysis and trial sequential analysis. Anaesthesia 2022;77(7):818–28.

45. Opperer M, Cozowicz C, Bugada D, et al. Does obstructive sleep apnea influence perioperative outcome? a qualitative systematic review for the society of anesthesia and sleep medicine task force on preoperative preparation of patients with sleep-disordered breathing. Anesth Analg 2016;122(5):1321–34.

46. Chan MTV, Wang CY, Seet E, et al. Association of unrecognized obstructive sleep apnea with postoperative cardiovascular events in patients undergoing major noncardiac surgery. JAMA 2019;321(18):1788–98.

47. Wong JK, Maxwell BG, Kushida CA, et al. Obstructive Sleep Apnea Is an Independent Predictor of Postoperative Atrial Fibrillation in Cardiac Surgery. J Cardiothorac Vasc Anesth 2015;29(5):1140–7.

48. Chung F, Waseem R, Wang CY, et al. Preoperative oximetry-derived hypoxemia predicts postoperative cardiovascular events in surgical patients with unrecognized obstructive sleep apnea. J Clin Anesth 2022;78:110653.

49. Ng KT, Lee ZX, Ang E, et al. Association of obstructive sleep apnea and postoperative cardiac complications: A systematic review and meta-analysis with trial sequential analysis. J Clin Anesth 2020;62:109731.

50. Young T, Peppard PE, Gottlieb DJ. Epidemiology of obstructive sleep apnea: a population health perspective. Am J Respir Crit Care Med 2002;165(9):1217–39.

51. Flegal KM, Carroll MD, Kit BK, et al. Prevalence of obesity and trends in the distribution of body mass index among US adults, 1999-2010. JAMA 2012;307(5):491–7.

52. Fietze I, Laharnar N, Obst A, et al. Prevalence and association analysis of obstructive sleep apnea with gender and age differences - Results of SHIP-Trend. J Sleep Res 2019;28(5):e12770.

53. Senaratna CV, Perret JL, Lodge CJ, et al. Prevalence of obstructive sleep apnea in the general population: A systematic review. Sleep Med Rev 2017;34:70–81.

54. Brennan M, McDonnell MJ, Walsh SM, et al. Review of the prevalence, pathogenesis and management of OSA-COPD overlap. Sleep Breath 2022;26(4):1551–60.

55. Kapur VK, Auckley DH, Chowdhuri S, et al. Clinical practice guideline for diagnostic testing for adult obstructive sleep apnea: an american academy of sleep medicine clinical practice guideline. J Clin Sleep Med 2017;13(3):479–504.

56. Chung F, Abdullah HR, Liao P. STOP-Bang questionnaire: a practical approach to screen for obstructive sleep apnea. Chest 2016;149(3):631–8.

57. Nagappa M, Liao P, Wong J, et al. Validation of the STOP-bang questionnaire as a screening tool for obstructive sleep apnea among different populations: a systematic review and meta-analysis. PLoS One 2015;10(12):e0143697.

58. Hwang M, Nagappa M, Guluzade N, et al. Validation of the STOP-Bang questionnaire as a preoperative screening tool for obstructive sleep apnea: a systematic review and meta-analysis. BMC Anesthesiol 2022;22(1):366.

59. Sankar A, Beattie WS, Tait G, et al. Response to 'OSA: innocent bystander or associate in crime?' (Br J Anaesth 2019; 123: e473-e474). Br J Anaesth 2019; 123(4):e474–5.

60. Chung F, Memtsoudis SG, Ramachandran SK, et al. Society of anesthesia and sleep medicine guidelines on preoperative screening and assessment of adult patients with obstructive sleep apnea. Anesth Analg 2016;123(2):452–73.

61. Kaw R, Wong J, Mokhlesi B. Obesity and obesity hypoventilation, sleep hypoventilation, and postoperative respiratory failure. Anesth Analg 2021;132(5):1265–73.

62. Golaz R, Tangel VE, Lui B, et al. Post-operative outcomes and anesthesia type in total hip arthroplasty in patients with obstructive sleep apnea: A retrospective analysis of the State Inpatient Databases. J Clin Anesth 2021;69:110159.

63. Habchi KM, Tangel VE, Weinberg RY, et al. Postoperative outcomes and anesthesia type in total knee arthroplasty in patients with obstructive sleep apnea. J Comp Eff Res 2022;11(17):1241–51.

64. Memtsoudis SG, Cozowicz C, Nagappa M, et al. Society of anesthesia and sleep medicine guideline on intraoperative management of adult patients with obstructive sleep apnea. Anesth Analg 2018;127(4):967–87.

65. Cozowicz C, Memtsoudis SG. Perioperative management of the patient with obstructive sleep apnea: a narrative review. Anesth Analg 2021;132(5):1231–43.

66. Writing Committee for the PCGotPVNftCTNotESoA, Bluth T, Serpa Neto A, et al. Effect of Intraoperative High Positive End-Expiratory Pressure (PEEP) With

Recruitment Maneuvers vs Low PEEP on Postoperative Pulmonary Complications in Obese Patients: A Randomized Clinical Trial. JAMA 2019;321(23):2292–305.

67. Chung F, Nagappa M, Singh M, et al. CPAP in the perioperative setting: evidence of support. Chest 2016;149(2):586–97.

68. Abdelsattar ZM, Hendren S, Wong SL, et al. The impact of untreated obstructive sleep apnea on cardiopulmonary complications in general and vascular surgery: a cohort study. Sleep 2015;38(8):1205–10.

69. Wong JK, Mariano ER, Doufas AG, et al. Preoperative treatment of obstructive sleep apnea with positive airway pressure is associated with decreased incidence of atrial fibrillation after cardiac surgery. J Cardiothorac Vasc Anesth 2017;31(4):1250–6.

70. Berezin L, Nagappa M, Poorzargar K, et al. The effectiveness of positive airway pressure therapy in reducing postoperative adverse outcomes in surgical patients with obstructive sleep apnea: A systematic review and meta-analysis. J Clin Anesth 2023;84:110993.

71. de Raaff CAL, Gorter-Stam MAW, de Vries N, et al. Perioperative management of obstructive sleep apnea in bariatric surgery: a consensus guideline. Surg Obes Relat Dis 2017;13(7):1095–109.

72. Jonsson Fagerlund M, Franklin KA. Perioperative continuous positive airway pressure therapy: a review with the emphasis on randomized controlled trials and obstructive sleep apnea. Anesth Analg 2021;132(5):1306–13.

73. Suen C, Wong J, Warsame K, et al. Perioperative adherence to continuous positive airway pressure and its effect on postoperative nocturnal hypoxemia in obstructive sleep apnea patients: a prospective cohort study. BMC Anesthesiol 2021;21(1):142.

74. Zaremba S, Shin CH, Hutter MM, et al. Continuous positive airway pressure mitigates opioid-induced worsening of sleep-disordered breathing early after bariatric surgery. Anesthesiology 2016;125(1):92–104.

75. Nagappa M, Mokhlesi B, Wong J, et al. The effects of continuous positive airway pressure on postoperative outcomes in obstructive sleep apnea patients undergoing surgery: a systematic review and Meta-analysis. Anesth Analg 2015; 120(5):1013–23.

The Geriatric Patient
Frailty, Prehabilitation, and Postoperative Delirium

Marcio Rotta Soares, MD[a,1,*],
Elizabeth Mahanna Gabrielli, MD, MSCTI[b,2],
Efrén C. Manjarrez, MD, SFHM[c,1]

KEYWORDS

- Older adult • Frailty • Prehabilitation • Postoperative delirium

KEY POINTS

- The population of people aged 65 and over has grown faster than any other group in the population. According to the US Census Bureau of 2022, 17.3% of the US population is above the age of 65 and this number is projected to reach 20.6% by 2030. By the year 2050 the population is expected to reach 89 million.
- Frailty increases risk of in hospital perioperative, short-term, and long-term mortality. Studies have also shown a direct association with increased postoperative complications, including delirium as well as hospital-based metrics such as increase length of stay and readmissions.
- Patient's needs should direct the required prehabilitation assessments and interventions. The general consensus is that at a minimum the screening should include an assessment on: cognitive, physical, functional, nutritional, emotional, and advanced care planning.
- Postoperative delirium carries significant morbidity and mortality. It is associated with falls, longer intensive care unit and hospital lengths of stay, nosocomial infections, and discharges to higher levels of care.

Historically and for ease of classification, the geriatric patient has received a chronologic definition of a person 65 years and older. As such, according to the US Census Bureau of 2022, 17.3% of the US population is above the age of 65 and this number is projected to reach 20.6% by 2030.[1,2] By the year 2050 this population is expected to

---

[a] University of Miami Miller School of Medicine; [b] Division Neuroanesthesiology, Critical Care Medicine, Neurocritical Care and Geriatric Anesthesiology, University of Miami Miller School of Medicine; [c] Division of Hospital Medicine, University of Miami Miller School of Medicine
[1] Present address: 1120 NW, 14 Street, CRB 1130, Miami, Florida 33136.
[2] Present address: 1611 NW 12th Avenue, Suite C300, Miami, FL 33136.
* Corresponding author. 5600 Maggiore Street, Coral Gables, FL 33146.
E-mail address: Msoares2@med.miami.edu
Twitter: @drefrenm (E.C.M.)

Med Clin N Am 108 (2024) 1101–1117
https://doi.org/10.1016/j.mcna.2024.06.001
medical.theclinics.com
0025-7125/24/© 2024 Elsevier Inc. All rights are reserved, including those for text and data mining, AI training, and similar technologies.

reach 89 million people.[3] As this subset of the population continues to grow, so too will their needs for surgical care. Chronologic age remains an independent risk of postoperative complications and adverse surgical outcomes. This is a reflection not of their chronologic age but of a combination of associated medical, cognitive, functional, and social factors. Physiologic changes which reduce the ability to tolerate the impact of the perioperative and postoperative burden, an increased number of comorbid conditions, and a declining functional and cognitive status are stronger predictors of surgical outcomes than age itself. Therefore, it becomes the role of the clinician to assess and identify those factors and determine their impact on perioperative risk. Best practice guidelines have been created by a collaborative effort between the American College of Surgeons National Surgical Quality Improvement Program and the American Geriatric Society (AGS). These guidelines provide recommendations on optimal perioperative assessment and management of the geriatric patients.[4,5] This goal of this article is to expand on 3 areas of great importance in the perioperative care of the older adult. These include Frailty, the concept of Prehabilitation, and Postoperative Delirium (POD).

FRAILTY

Frailty is a multi-dimensional syndrome that results from increased vulnerability, at any age, to adverse outcomes related to the demand of physiologic, medical, surgical, and psychological stress.[6] Frailty is not the equivalent of chronologic age but rather biological age. Clinicians should consider 4 contributors to frailty: physical performance, cognition, malnutrition, and mental health to interplay with the aging patient's comorbidities leading to increased perioperative vulnerability. There are 2 major conceptual frameworks of frailty: the frailty phenotype related to individual cellular function. This has 5 measures: gait speed, weakness (measured by grip strength), energy level, unintentional weight loss, and falls.[7] The second type is the deficits accumulation variety. This version of frailty relates to biologic, not chronologic, aging related to accumulation of performance deficits across multiple domains along with presence of high-risk comorbidities. In this framework, there are 40 potential deficits.[8]

Many practice guidelines require practitioners to assess frailty preoperatively. However, practice patterns do not routinely result in frailty assessments. There are multiple barriers to frailty assessment. The first is that there is no consensus on which frailty instrument is the best. Many of these instruments can be cumbersome and add to the workflow of the routine preop visit, the instruments needed to perform such measurements are not routinely used in a preop visit, and many preop assessments are now done virtually—not in person.[6,9]

Instruments

To date, there are over 40 instruments used to assess frailty with few head-to-head comparison studies. These instruments typically have an area under the curve between 0.65 and 0.85, depending on outcome measured, suggesting good reliability.[6] Some of the most commonly studied instruments are shown in **Table 1**. Preoperative clinicians should get familiar with one tool that works best for them in their work flow, preferably one that can automate as much information from their electronic medical record. Some of these instruments require extra time. According to the table provided, it is suggested that the Clinical Frailty Scale takes less than 1 minute to administer, whereas the EFS takes 5 minutes, the FI takes 10 minutes, and the FP could take between 5 minutes and 20 minutes.[6] The 5-Factor Modified Frailty Index from the National Surgical Quality Improvement Program has been proven to be accurate and

Table 1
Composition of frailty instruments commonly studied in the perioperative setting

Frailty Index Variable	Fried Phenotype	Clinical Frailty Scale	Edmonton Frail Scale
Anemia Albumin Sodium	Weight loss: >10 lbs unintentionally in the previous y	1. Very fit: People who are robust, very active, and motivated. These people commonly exercise regularly. They are among the fittest of their age	Cognition: Clock draw test
Low body mass index Obstructive sleep apnea Cerebrovascular disease	Grip strength: Lowest 20% (by sex and body mass index)	2. Well: People who have no active disease symptoms but are less fit than category 1. Often, they exercise or are very active occasionally	General health: Number of hospital admissions in the past y
Cancer Diabetes mellitus Cognitive impairment	Exhaustion: Self-report	3. Managing well: People whose medical problems are well controlled, but they are rarely active beyond walking	Functional independence: Number of activities of daily living requiring assistance
Alcohol abuse Falls history Heart failure Insulin use	Slowness: 15-foot walking speed (by sex and height) Low activity: Kilocalories per wk (males <383, females <270)	4. Vulnerable: While not dependent on others for daily help, often symptoms limit activities. A common complaint is being "slowed up," and/or being tired during the d	Social support: Availability of reliable help Medication use: Presence of polypharmacy
Liver disease Coronary artery disease Peptic ulcer disease Peripheral vascular disease Renal disease		5. Mildly frail: These people often have more evident slowing and need help in high order IADLs. Typically, this impairs shopping and walking outside alone, meal preparation, and housework	Medication use: Forgetting to take prescribed medications

(continued on next page)

Table 1
(continued)

Frailty Index Variable	Fried Phenotype	Clinical Frailty Scale	Edmonton Frail Scale
Rheumatic disease Smoker Visual impairment Hearing impairment		6. Moderately frail: People need help with all outside activities and with keeping house. Inside, they often have problems with stairs and need help with bathing and might need minimal help with dressing	Nutrition: Unintentional weight loss Mood: Feelings of sadness or depression
Assistance needed dressing Assistance needed meals Assistance needed shopping Weight loss		7. Severely frail: Completely dependent for all personal care from whatever cause (physical or cognitive). Even so, they seem stable and not at high risk of dying (within ~6 mo)	Continence: Presence of urinary incontinence
Multimorbidity Depression Possibly inappropriate medication Polypharmacy		9. Terminally ill: Approaching the end of life. This category applies to people with a life expectancy <6 mo, who are not evidently frail	Functional performance: Timed up and go test

AD8-Alzheimer's Disease in 8 questions questionnaire[57]; PHQ-2-Patient Health Questionnaire[56]; CAGE[58]. The Frailty Index is calculated as a number from 0 to 1 by dividing the number of deficits present by the number of deficits measured (ie, 30) as recommended by Searle et al.[20] One point is assigned for the presence of each feature of the phenotype, resulting in a score from 0 to 5. Following assessment, an individual is assigned a score on the scale. 0 to 2 points are assigned to each question, creating a score that ranges from 0 to 17.

Abbreviations: CAGE, cut down, annoyed, guilty, eye-opener; IADL, instrumental activities of daily living; PHQ-2, 2 questions personal health questionnaire.

From McIsaac DI, MacDonald DB, Aucoin SD. Frailty for Perioperative Clinicians: A Narrative Review. Anesthesia & Analgesia130(6):1450-1460, June 2020. https://doi.org/10.1213/ANE.0000000000004602.

easy to use. The 5 factors used are: functional status, Diabetes Mellitus, COPD, CHF, and Hypertension on medicines.[10] A tool gaining momentum for its simplicity of use has been proposed by the Geriatric Advisory Panel is the Frail Scale.[11] See **Box 1**. This scale has been proposed for use to identify patients who need a more comprehensive geriatric assessment (CGA) to modify reversible factors.[12,13]

Framework for Practitioners to Assess Frailty

Mc Isaac and colleagues proposed a framework for practitioners to assess frailty moving away from a strictly physical strength and comorbidities framework.[6] In this model, they propose 4 pillars of frailty: physical performance, cognition, malnutrition, and mental health. See **Fig. 1**. These 4 pillars can be assessed by 2 main conceptual frameworks. The frailty phenotype consists of weakness, low energy, slow velocity, weight loss, and falls. The accumulating deficits phenotype consists of comorbidities, depression, nutrition, social stressors, cognitive dysfunction, and physical decline. Each of these 2 main conceptual frameworks has examples of selected risk assessment tools.

In an aging population, frailty worsens perioperative outcomes. See **Table 2**.

Frailty increases risk of in hospital perioperative, short-term, and long-term mortality. There were 4 studies of database reviews resulting in increased risk of in hospital mortality for highest risk frail patients. The adjusted odds ratios (aOR) increased depending on the severity of frailty: 2.27 in lung cancer resection,[14] 7.1 to 10.68,[15] and 6.99 to 9.67[16] in noncardiac surgery after cardiac arrest. There were multiple systematic reviews and meta-analyses showing an increased risk of in hospital and 30-day mortality. One systematic review and meta-analysis of 45 articles showed the highest association with short term mortality was the Clinical Frailty Scale OR = 4.89 followed by the Fried Phenotype OR-3.95.[17] A large systematic review and meta-analysis in the Netherlands of over 1.1 million patients showed frailty had a 30 day mortality relative risk of 3.71 using 12 frailty instruments and a 1 year mortality relative risk of 3.41 in a comparison of 6 instruments.[18] In cancer patients, the data were similar with an aOR 3.02.[14]

Frailty is also associated with postoperative complications, perioperative delirium, and prolonged length of stay (LOS).

Box 1
FRAIL scale

- *Fatigue: Are you fatigued?*
- *Resistance: Cannot walk up 1 flight of stairs?*
- *Aerobic: Cannot walk 1 block?*
- *Illnesses: Do you have more than 5 illnesses?*
- *Loss of weight: Have you lost more than 5% of your weight in the past 6 months?*
- 1 point for each
- ≥ 3 = frailty
- 1 or 2 = prefrail
- 0 = robust

John E. Morley et al., Frailty Consensus: A Call to Action, Journal of the American Medical Directors Association, 14 (6), 2013, 392-397, https://doi.org/10.1016/j.jamda.2013.03.022.

Relationship between recognized contributors to frailty, conceptual frameworks for frailty and assessment tools

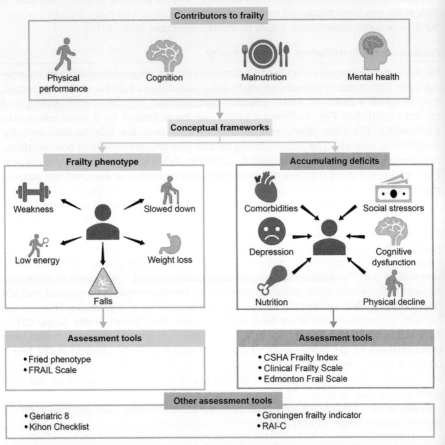

Fig. 1. The relationship between domains contributing to frailty, conceptual frameworks, and commonly used frailty instruments (CSHA, FRAIL, RAI). (Terms of Use: This work is licensed under a Creative Commons Attribution-ShareAlike 4.0 International License. It is attributed to Daniel McIsaac.). CSHA, Canadian study of health and aging; FRAIL, fatigue, resistance, ambulation, illnesses, and loss of weight; RAI, risk analysis index. (*From* McIsaac DI, MacDonald DB, Aucoin SD. Frailty for Perioperative Clinicians: A Narrative Review. Anesthesia & Analgesia130(6):1450-1460, June 2020. https://doi.org/10.1213/ANE.0000000000004602.)

Because patients with frailty have decreased reserve, these patients have an increased risk for postoperative complications. In a same study mentioned above by Tjeertes, frailty was associated with a relative risk of 2.39 for postoperative complications. This study compared 9 different frailty instruments with over 50,000 patients.[18]

3 systematic reviews and meta-analyses found an association between preoperative frailty and POD. In 1 report of 45 studies with multiple instruments and over 42,000 total subjects, the frailty phenotype had the highest association with POD OR-3.79.[17] Another study reported a relative risk of 2.13.[18] With the association of frailty with postoperative complications and delirium, it is no surprise to find frailty

Table 2 Association of frailty and outcomes associated with major noncardiac surgery from selected studies			
Outcome	In Hospital	30 d	1 y
Mortality	•	•	•
Serious Complications	•	•	•
Length of Stay	•		
Readmission		•	
Institutional Discharge	•		
Cost	•		
Postoperative Delirium	•		

associated with a prolonged hospital LOS. In one study of over 70,000 patients, the Hospital Frailty Risk Score predicted prolonged LOS, medium risk patients had an aOR 2.08 and high-risk patients an aOR of 2.59.[16] Another study in cancer surgery patients found frailty associated with a longer LOS by 3 days.[19] The same authors in a meta-analysis of 71 studies showed a prolonged LOS in cancer surgeries of 2.3 days.[20]

As a result of the impact of frailty on the above perioperative outcomes, frail patients are more likely than non-frail patients to experience a non-home hospital discharge. Multiple studies across multiple frailty instruments have shown an association with frailty and institutional discharge in noncardiac surgeries, including cancer (aOR to skilled nursing facility = 2.38)[19] and in another large database 63.5% of high-risk frail patients versus 17.6% low-risk patients went to skilled nursing facility on discharge.[21] A large meta-analysis with OR 1.52 to 6.31 of admission to nursing home. In this study, the Clinical Frailty Scale was the best predictor of institutional discharge.[17]

In summary, frailty is not chronologic age, nor does it encompass one disease state. Frailty is a state of reduced reserve to tolerate surgical stress. Frailty, as measured by multiple instruments, is consistently associated with poor short-term and long-term outcomes, including postoperative mortality. Office based internists and hospitalists would be best to screen all surgical patients for frailty. In frail patients, this information should be used to initiate goals of care conversations, including whether surgery is the right next step outlining the above perioperative outcomes. If so, then guide the preoperative optimization program toward modifiable risk factors per **Fig. 1**. Secondly, practitioners should discuss the likelihood for a potential post discharge stay in a skilled nursing facility or other rehabilitation setting.

PREHABILITATION

The concept of Prehabilitation emerged from protocols known as Enhanced Recovery After Surgery programs. These programs revealed that modifying the physiologic and psychological responses to major surgery can lead to a reduction in complications and earlier return to pre-surgical functional levels. They have further revealed that the patient's baseline health and functional status at the time of surgery are important predictors of postoperative outcomes.[22,23] Prehabilitation focuses on optimizing an individual's functional capacity prior to a surgical procedure. It focuses on patients identified as frail, decreasing the physiologic impact of surgery and consequently reducing the surgical complications and avoiding a prolonged recovery phase. It is estimated that patients can experience up to a 40% reduction in the physiologic and functional capacity after a major surgery.[24] In some instances, perioperative stress can reveal previously unidentified preexisting frail or pre-frail states. Consequently, it is thought that these patients can gain the most benefit from the prehabilitation strategies.

Cardiac and colorectal cancer surgery have been instrumental in the field of prehabilitation. Leaders in these surgical specialties have pioneered the development and implementation of prehabilitation programs. The PREHAB trial concluded that patients who were submitted to a 4-week prehabilitation program prior to elective colorectal cancer surgery had lower rates of severe complications and medical complications. There was no difference in surgical complications. The prehabilitation program resulted in improved functional recovery after surgery.[22,25] A systematic review and meta-analysis that looked at studies measuring the impact of exercise based prehabilitation on patients awaiting cardiac surgery revealed that participation in exercise based prehabilitation programs had positive responses. These studies showed an improvement in postoperative 6-min walking distance, LOS as well as a decreased risk in the development of postoperative atrial fibrillation in younger patients. The importance of the incidence of atrial fibrillation is compacted by its association to an increase in postoperative mortality.[26]

Standardization regarding which domains of care should be the focus of a prehabilitation strategy is still lacking. Even though patient's needs should direct the required interventions, the general consensus is that at a minimum the screening should include an assessment on: cognitive, physical, functional, nutritional, emotional, and advanced care planning. An attempt to create a framework for prehab protocol has been the concept of the NEW approach to Prehabilitation. This 3-way strategy focuses on *Nutritional* optimization, improvement of physical capacity through *Exercise* modalities, and addressing the fear and *Worry* associated to surgery through interventions directed and reducing anxiety.[27] The appropriate duration of prehabilitation interventions poses another challenge. Programs with durations of 4 weeks or less have been shown to be ineffective, whereas programs that exceed 3 months have been associated to poor adherence by patients. It has been proposed that prehab programs with duration of 6 to 8 weeks have the highest probability to deliver expected benefits and maintain patients engaged and adherent to the treatment plan.[22,26,27]

Prehabilitation focuses on a proactive preoperative optimization prior to surgery. General consensus dictates that the more functionally declined the individual, the more they stand to benefit from participation in these programs. Patient's areas of decline should guide the strategic components of the patient's protocol. An assessment of the individuals cognitive, physical, functional, nutritional, emotional, and advanced care planning should be considered the standard. The duration of these programs should be based on time in which a desired improvement can be achieved while still maintaining adherence to the program. Further research is needed to determine which areas should have the major focus as well as all potential benefits associated to these interventions.

POSTOPERATIVE DELIRIUM

Neurocognitive recovery is of major importance to older adults undergoing surgery and procedures. POD is the most common neuropsychological complication after surgery. It along with postoperative cognitive decline comprise the perioperative neurocognitive disorders (NCD).[28] POD is defined as delirium whose onset occurs within 7 days of a procedure, usually after a lucid interval after recovery from anesthesia.

Delirium is an acute onset and often fluctuating presentation of disturbance in attention, awareness, and cognition not explained by dementia or coma with evidence of an underlying disease or process.[29] The incidence of POD varies by surgical type, setting, anesthesia, and patient comorbidities.[30,31] The reported incidence in hip fracture repair surgery averages 33% (range 20%–79%) and hip and knee arthroplasty averages 17% (range 0%–80%) in meta-analyses.[32,33] The reported incidence of POD after open cardiac surgery averages 28% (range 4.1%–54.4%).[34]

Postoperative cognitive dysfunction (POCD), a research diagnosis, has had variable definitions but entails a condition of a decrease in cognitive ability, usually at least 1 standard deviation, compared to controls within 1 year after surgery or anesthesia. In 2018, there was a call to standardize the nomenclature and to align it with the NCDs in the Diagnostic and Statistical Manual 5th Edition (DSM-V).[28] Evered and colleagues suggested a continuum of perioperative NCDs. Delayed neurocognitive recovery may be diagnosed within a week of surgery if delirium is ruled out and continues until 6 weeks. After 6 weeks, the patient should be classified as mild or major NCD (postoperative) with the same DSM-V criteria as other mild and major NCD.[28,29] Incidences of POCD for non-cardiac surgery have been found to be 17% to 26% at 7 days but only 10% to 17% at 3 months.[35,36] Similarly, POCD for cardiac surgery has been found to be 43% at 7 days but only 17% at 3 months.[9] It is because the vast majority of patients do end up recovering their cognitive function that the term delayed neurocognitive function is used for this subacute time after surgery and anesthesia.

The pathophysiology of POD and POCD has not been completely elucidated given the complex interplay and heterogeneity of precipitating factors and subtypes. There are multiple pathophysiological hypotheses that have been presented primarily for POD but also for POCD and likely there is truth behind each of these with complex interactions in the individual patients.[37] Altered oxidative cellular metabolism is hypothesized to play a role and could lead to neurotransmitter alterations and imbalances including acetylcholine deficits and dopamine excess.[38–40] Another hypothesis focuses on the sympathetic stress response system leading to the release proinflammatory cytokine and altered neurotransmitters.[41] Evidence of perioperative neuroinflammation after surgery and anesthesia has been found with numerous studies showing elevated neuroinflammatory markers postoperatively.[42–45] In addition, there is evidence that systemic inflammation is also associated with POD, especially when there is evidence of disruption in the blood brain barrier.[46,47] All of these may lead to disruption of neuronal connectivity manifesting in symptoms of POD and cognitive impairment. Finally, another hypothesis states that POD and POCD may be the first manifestation of dementia or pre-existing neurodegeneration with an accelerated course after the stress response from the surgery.[48–52]

Risk factors for POD, POCD, and postoperative NCD include both nonmodifiable, predisposing factors and modifiable precipitating factors.[37] In 2016, the AGS jointly with the American College of Surgeons published guidelines recommending to screen patients for major predisposing risk factors.[5] These nonmodifiable risk factors include older age (65 years and older), pre-existing cognitive impairment and dementia, vision and hearing impairment, critical illness, and active infection.[5] Age caries a mean difference of 4.94 per year (CI 2.93–6.94) in a recent meta-analysis.[53] Pre-existing dementia increases the risk of delirium by 2 to 3 fold compared to patients without dementia.[46] Critical illness and active infection, often measured with the Charlson Comorbidity Index, has been consistently associated with delirium.[53] Subsequent expert consensus and guidelines by the American Society of Anesthesiology Brain Health Initiative, the American Society for Enhanced Recovery, the Perioperative Quality Initiative, and the

World Society of Emergency Surgery have recommended additionally screening for frailty as a risk factor.[54–56] Frailty in patients undergoing urgent or emergent surgery is a nonmodifiable risk factor. However, in elective surgery, it has the potential to be modifiable and improved through prehabilitation. Preoperative frailty in older, surgical patients carries a 2 to 3-fold increased incidence of POD.[57–59] However, frailty has not been associated with increased POCD.[58,60,61]

Modifiable or precipitating factors have been an important area of inquiry as this is where we can target preventative measures. Possible modifiable precipitators which have been studied include medications, intraoperative anesthetics, the depth of anesthesia, and intraoperative hemodynamics. The AGS publishes the Beers Criteria medications of medications that should generally be avoided in older patients given the risk of adverse effects and complications. Amongst these are benzodiazepines, first-generation antihistamines, anticholinergics.[62] The majority of studies have found that benzodiazepines used for sedation in the intensive care unit significantly increase the risk of delirium.[63] However, recent studies have shown that a preoperative dose of benzodiazepine for anxiolysis prior to surgery was not associated with an increase in POD nor POCD.[64–67] Further large scale, randomized studies are needed to determine if benzodiazepine for perioperative anxiolysis in older patients increases the risk of perioperative cognitive complications.[66,67] Anesthetic type, general anesthesia versus neuraxial anesthesia with sedation, has not been shown to affect the risk of delirium.[68] Increased anesthetic depth has not consistently been shown to increase the risk of delirium, except possibly when the patient enters very deep, burst suppression patterns, which has been associated with increased incidences of POD.[69–71] Intraoperative hemodynamics have been associated with delirium. There is equipoise in the literature on whether intraoperative hypotension increases incidence of POD.[72–76] This may be not only be due to variable definitions of hypotension but that patients with different comorbidities may have variable abilities to autoregulate to maintain cerebral perfusion in the setting of hypotension. One study found that not hypotension but volatile blood pressure was associated with increased delirium.[77] Near infrared spectroscopy cerebral oximetry has been used to trend cerebral perfusion intraoperatively and lower baseline values or intraoperative reductions are associated with increased POD.[78–80]

There are multiple prevention measures that have been studied and few treatment measures. CGA develops a detailed, personalized plan for optimization and mitigation of risk factors for postoperative complications. Expert consensus for geriatric care of surgical patients recommends CGA in patients at risk for POD.[5,54–56] However, equipoise exists in the literature as to whether a CGA reliably reduces older patients' risk of POD.[81] Prior negative studies may have resulted from including robust subjects, who may not have substantial benefit from a CGA. The most robust preventions measures are bundled multidisciplinary care plans. These include the ABCDEF bundle in the intensive care unit (ICU) that incorporates assessment of pain and delirium, daily awakening and breathing trials for ventilated patients, sedation that avoids benzodiazepines and gives preferences to treatment of pain and light sedation, early mobility, and family involvement.[82] Light sedation with dexmedetomidine in the ICU has been shown to reduce delirium in multiple studies, and a meta-analysis odds of having delirium was reduced by over 60% in patients who received dexmedetomidine.[83] The ABCDEF bundle led to both more days alive and free of delirium or coma with partial and total bundle compliance.[82] The Hospital Elder Life Program (HELP) is a multidisciplinary bundle employed in non-Intensive care settings. Similarly, HELP reduced delirium by half in a recent meta-analysis of 14 studies.[84] These multidisciplinary bundles have also been applied as treatment for delirium. While studies on this are lacking as these bundles are started prior to the onset of delirium, it is reasonable to think they may also reduce delirium severity or duration. Antipsychotics historically have been used to treat agitated delirium. High-quality evidence shows that neither haloperidol nor atypical antipsychotics reduce the severity nor length of delirium.[85] The use of antipsychotics should be reserved for when patients need to be sedated as they are a danger to themselves, the staff, or risk interrupting vital medical care. Melatonin or ramelteon may reduce the duration of delirium, but current evidence is limited and high quality studies are needed.[86] Valproic acid has also been used in the treatment of delirium, but current studies are limited to retrospective or cases series and have had variable results.[87,88] Thus, the primary treatment for delirium remains preventative strategies.

POD and cognitive impairment carry significant morbidity and mortality. During the hospital stay POD is associated with falls, longer ICU lengths of stay, longer hospital lengths of stay, nosocomial infections, discharges to higher levels of care than they were preoperatively, and higher mortality.[37,82,84,89] Posthospital, POD has consistently been shown to increase the risk of cognitive impairment, dementia or worsen the trajectory in patients with pre-existing cognitive impairment.[46,90–95] Understanding whether or not POD simply reveals preexisting vulnerable pathophysiology or is a causative precipitant is an area of ongoing investigation as is understanding if delirium prevention strategies can affect term cognitive function. Patients experiencing POD are at risk for subsequent delirium in after any future surgery or hospitalization. Postoperative cognitive impairment has been associated with long-term complications including lower functional status, increased rates of depression, lower overall general health and possible dementia and mortality.[96–101] Patients experiencing any cognitive changes postoperatively should be followed closely after surgery.

The physiologic changes experienced by the aging individual reduce their ability to tolerate the impact of the perioperative and postoperative burden. Increased comorbid conditions, functional decline and cognitive functions become strong predictors of surgical outcomes in the older patient. Frailty conceptualizes this reduced physiologic reserve. Similarly, POD and cognitive impairment lead to poorer surgical outcomes and negative hospital-based metrics. Prehabilitation, a proactive approach to preoperative optimization, may help to mitigate some of these outcomes. Further studies should focus on strategic components of its assessment as well as the duration of this intervention.

CLINICS CARE POINTS

- Frailty is a multi-dimensional syndrome that results from increased vulnerability, at any age, to adverse outcomes related to the demand of physiologic, medical, surgical, and psychological stress.

- It is estimated that patients can experience up to a 40% reduction in physiologic and functional capacity after a major surgery.

- An accepted framework for Prehabilitation has been the concept of NEW. This 3-way strategy focuses on *Nutritional* optimization, improvement of physical capacity through *Exercise* modalities, and addressing the fear and *Worry* associated to surgery through interventions directed and reducing anxiety.

- POD is defined as delirium whose onset occurs within 7 days of a procedure, usually after a lucid interval after recovery from anesthesia. Delirium is an acute onset and often fluctuating presentation of disturbance in attention, awareness, and cognition not explained by dementia or coma with evidence of an underlying disease or process.

DISCLOSURE

The authors have nothing to disclose.

REFERENCES

1. Bureau USC. ACS 1-Year Estimates Subject Tables: Age and Sex. American Community Survey; 2022.
2. Health care visits to doctor offices, emergency departments, and home visits within the past 12 months, by selected characteristics: United States, selected years 1997-2018. Available at: https://www.cdc.gov/nchs/hus/contents2019.htm#Table-030. (Accessed April 4 2024). 2019.
3. Dall TM, Gallo PD, Chakrabarti R, et al. An aging population and growing disease burden will require a large and specialized health care workforce by 2025. Health Aff 2013;32(11):2013-20.
4. Wolfe JD, Wolfe NK, Rich MW. Perioperative care of the geriatric patient for noncardiac surgery. Clin Cardiol 2020;43(2):127-36.
5. Mohanty S, Rosenthal RA, Russell MM, et al. Optimal perioperative management of the geriatric patient: a best practices guideline from the american college of surgeons nsqip and the american geriatrics society. J Am Coll Surg 2016;222(5):930-47.
6. McIsaac DI, MacDonald DB, Aucoin SD. Frailty for perioperative clinicians: a narrative review. Anesth Analg 2020;130(6):1450-60.
7. Fried LP, Tangen CM, Walston J, et al. Frailty in older adults: evidence for a phenotype. J Gerontol A Biol Sci Med Sci 2001;56(3):M146-56.
8. Searle SD, Mitnitski A, Gahbauer EA, et al. A standard procedure for creating a frailty index. BMC Geriatr 2008;8:24.
9. Alkadri J, Hage D, Nickerson LH, et al. A systematic review and meta-analysis of preoperative frailty instruments derived from electronic health data. Anesth Analg 2021;133(5):1094-106.
10. Subramaniam S, Aalberg JJ, Soriano RP, et al. New 5-factor modified frailty index using american college of surgeons NSQIP data. J Am Coll Surg 2018; 226(2):173-181 e178.
11. Abellan van Kan G, Rolland YM, Morley JE, et al. Frailty: toward a clinical definition. J Am Med Dir Assoc 2008;9(2):71-2.
12. Morley JE, Malmstrom TK, Miller DK. A simple frailty questionnaire (FRAIL) predicts outcomes in middle aged African Americans. J Nutr Health Aging 2012; 16(7):601-8.
13. Morley JE, Vellas B, van Kan GA, et al. Frailty consensus: a call to action. J Am Med Dir Assoc 2013;14(6):392-7.
14. Lee ACH, Lee SM, Ferguson MK. Frailty is associated with adverse postoperative outcomes after lung cancer resection. JTO Clin Res Rep 2022;3(11): 100414.
15. Wu KY, Gouda P, Wang X, et al. Association of frailty, age, socioeconomic status, and type of surgery with perioperative outcomes in patients undergoing noncardiac surgery. JAMA Netw Open 2022;5(7):e2224625.
16. Gouda P, Wang X, Youngson E, et al. Beyond the revised cardiac risk index: Validation of the hospital frailty risk score in non-cardiac surgery. PLoS One 2022;17(1):e0262322.
17. Aucoin SD, Hao M, Sohi R, et al. Accuracy and feasibility of clinically applied frailty instruments before surgery: a systematic review and meta-analysis. Anesthesiology 2020;133(1):78-95.

18. Tjeertes EKM, van Fessem JMK, Mattace-Raso FUS, et al. Influence of frailty on outcome in older patients undergoing non-cardiac surgery - a systematic review and meta-analysis. Aging Dis 2020;11(5):1276–90.
19. Shaw JF, Mulpuru S, Kendzerska T, et al. Association between frailty and patient outcomes after cancer surgery: a population-based cohort study. Br J Anaesth 2022;128(3):457–64.
20. Shaw JF, Budiansky D, Sharif F, et al. The association of frailty with outcomes after cancer surgery: a systematic review and metaanalysis. Ann Surg Oncol 2022;29(8):4690–704.
21. Siddiqui E, Banco D, Berger JS, et al. Frailty assessment and perioperative major adverse cardiovascular events after noncardiac surgery. Am J Med 2023; 136(4):372–379 e375.
22. Kow AW. Prehabilitation and its role in geriatric surgery. Ann Acad Med Singap 2019;48(11):386–92.
23. Melnyk M, Casey RG, Black P, et al. Enhanced recovery after surgery (ERAS) protocols: time to change practice? Can Urol Assoc J 2011;5(5):342–8.
24. Christensen T, Kehlet H. Postoperative fatigue. World J Surg 1993;17(2):220–5.
25. Stammers AN, Kehler DS, Afilalo J, et al. Protocol for the PREHAB study-preoperative rehabilitation for reduction of hospitalization after coronary bypass and valvular surgery: a randomised controlled trial. BMJ Open 2015;5(3): e007250.
26. Steinmetz C, Bjarnason-Wehrens B, Walther T, et al. Efficacy of prehabilitation before cardiac surgery: a systematic review and meta-analysis. Am J Phys Med Rehabil 2023;102(4):323–30.
27. Arora RC, Brown CHt, Sanjanwala RM, et al. "NEW" prehabilitation: a 3-way approach to improve postoperative survival and health-related quality of life in cardiac surgery patients. Can J Cardiol 2018;34(7):839–49.
28. Evered L, Silbert B, Knopman DS, et al. Recommendations for the nomenclature of cognitive change associated with anaesthesia and surgery-2018. Anesth Analg 2018;127(5):1189–95.
29. American Psychiatry Association A. Neurocognitive Disoder. Diagnostic and Statistical Manual of Mental Disorder. 5th Edition, Text Revision DSM-V-TR ed. Washington, DC: American Psychiatric Association Publishing; 2022.
30. Berian JR, Zhou L, Russell MM, et al. Postoperative delirium as a target for surgical quality improvement. Ann Surg 2018;268(1):93–9.
31. American Geriatrics Society Expert Panel on Postoperative Delirium in Older A. Postoperative delirium in older adults: best practice statement from the American Geriatrics Society. J Am Coll Surg 2015;220(2):136–148 e131.
32. Smith TO, Cooper A, Peryer G, et al. Factors predicting incidence of postoperative delirium in older people following hip fracture surgery: a systematic review and meta-analysis. Int J Geriatr Psychiatry 2017;32(4):386–96.
33. Scott JE, Mathias JL, Kneebone AC. Incidence of delirium following total joint replacement in older adults: a meta-analysis. Gen Hosp Psychiatry 2015; 37(3):223–9.
34. Chen H, Mo L, Hu H, et al. Risk factors of postoperative delirium after cardiac surgery: a meta-analysis. J Cardiothorac Surg 2021;16(1):113.
35. Moller JT, Cluitmans P, Rasmussen LS, et al. Long-term postoperative cognitive dysfunction in the elderly ISPOCD1 study. ISPOCD investigators. International Study of Post-Operative Cognitive Dysfunction. Lancet 1998;351(9106):857–61.
36. Evered L, Scott DA, Silbert B, et al. Postoperative cognitive dysfunction is independent of type of surgery and anesthetic. Anesth Analg 2011;112(5):1179–85.

37. Mahanna-Gabrielli E, Schenning KJ, Eriksson LI, et al. State of the clinical science of perioperative brain health: report from the American Society of Anesthesiologists Brain Health Initiative Summit 2018. Br J Anaesth 2019;123(4):464–78.

38. Hshieh TT, Fong TG, Marcantonio ER, et al. Cholinergic deficiency hypothesis in delirium: a synthesis of current evidence. J Gerontol A Biol Sci Med Sci 2008; 63(7):764–72.

39. Inouye SK, Westendorp RG, Saczynski JS. Delirium in elderly people. Lancet 2014;383(9920):911–22.

40. Young BK, Camicioli R, Ganzini L. Neuropsychiatric adverse effects of antiparkinsonian drugs. Characteristics, evaluation and treatment. Drugs Aging 1997; 10(5):367–83.

41. van der Mast RC. Pathophysiology of delirium. J Geriatr Psychiatry Neurol 1998; 11(3):138–45 ; discussion 157-138.

42. Hirsch J, Vacas S, Terrando N, et al. Perioperative cerebrospinal fluid and plasma inflammatory markers after orthopedic surgery. J Neuroinflammation 2016;13(1):211.

43. Buvanendran A, Kroin JS, Berger RA, et al. Upregulation of prostaglandin E2 and interleukins in the central nervous system and peripheral tissue during and after surgery in humans. Anesthesiology 2006;104(3):403–10.

44. Berger M, Ponnusamy V, Greene N, et al. The effect of propofol vs. isoflurane anesthesia on postoperative changes in cerebrospinal fluid cytokine levels: results from a randomized trial. Front Immunol 2017;8:1528.

45. Berger M, Murdoch DM, Staats JS, et al. Flow cytometry characterization of cerebrospinal fluid monocytes in patients with postoperative cognitive dysfunction: a pilot study. Anesth Analg 2019;129(5):e150–4.

46. Fong TG, Inouye SK. The inter-relationship between delirium and dementia: the importance of delirium prevention. Nat Rev Neurol 2022;18(10):579–96.

47. Hov KR, Berg JP, Frihagen F, et al. Blood-cerebrospinal fluid barrier integrity in delirium determined by Q-Albumin. Dement Geriatr Cogn Disord 2016;41(3–4): 192–8.

48. Berger M, Nadler JW, Friedman A, et al. The effect of propofol versus isoflurane anesthesia on human cerebrospinal fluid markers of alzheimer's disease: results of a randomized trial. J Alzheimers Dis 2016;52(4):1299–310.

49. Palotas A, Reis HJ, Bogats G, et al. Coronary artery bypass surgery provokes Alzheimer's disease-like changes in the cerebrospinal fluid. J Alzheimers Dis 2010;21(4):1153–64.

50. Reinsfelt B, Westerlind A, Blennow K, et al. Open-heart surgery increases cerebrospinal fluid levels of Alzheimer-associated amyloid beta. Acta Anaesthesiol Scand 2013;57(1):82–8.

51. Evered L, Silbert B, Scott DA, et al. Cerebrospinal fluid biomarker for alzheimer disease predicts postoperative cognitive dysfunction. Anesthesiology 2016; 124(2):353–61.

52. Xie Z, Swain CA, Ward SA, et al. Preoperative cerebrospinal fluid beta-Amyloid/ Tau ratio and postoperative delirium. Ann Clin Transl Neurol 2014;1(5):319–28.

53. Mevorach L, Forookhi A, Farcomeni A, et al. Perioperative risk factors associated with increased incidence of postoperative delirium: systematic review, meta-analysis, and grading of recommendations assessment, development, and evaluation system report of clinical literature. Br J Anaesth 2023;130(2): e254–62.

54. Peden CJ, Miller TR, Deiner SG, et al. Members of the perioperative brain health expert P. improving perioperative brain health: an expert consensus review of key actions for the perioperative care team. Br J Anaesth 2021;126(2):423–32.

55. Hughes CG, Boncyk CS, Culley DJ, et al. American society for enhanced recovery and perioperative quality initiative joint consensus statement on postoperative delirium prevention. Anesth Analg 2020;130(6):1572–90.

56. Tian B, Stahel PF, Picetti E, et al. Assessing and managing frailty in emergency laparotomy: a WSES position paper. World J Emerg Surg 2023;18(1):38.

57. Gracie TJ, Caufield-Noll C, Wang NY, et al. The association of preoperative frailty and postoperative delirium: a meta-analysis. Anesth Analg 2021;133(2):314–23.

58. Mahanna-Gabrielli E, Zhang K, Sieber FE, et al. Frailty is associated with postoperative delirium but not with postoperative cognitive decline in older noncardiac surgery patients. Anesth Analg 2020;130(6):1516–23.

59. Fu D, Tan X, Zhang M, et al. Association between frailty and postoperative delirium: a meta-analysis of cohort study. Aging Clin Exp Res 2022;34(1):25–37.

60. Nomura Y, Nakano M, Bush B, et al. Observational study examining the association of baseline frailty and postcardiac surgery delirium and cognitive change. Anesth Analg 2019;129(2):507–14.

61. Evered LA, Vitug S, Scott DA, et al. Preoperative frailty predicts postoperative neurocognitive disorders after total hip joint replacement surgery. Anesth Analg 2020;131(5):1582–8.

62. By the American Geriatrics Society Beers Criteria Update Expert P. American geriatrics society 2019 updated ags beers criteria(r) for potentially inappropriate medication use in older adults. J Am Geriatr Soc 2019;67(4):674–94.

63. Kok L, Slooter AJ, Hillegers MH, et al. Benzodiazepine use and neuropsychiatric outcomes in the ICU: a systematic review. Crit Care Med 2018;46(10):1673–80.

64. Spence J, Belley-Cote E, Jacobsohn E, et al. Restricted versus liberal intraoperative benzodiazepine use in cardiac anaesthesia for reducing delirium (B-Free Pilot): a pilot, multicentre, randomised, cluster crossover trial. Br J Anaesth 2020;125(1):38–46.

65. Wang ML, Min J, Sands LP, et al. The perioperative medicine research g. midazolam premedication immediately before surgery is not associated with early postoperative delirium. Anesth Analg 2021;133(3):765–71.

66. Mahanna-Gabrielli E, Schenning KJ, Deiner SG, et al. Pro-con debate: judicious benzodiazepine administration for preoperative anxiolysis in older patients. Anesth Analg 2023;137(2):280–8.

67. Heinrich M, Nottbrock A, Borchers F, et al. Preoperative medication use and development of postoperative delirium and cognitive dysfunction. Clin Transl Sci 2021;14(5):1830–40.

68. Neuman MD, Feng R, Carson JL, et al. Spinal anesthesia or general anesthesia for hip surgery in older adults. N Engl J Med 2021;385(22):2025–35.

69. Wildes TS, Mickle AM, Ben Abdallah A, et al. Effect of electroencephalography-guided anesthetic administration on postoperative delirium among older adults undergoing major surgery: the engages randomized clinical trial. JAMA 2019;321(5):473–83.

70. Chan MT, Cheng BC, Lee TM, et al. BIS-guided anesthesia decreases postoperative delirium and cognitive decline. J Neurosurg Anesthesiol 2013;25(1):33–42.

71. Sieber FE, Neufeld KJ, Gottschalk A, et al. Effect of depth of sedation in older patients undergoing hip fracture repair on postoperative delirium: the STRIDE randomized clinical trial. JAMA Surg 2018;153(11):987–95.

72. Wang J, Li Z, Yu Y, et al. Risk factors contributing to postoperative delirium in geriatric patients postorthopedic surgery. Asia Pac Psychiatry 2015;7(4): 375–82.

73. Siepe M, Pfeiffer T, Gieringer A, et al. Increased systemic perfusion pressure during cardiopulmonary bypass is associated with less early postoperative cognitive dysfunction and delirium. Eur J Cardio Thorac Surg 2011;40(1):200–7.

74. Yocum GT, Gaudet JG, Teverbaugh LA, et al. Neurocognitive performance in hypertensive patients after spine surgery. Anesthesiology 2009;110(2):254–61.

75. Williams-Russo P, Sharrock NE, Mattis S, et al. Randomized trial of hypotensive epidural anesthesia in older adults. Anesthesiology 1999;91(4):926–35.

76. Wesselink EM, Kappen TH, van Klei WA, et al. Intraoperative hypotension and delirium after on-pump cardiac surgery. Br J Anaesth 2015;115(3):427–33.

77. Hirsch J, DePalma G, Tsai TT, et al. Impact of intraoperative hypotension and blood pressure fluctuations on early postoperative delirium after non-cardiac surgery. Br J Anaesth 2015;115(3):418–26.

78. Schoen J, Meyerrose J, Paarmann H, et al. Preoperative regional cerebral oxygen saturation is a predictor of postoperative delirium in on-pump cardiac surgery patients: a prospective observational trial. Crit Care 2011;15(5):R218.

79. Wang X, Feng K, Liu H, et al. Regional cerebral oxygen saturation and postoperative delirium in endovascular surgery: a prospective cohort study. Trials 2019;20(1):504.

80. Lei L, Katznelson R, Fedorko L, et al. Cerebral oximetry and postoperative delirium after cardiac surgery: a randomised, controlled trial. Anaesthesia 2017;72(12):1456–66.

81. Saripella A, Wasef S, Nagappa M, et al. Effects of comprehensive geriatric care models on postoperative outcomes in geriatric surgical patients: a systematic review and meta-analysis. BMC Anesthesiol 2021;21(1):127.

82. Barnes-Daly MA, Phillips G, Ely EW. Improving hospital survival and reducing brain dysfunction at seven california community hospitals: implementing PAD guidelines via the ABCDEF bundle in 6,064 patients. Crit Care Med 2017; 45(2):171–8.

83. Ng KT, Shubash CJ, Chong JS. The effect of dexmedetomidine on delirium and agitation in patients in intensive care: systematic review and meta-analysis with trial sequential analysis. Anaesthesia 2019;74(3):380–92.

84. Hshieh TT, Yang T, Gartaganis SL, et al. Hospital elder life program: systematic review and meta-analysis of effectiveness. Am J Geriatr Psychiatry 2018;26(10): 1015–33.

85. Girard TD, Exline MC, Carson SS, et al. Haloperidol and ziprasidone for treatment of delirium in critical illness. N Engl J Med 2018;379(26):2506–16.

86. Beaucage-Charron J, Rinfret J, Coveney R, et al. Melatonin and Ramelteon for the treatment of delirium: a systematic review and meta-analysis. J Psychosom Res 2023;170:111345.

87. Cuartas CF, Davis M. Valproic acid in the management of delirium. Am J Hosp Palliat Care 2022;39(5):562–9.

88. Swayngim R, Preslaski C, Dawson J. Use of valproic acid for the management of delirium and agitation in the intensive care unit. J Pharm Pract 2024;37(1): 118–22.

89. Gleason LJ, Schmitt EM, Kosar CM, et al. Effect of delirium and other major complications on outcomes after elective surgery in older adults. JAMA Surg 2015;150(12):1134–40.
90. Saczynski JS, Marcantonio ER, Quach L, et al. Cognitive trajectories after postoperative delirium. N Engl J Med 2012;367(1):30–9.
91. Brown CHt, Probert J, Healy R, et al. Cognitive decline after delirium in patients undergoing cardiac surgery. Anesthesiology 2018;129(3):406–16.
92. Sauer AC, Veldhuijzen DS, Ottens TH, et al. Association between delirium and cognitive change after cardiac surgery. Br J Anaesth 2017;119(2):308–15.
93. Inouye SK, Marcantonio ER, Kosar CM, et al. The short-term and long-term relationship between delirium and cognitive trajectory in older surgical patients. Alzheimers Dement 2016;12(7):766–75.
94. Vasunilashorn SM, Fong TG, Albuquerque A, et al. Delirium severity postsurgery and its relationship with long-term cognitive decline in a cohort of patients without dementia. J Alzheimers Dis 2018;61(1):347–58.
95. Goldberg TE, Chen C, Wang Y, et al. Association of delirium with long-term cognitive decline: a meta-analysis. JAMA Neurol 2020;77(11):1373–81.
96. Phillips-Bute B, Mathew JP, Blumenthal JA, et al. Association of neurocognitive function and quality of life 1 year after coronary artery bypass graft (CABG) surgery. Psychosom Med 2006;68(3):369–75.
97. Steinmetz J, Christensen KB, Lund T, et al. Long-term consequences of postoperative cognitive dysfunction. Anesthesiology 2009;110(3):548–55.
98. Abildstrom H, Rasmussen LS, Rentowl P, et al. Cognitive dysfunction 1-2 years after non-cardiac surgery in the elderly. ISPOCD group. International Study of Post-Operative Cognitive Dysfunction. Acta Anaesthesiol Scand 2000;44(10):1246–51.
99. Steinmetz J, Siersma V, Kessing LV, et al. Is postoperative cognitive dysfunction a risk factor for dementia? a cohort follow-up study. Br J Anaesth 2013;110(Suppl 1):i92–7.
100. Monk TG, Weldon BC, Garvan CW, et al. Predictors of cognitive dysfunction after major noncardiac surgery. Anesthesiology 2008;108(1):18–30.
101. Evered LA, Silbert BS, Scott DA, et al. Prevalence of dementia 7.5 years after coronary artery bypass graft surgery. Anesthesiology 2016;125(1):62–71.

Perioperative Liver and Kidney Diseases

Jeffrey W. Redinger, MD[a,b,]*, Kay M. Johnson, MD, MPH[a,b],
Barbara A. Slawski, MD, MS[c]

KEYWORDS

- Liver disease • Kidney disease • Postoperative • Acute kidney injury • Cirrhosis
- Perioperative • Perioperative risk • Optimization

KEY POINTS

- Preoperative risk assessment for patients with chronic liver disease should focus on severity of liver disease, including the presence of cirrhosis and portal hypertension that may warrant preoperative optimization.
- The Veterans Outcomes and Costs Associated with Liver Disease-Penn risk score has superior accuracy compared with traditional perioperative risk prediction models in patients with cirrhosis and incorporates type and urgency of surgical procedure.
- Chronic kidney disease is the most potent risk factor for postoperative acute kidney injury (AKI) and a strong predictor of adverse perioperative outcomes including mortality.
- Postoperative AKI can be classified via Kidney Disease Improving Global Outcomes (KDIGO) definitions, and its prevention and management should include implementation of the KDIGO guideline bundle of care.
- Restrictive fluid therapy during and after major elective surgery is associated with a higher rate of postoperative AKI and should be avoided.

INTRODUCTION

Renal and hepatic diseases are challenging to manage perioperatively given the myriad of associated comorbidities in this population. Despite substantial postoperative risk associated with cirrhosis and chronic kidney disease (CKD) and increasing prevalence in surgical populations, perioperative research and clinical care in these important

[a] Division of General Internal Medicine, Department of Medicine, University of Washington School of Medicine, 1959 NE Pacific Street, Seattle, WA 98195, USA; [b] Hospital and Specialty Medicine, VA Puget Sound Healthcare System, 1660 South Columbian Way (S-111-MED), Seattle, WA 98108, USA; [c] Division of General Internal Medicine, Department of Medicine, Medical College of Wisconsin, The Hub for Collaborative Medicine, 8701 Watertown Plank Road, Milwaukee, WI 53226, USA
* Corresponding author. VA Puget Sound Health Care System, 1660 South Columbian Way (S-111-MED), Seattle, WA 98108.
E-mail address: jrednger@uw.edu

Med Clin N Am 108 (2024) 1119–1134
https://doi.org/10.1016/j.mcna.2024.04.001   medical.theclinics.com
0025-7125/24/Published by Elsevier Inc.

fields have traditionally had less focus in comparison with cardiac disease. Optimal perioperative management relies on a thorough understanding of hepatic and renal disease pathophysiology, a targeted preoperative evaluation, accurate estimation of perioperative risk, and facility in managing common postoperative complications.

DISCUSSION: PERIOPERATIVE LIVER DISEASE

Acute hepatitis is considered a contraindication to all but the most urgent surgery[1] based on older studies that observed increased mortality after laparotomy in patients with acute viral or medication-induced hepatitis[2] or acute alcohol-associated hepatitis.[3] Acute liver failure (rapid deterioration of liver function resulting in encephalopathy and impaired synthetic function, where internation normalised ratio [INR] is > 1.5, in patients without known pre-existing liver disease) and acute on chronic liver failure are also contraindications to surgery other than liver transplant.[4,5] Patients with chronic hepatitis comprise of a heterogenous population with a wide range of inflammation and fibrosis because of many potential causes (eg, chronic hepatitis B or C, [metabolic dysfunction-associated steatohepatitis [MASH], formerly known as non-alcoholic steatohepatitis], hemochromatosis and many others)[6] and tolerate surgery well as long as it has not progressed to cirrhosis. Therefore, the authors will focus on recognizing cirrhosis, assessing its severity, perioperative risk stratification, and optimization in non-hepatic and non-cardiac surgery settings.

Cirrhosis is a major risk factor for perioperative morbidity and mortality. The prevalence of cirrhosis in the United States (US) has roughly doubled over the past 2 decades, driven by increased prevalence of hepatitis C-related cirrhosis, alcohol-related liver disease[7], and MASH.[8] Concurrently, the volume of elective surgeries in patients with cirrhosis has risen steadily in recent years, particularly for hernia repairs and total knee and hip replacements.[9]

In patients with cirrhosis, overall perioperative mortality is at least twice that of the general population and correlates with the degree of hepatic dysfunction and portal hypertension.[10–12] Complications include infection, bleeding, liver failure, renal failure, venous thromboembolism, impaired wound healing, and encephalopathy, some of which may present in a delayed fashion, making 30-day or 90-day mortality a more robust research outcome than in-hospital mortality. The mechanisms of increased morbidity and mortality are numerous and relate to the hematologic, immunologic, metabolic, and circulatory consequences of cirrhosis, while the presence of portal hypertension is a significant risk factor because of its potential to precipitate esophageal varices (EV) formation, ascites, or hepatic encephalopathy (HE) and its impact on intraoperative hepatic perfusion.[11,13]

PERIOPERATIVE RISK IN CIRRHOSIS

Perioperative risk in patients with cirrhosis is affected by severity of cirrhosis, type and anatomic site of surgery, and surgical urgency, as well as comorbidities like heart disease or frailty.[10] Perioperative mortality for emergent procedures is 4 to 10 times higher than for elective procedures.[1,11] For instance, among 8193 patients with cirrhosis undergoing abdominal surgery in the Veterans Health Administration, 30-day mortality was almost 6 times higher after emergent than elective surgery.[14] A large retrospective study of cirrhosis patient hospitalizations in the 2005 to 2014 National Inpatient Sample reported consistently higher in-hospital mortality for non-elective versus elective admissions involving hernia repair or major abdominal, cardiovascular, or orthopedic surgery[9]; mortality after non-elective major abdominal surgery exceeded 20%. Surgical complexity and anatomic location also significantly influence postoperative mortality, with the greatest risk associated with open abdominal surgery, followed by cardiothoracic surgery, major orthopedic surgery, vascular surgery, and hernia repair.[10] Hepatic surgeries, such as liver transplantation or hepatic resection, are outside the scope of this article, and generally confer even larger risk than the aforementioned surgical categories.

Severity of cirrhosis is strongly associated with perioperative risk. As hepatocellular synthetic function decreases, impaired protein synthesis (including albumin and complement) leads to malnutrition, relative immune deficiency, and contributes to extracellular fluid accumulation. If cirrhosis has progressed to the point of clinically significant portal hypertension (CSPH), this reduction in portal blood flow predisposes the liver to intraoperative hypoperfusion and hypoxemia.[15] Decompensated cirrhosis, defined by a history of ascites, variceal hemorrhage, or HE, is associated with higher risk of death in all elective inpatient surgical categories compared with compensated cohorts.[9] Surgery-specific factors, including intermittent positive-pressure ventilation, pneumoperitoneum during laparoscopy, and traction on abdominal viscera can further lower hepatic blood flow.[16]

RECOGNIZING CIRRHOSIS AND QUANTIFYING SEVERITY

Chronic liver inflammation of any cause can lead to progressive stages of fibrosis (ie, scarring) defined histologically from F0 (no scarring) then F1, F2, F3 and finally F4 (ie, cirrhosis), where broad fibrous bands and regenerative nodules have formed in response to chronic liver inflammation.[17] Cirrhosis can be further categorized clinically into compensated or decompensated forms (**Fig. 1**). Decompensated cirrhosis is usually easy to recognize but compensated cirrhosis, even in the presence of significant

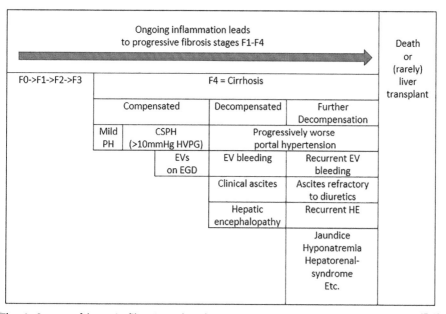

Fig. 1. Stages of hepatic fibrosis and cirrhosis in patients with chronic liver disease.[17–19] CSPH, clinically significant portal hypertension; EGD, esophagogastroduodenoscopy; EV, esophageal varices; F, fibrosis; HE, hepatic encephalopathy; HVPG, hepatic venous pressure gradient; PH, portal hypertension.

portal hypertension, is often missed. Though liver biopsy is considered the gold standard for diagnosis of cirrhosis, a combination of history, physical examination, laboratory and imaging features, and other non-invasive tools are generally used to make the diagnosis. For instance, in patients with risk factors for chronic hepatitis, compensated cirrhosis should be suspected if the platelet count is below normal or imaging suggests a nodular liver, especially, if there are other signs of portal hypertension such as splenomegaly or porto-systemic collateral circulation on cross-sectional imaging. Physical examination findings such as spider angiomas or palmar erythema can also provide clues. Non-invasive tests to estimate level of fibrosis are available including the Non-Alchoholic Fatty Liver Disease Fibrosis Score, the aspartate aminotransferase to platelet ratio, and the Fibrosis-4 (FIB-4) score.[20] The FIB-4 score, which incorporates age, transaminases, and platelet count, is a key element of national metabolic dysfunction-associated steatotic liver disease (MASLD) management guidelines, where a FIB-4 greater than 1.3 warrants further evaluation for presence of cirrhosis, especially if greater than 2.67.[21,22]

Image-based elastography modalities can confirm suspected cirrhosis, taking advantage of the fact that livers become less elastic as fibrosis progresses. Transient elastography (FibroScan) was approved by the US Food and Drug Administration (FDA) for use in diagnosing cirrhosis, with a reported sensitivity of 87% and specificity of 91%.[23] Liver stiffness less than 7 kPa to 8 kPa by transient elastography reliably rules out cirrhosis while values greater than 12 kPa to 15 kPa confirm disease with a few caveats: inflammation and venous congestion can increase liver stiffness, so transient elastography should be deferred in the presence of acute hepatitis, heavy alcohol use, ascites, and heart failure. Magnetic resonance elastography (MRE) quantifies liver stiffness by capturing images while low-frequency vibrations are sent through the liver.[24] MRE measures stiffness of the entire liver and simultaneously estimates hepatic iron levels, but it is less widely available and much more expensive.

PREOPERATIVE EVALUATION OF CIRRHOSIS

An approach to preoperative evaluation of patients with known or suspected liver disease is summarized in **Box 1**. All patients should first be assessed for non-hepatic comorbidities, especially cardiopulmonary disease, as well as frailty.[26] Alcohol use screening is recommended given the high prevalence of alcohol use disorder in patients with liver disease; need to assess risk of postoperative alcohol withdrawal, and importance of letting patients know there is no safe level of alcohol use in the setting of cirrhosis.

Preoperative laboratories should include a complete blood count and serum sodium, creatinine, transaminases, alkaline phosphatase, total bilirubin, albumin, and INR. Transaminases above 3 times the upper limit of normal are not typical of cirrhosis and should prompt a search for an underlying cause of ongoing inflammation, such as alcohol-related hepatitis, drug induced liver injury, or untreated viral hepatitis. If the etiology of cirrhosis is unknown preoperatively, referral to hepatologist or gastroenterologist is warranted if time permits.

Prior imaging and upper endoscopies should be reviewed. The presence of significant portal hypertension is confirmed by endoscopically visualized varices, porto-systemic collateral vessel formation on cross-sectional imaging, or reversed portal vein flow seen on Doppler ultrasound. Portal hypertension is likely when liver stiffness is above 20 kPa to 25 kPa by transient elastography.[19] Before very high-risk procedures, the hepatic venous pressure gradient can be directly measured by experienced interventional radiologists, where values more than 10 mm Hg indicate CSPH.[27]

Box 1
Preoperative considerations in cirrhosis[20,21,25]

Preoperative Evaluation
- Identify comorbidities including frailty or non-hepatic "deal breakers", like unstable or severe cardiac or pulmonary conditions.
- Rule out acute hepatitis (such as alcohol-related hepatitis, drug-induced liver injury, or viral hepatitis) in patients with transaminases greater than 3 times the upper limit of normal. Strongly consider delaying surgery, if present.
- Review evidence for cirrhosis based on history, examination, laboratories including FIB-4, imaging, prior EGD, and so forth.
- Is the cause of cirrhosis known? If not, consider referral to Hepatology before surgery.
- Assess severity of cirrhosis
  - History of decompensation? (Ascites, EV bleeding, or encephalopathy). How well controlled are these currently?
  - On diuretics? Non-selective beta blockers (NSBB)? Lactulose and/or rifaximin?
  - If cirrhosis is still compensated, is there evidence of portal hypertension?
  - Review platelet count and synthetic function (INR, albumin).
  - Determine MELD score and/or Child-Pugh class.
- If EV screening is indicated, is screening up to date?
- Up to date on HCC screening? (The presence and treatment of HCC would take precedence over most elective surgeries)

Risk Prediction
- Use VOCAL-Penn model if abdominal, abdominal wall (hernia), cardiac/pulmonary, vascular, or major orthopedic surgery.
- In general, MELD less than 9 indicates low risk for surgery. If MELD greater than 15 or Child-Pugh C, consider whether liver transplant workup may be indicated before surgery.

Optimization
- Can the cause of cirrhosis be treated relatively quickly (alcohol, HCV treatment)? Treatment may decrease inflammation and portal hypertension. Platelet count can improve with alcohol cessation because alcohol suppresses bone marrow activity.
- If applicable, continue NSBB perioperatively, unless contraindicated by hypotension or bradycardia.
- If EV screening is indicated but past due, is there time to do this before surgery? If no time to do EGD before surgery, consider starting an NSBB or switching a current selective BB (eg, atenolol, metoprolol) to an NSBB, collaborating with Cardiology as needed. Though not studied in perioperative settings, NSBB can reduce portal hypertension and decrease risk of decompensation. Carvedilol is preferred but propranolol or nadolol are also options.
- Avoid routine blood products in an attempt to normalize a high INR, especially fresh frozen plasma, which can lead to volume expansion
- Advise minimizing use of opiates and benzodiazepines, which may worsen or precipitate HE
- Advise avoiding NSAIDs. Acetaminophen is OK up to 2 g/day.
- If the platelet count is unacceptable, consider transfusion or TPO agonist.
- HE secondary prevention: Continue lactulose ± rifaximin, if applicable. Plan how to prevent constipation, recommend documentation of number bowel movements per day. Do not restrict protein intake.
- Volume status: Generally plan to continue diuretics, if applicable. Plan to document daily weights postoperatively.

Abbreviations: EGD, esophagogastroduodenoscopy; EV, esophageal varices; FIB-4, fibrosis-4 score; HCC, hepatocellular carcinoma; HCV, hepatitis C virus; HE, hepatic encephalopathy; INR, prothrombin time-international normalized ratio; MASLD, metabolic dysfunction-associated steatotic liver disease; MELD, model for end-stage liver disease; NSBB, non-specific beta-blocker; TPO, thrombopoeitin.

PREOPERATIVE RISK ESTIMATION IN CHRONIC LIVER DISEASE

Accurate perioperative risk assessment is vital for weighing the risks versus benefits of surgery in a patient with cirrhosis and may facilitate informed consent discussions. Four models are primarily used: the Child-Turcotte-Pugh (CTP) score, the Model for End-stage Liver Disease (MELD) score, the Mayo Risk Score (MRS), and the Veterans Outcomes and Costs Associated with Liver Disease-Penn (VOCAL-Penn) score (**Table 1**).

The CTP score was developed in 1964 and is still used to categorize severity of cirrhosis into Class A, B or C.[28] Though CTP class does correlate with perioperative risk, each of its 3 categories are very broad, encompassing a wide range of risk. The MELD score is also associated with postoperative mortality and in 2007 was incorporated into the MRS along with, age, American Society of Anesthesiologists (ASA) class and etiology of cirrhosis.[12] The predictive accuracy of the MRS has diminished since its development, showing a trend of overestimating postoperative risk in cirrhosis.[10] Like the CTP and MELD scores, the MRS does not include surgery type or urgency, which is a major limitation.

The VOCAL-Penn score was derived in 2020 from a large national cohort of patients within the Veterans Health Administration and incorporates age, ASA score, albumin, total bilirubin, platelet count, body mass index, cirrhosis etiology (MASLD vs other), emergency indication, and 6 anatomic categories of surgery (open and laparoscopic abdominal, abdominal wall, cardiac/thoracic, vascular, and major orthopedic).[10]

Table 1
Perioperative risk scores in cirrhosis

Risk Score	Components	Notes
Child-Turcotte-Pugh (CTP) Score	Albumin Ascites Bilirubin Encephalopathy INR	Originally developed for prognostic evaluation in cirrhosis. Presence of ascites or encephalopathy may be more subjective than laboratory-based models.
Model for End-stage Liver Disease (MELD) score	Bilirubin Creatinine INR	Originally designed to predict survival after transjugular intrahepatic portosystemic shunt (TIPS)
Mayo Risk Score (MRS)	Age ASA class Bilirubin Creatinine INR Etiology of Disease (alcohol, cholestasis, viral, other)	Combines MELD with age, ASA class, and disease etiology
VOCAL-Penn Score	Age Albumin ASA score Bilirubin Body Mass Index>30 (Yes/No) MASLD (Yes/No) Platelet count Surgery Type Surgical Emergency (Yes/No)	Only risk score to incorporate surgical type and urgency

Abbreviations: ASA, American Society of Anesthesiologists; INR, International Normalized Ratio; MASLD, metabolic dysfunction-associated steatotic liver disease.

Areas under the receiver-operator curve for the VOCAL-Penn score were superior to MELD, CTP, and the MRS in predicting postoperative mortality, and the score was subsequently externally validated in non-Veteran populations.[29] Though its surgical categories are still broad, this represents the first risk predictor in cirrhosis that incorporates surgical type and circumstance rather than patient factors alone. The VOCAL-Penn score has become an important tool to prevent overestimation of surgical risk in this population and allow for consideration of surgery in certain patients who would previously be deemed too high risk in older models. Not all types of surgery fall into the 6 VOCAL-Penn surgical categories, and because it is based only on outcomes in patients who were deemed surgical candidates, it may underestimate risk when applied to all patients with cirrhosis who are interested in surgery so clinical judgment is still vital.

COMMON PREOPERATIVE SCENARIOS

The demand for bariatric surgery has escalated because of the obesity epidemic. Because obesity is a major risk factor for MASH-induced fibrosis, patients presenting for bariatric surgery often already have cirrhosis, though not always clinically recognized.[30] In a large US population-based study, mortality risk was somewhat higher after bariatric surgery in compensated cirrhosis (0.9% vs 0.3% in patients without cirrhosis) but vastly higher (16.3%) in those with a history of decompensation.[31] The American Gastroenterological Association (AGA) Clinical Practice Update on Bariatric Surgery in Cirrhosis recommends identification of CSPH via cross-sectional imaging and upper endoscopy before undergoing bariatric surgery.[30] In patients with CSPH, bariatric surgery was not recommended, or should be restricted to centers with a high level of surgical and anesthesia experience with this population.

Umbilical hernias are common among patients with cirrhosis, especially in the setting of ascites. The largest study of umbilical hernia repair in this population found that 30-day postoperative mortality was significantly higher in the emergent (12.2%) versus nonemergent setting (1.2%).[32] To mitigate the possibility of emergent repair, patients with symptomatic umbilical hernia and cirrhosis should at least be considered for elective repair. Episodes of painful incarceration or thin, ulcerated skin at the hernia site warrant urgent surgical referral because they are at high risk for emergency repair in the future. Decision analytic models can help weigh not only risks but also benefits of repair.[33]

PERIOPERATIVE OPTIMIZATION OF CIRRHOSIS

Non-emergent surgery should be delayed until complications of cirrhosis can be optimized (ie, HE, EV bleeding risk, ascites, hepatorenal syndrome, and so forth.). Pausing to treat the underlying etiology of liver disease can sometimes improve portal hypertension and synthetic function. An AGA Clinical Practice Update recommends that bleeding risk from EV be minimized before surgery in patients with cirrhosis[25]; though these guidelines do not provide details, this generally means ensuring screening endoscopy is up-to-date[34] and treatment with a nonselective beta-blocker (ideally carvedilol) or endoscopic variceal ligation in those with medium or large varices. Initiation of nonselective beta-blockade should occur far enough before surgery to ensure tolerability and allow dose titration. Notably, patients with liver stiffness less than 20 kPa on transient elastography and a platelet count greater than 150,000 have a very low probability (<5%) of high-risk varices, so the 2016 American Association for the Study of Liver Disease portal hypertensive bleeding guidelines endorsed deferring esophagogastroduodenoscopy in these patients.[35]

Ascites is particularly important to minimize before non-emergent abdominal or abdominal wall procedures to prevent wound dehiscence. Ascites should be managed by using potassium-sparing and loop diuretics and, if needed, by large-volume paracentesis, while a plan should also be formed to adequately manage ascites postoperatively.

Preoperative transjugular intrahepatic portosystemic shunt (TIPS) to manage refractory ascites or reduce perioperative variceal bleeding risk lacks evidence for routine preoperative use, with a preponderance of observational data, small case studies, and uncontrolled series.[25] A meta-analysis found a possible beneficial effect of preoperative TIPS on incidence of postoperative ascites, but no significant effect on perioperative transfusions, HE, liver failure, or 90-day mortality.[36] When considering preoperative TIPS, a multidisciplinary discussion should occur with an assessment of possible risks, which include deteriorating liver synthetic function, new-onset or worsening HE, and altered cardiopulmonary or renal hemodynamics. TIPS should be avoided with left ventricular ejection fracture less than 50% or grade III diastolic dysfunction.

In patients undergoing treatment for hepatitis C, missed doses increase the likelihood of treatment failure and the development of viral resistance. Elective surgeries should be delayed in favor of completing treatment, since modern hepatitis C regimens now require only 8 weeks to 12 weeks for viral eradication.[25]

High-risk procedures in patients with advanced cirrhosis should ideally be performed in highly experienced surgical centers, and for patients who are potential liver transplantation candidates a preoperative transplantation evaluation should be initiated to determine optimal timing of surgery and to facilitate rescue transplantation in case of postoperative hepatic failure. AGA guidelines recommend preoperative evaluation for liver transplantation for a MELD score more than 15-month or 3-month postoperative mortality risk above 15%.[25]

Impaired protein synthesis in patients with cirrhosis leads to a mixture of procoagulant and anticoagulant effects, so an elevated INR is an unreliable marker of either bleeding risk or protection from venous thromboembolism.[34] This complicates decisions regarding blood product administration. Aggressive transfusion protocols using fresh frozen plasma to target a specific INR are ineffective in reducing perioperative bleeding and can lead to volume expansion and increased portal venous pressure.[37] Commonly used preoperative transfusion thresholds include platelets less than 50,000/μL and low-volume cryoprecipitate for fibrinogen less than 100 mg/dL. Avatrombopag and lusutrombopag are FDA-approved thrombopoietin receptor agonists that stimulate bone marrow production of platelets, though require up to 10 days to increase the platelet count.[38,39] These agents are a reasonable alternative to platelet transfusion in many patients with cirrhosis.

DISCUSSION: PERIOPERATIVE RENAL DISEASE

CKD affects at least 14% of adults in the US and is associated with a myriad of adverse perioperative outcomes, including postoperative AKI.[40] The categorization of CKD severity is common across all etiologies of CKD and based upon a widely accepted set of definitions outlined by the Kidney Disease Improving Global Outcomes (KDIGO) program in 2012[41] (**Table 2**). These definitions assist in the perioperative optimization of CKD by way of viewing disease as an age- and risk-factor related progression, with CKD affecting over 30% of US adults aged above 65. Accordingly, CKD is common in patients undergoing surgery and its identification provides an opportunity to decrease risk of postoperative AKI and improve perioperative outcomes.

Table 2	
Stages of chronic kidney disease	
CKD Stage	**Estimated Glomerular Filtration Rate (mL/min/1.73m2)**
G1	$\geq$90
G2	60–89
G3a	45–59
G3b	30–44
G4	15–29
G5	<15

From Kidney Disease: KDIGO 2012 clinical practice guideline for the evaluation and management of chronic kidney disease. Kidney Inter Suppl. 2013;3(1):1-136.

PERIOPERATIVE OUTCOMES IN CHRONIC KIDNEY DISEASE

CKD is an interconnected risk factor for AKI[42] and is one of the most significant risk factors for postoperative AKI.[43] In a large heterogenous observational cohort study of 3.6 million US Veterans from 2004 to 2011, each increase in estimated glomerular filtration rate (eGFR) by 10 mL/min/1.73 m^2 was associated with a 20% risk reduction for postoperative AKI across all surgery subtypes.[44] Cardiac surgery is a potent risk factor for postoperative AKI compared with noncardiac surgery, with a rate of AKI after cardiac surgery of more than 20% of patients, and up to 40% in some studies depending on the definition of AKI used.[45,46] Nonetheless, the rate of AKI after noncardiac surgery remains significant, with especially high rates after vascular surgery and liver transplantation.[47,48] Though the large evidence base describing postsurgical AKI is predominantly based on retrospective data, CKD is a clear and potent risk factor.

Amongst patients undergoing cardiac surgery, CKD is correlated with postoperative mortality with the most common causes being sepsis and cardiovascular death. A recent retrospective study of more than 1300 patients undergoing coronary artery bypass grafting demonstrating a roughly 40% increased risk of death for every decrease in eGFR by 10 mL/min/1.73 m^2.[49] Similarly, noncardiac surgeries pose an increased risk of morbidity and mortality in the CKD population. In a meta-analysis of 31 cohort studies, patients with CKD were found to have 2- to 5-fold higher risks of postoperative mortality and cardiovascular events compared with patients with normal kidney function. This relationship was found to be graded with an association between severity of preoperative CKD and incidence of postoperative adverse events independent of age.

Patients with end-stage kidney disease (ESKD) on dialysis frequently require disease-related surgeries, including vascular procedures and parathyroidectomy, and warrant particular consideration of perioperative risks. Compared with patients without ESKD, this cohort has a higher likelihood of cardiovascular complications, fluid and electrolyte derangements, bleeding complications, and hemodynamic instability. As a result, these patients have a higher risk of perioperative morbidity and all-cause mortality spanning a wide range of surgery types, with increased rates of postoperative unplanned intubation, ventilator dependence, reoperation, stroke, myocardial infarction, and death within 30 days.[50,51]

PREOPERATIVE EVALUATION OF CHRONIC KIDNEY DISEASE

Given the association of CKD with adverse perioperative outcomes, the identification of CKD is vital preoperatively. As many as 90% of patients with eGFR between

15 mL/min/1.73 m^2 to 59 mL/min/1.73 m^2 are unaware of their kidney disease, perhaps because of the paucity of clinical signs or symptoms until significant disease has developed.[52] As a result, familiarity with CKD risk factors should guide clinicians in determining which patients should have baseline kidney function assessed. Potent risk factors for CKD include age, diabetes, hypertension, cardiovascular disease, current or prior history of malignancy, sickle cell disease or trait, chronic viral infection including HIV and hepatitis C, family history of kidney disease, and chronic use of nephrotoxic medications including nonsteroidal anti-inflammatories (NSAIDs).[53] In at-risk populations, assessment of CKD stage by serum creatinine and urine albumin is warranted.

Several risk prediction tools have been developed to estimate risk for postoperative AKI, with most incorporating preoperative kidney function via either preoperative eGFR or serum creatinine. These tools include, among others the Cleveland Clinic Foundation Risk Score, the Society of Thoracic Surgeons Risk Model, the Simplified Renal Index Score, and the General Surgery AKI Risk Index.[54] In each tool, preexisting CKD is a highly dominant component of risk. Though these models are useful instruments in population analysis, their utility on an individual patient level has been questioned and they are not commonly used in clinical settings.

In patients with established CKD, no formal guidelines exist to guide preoperative evaluation. The authors recommend that the preoperative visit focus on identifying patients at risk for postsurgical AKI, implementing a plan to decrease the probability of AKI, and determining interventions needed when AKI develops. The severity, chronicity, and etiology of kidney disease should be documented, and in patients for whom the cause is unclear or untreated a preoperative nephrologist referral may be considered. Comorbidities that affect the risk of postoperative complications and AKI should be assessed including hypertension, cardiovascular disease, heart failure, diabetes mellitus, chronic pulmonary disease, chronic liver disease, and anemia. Perioperative cardiovascular risk should be estimated and optimized. Pertinent preoperative laboratory indices include blood urea nitrogen, serum creatinine with accompanying estimation of eGFR, serum potassium and sodium, and hemoglobin. Renally metabolized medications and medications that affect renal function should be reviewed and their necessity should be carefully considered, particularly NSAIDs, antibiotics, and medications that act on the renin-angiotensin system. Lastly, vascular access needed for surgical planning should be reviewed, with avoidance of peripherally inserted central catheter (PICC) lines in cephalic, brachial, or basilic veins depending on the future need for dialysis access.

For patients with ESKD on dialysis, the preoperative visit should carefully plan several aspects of perioperative care unique to this population. A recent retrospective cohort study of almost 350,000 Medicare beneficiaries with ESKD undergoing surgery found that longer intervals between hemodialysis and surgery are associated with higher postoperative mortality in a dose-dependent manner.[55] Thus, it is recommended that patients should be dialyzed on the day before surgery. Ideally, ultrafiltration and clearance achieved via hemodialysis should yield euvolemia and electrolyte status that is normal or close to normal. For elective surgeries, consider checking serum potassium on the morning of surgery to determine if presurgical dialysis is indicated. If dialysis is performed on the day of surgery, heparin should be minimized or avoided completely to prevent prolonged anticoagulation which may affect surgery. Clinicians should consult with the patient's nephrology team in order to coordinate timing and parameters of presurgical dialysis. Lastly, PICC lines should be avoided while blood draws and blood pressure measurements should occur in the arm not designated for current or future arteriovenous fistulas.

POSTOPERATIVE ACUTE KIDNEY INJURY

AKI is a heterogenous syndrome characterized by an eGFR decline over hours to days, resulting in retention of metabolic waste products and fluid, electrolyte, and acid-base dysregulation.[56] As in CKD, KDIGO criteria have supplanted older definitions of AKI and include AKI stages 1 to 3 (**Table 3**).[57] Even small decreases in postoperative kidney function have important long-term implications: a 2021 multicenter retrospective cohort study of 6637 patients treated for postoperative AKI within 72 hours of cardiac surgery found that all severities of AKI were associated with increased risk of death, ongoing dialysis requirement, and persistently decreased eGFR 6 months after surgery, while even stage 1 oliguria was associated with persistent renal dysfunction.[58]

Numerous factors before, during, and after surgery contribute to postoperative AKI. Preoperatively, CKD remains a seminal risk factor for both cardiac and noncardiac surgeries, while antecedent volume depletion, exposure to nephrotoxins, and infection can increase AKI risk. Intraoperatively, renal blood flow may be decreased by anesthesia-related symphatholysis and intraoperative hypotension.[59] Catecholamine response to noxious stimuli during surgery constricts renal circulation and stimulates the renin-angiotensin system, further decreasing renal blood flow. Postoperative factors include sepsis, hemodynamic instability, decreased cardiac output, hypovolemia, urinary obstruction, and medications that are nephrotoxic or decrease renal function.

AKI is common after cardiac surgery, with postoperative dialysis required in roughly 2% of patients.[60] Acute tubular necrosis and prerenal azotemia are the most frequent etiologies of AKI, with operative factors including prolonged cardiopulmonary bypass, intra-aortic balloon pump insertion, and redo coronary artery bypass grafting all associated with elevated AKI risk.[45] Postoperative factors after cardiac surgery that can lead to AKI include bleeding, reduced cardiac output, vasodilatory shock, and the use of diuretics or afterload reducing medications. Administration of iodinated contrast, antibiotic-associated acute interstitial nephritis, or atheroembolic disease are alternative causes that are important to consider. "Off pump" cardiac surgery conducted without bypass may possibly reduce AKI rates, though this has not improved dialysis requirements or mortality.[61]

MANAGEMENT OF POSTOPERATIVE ACUTE KIDNEY INJURY

A range of prophylactic and therapeutic pharmacologic therapies has been studied in postoperative AKI, including statins, N-acetylcysteine, and levosimendan, among others.[45] No definitive evidence exists to support pharmacologic therapy to prevent or treat AKI. Alternatively, KDIGO guidelines proposed a bundle of strategies in 2012 for the perioperative prevention and management of AKI (**Box 2**), which largely consists

Table 3
Staging of acute kidney injury

AKI Stage	Serum Creatinine	Urine Output
1	1.5–1.9 times baseline or increase by $\geq$ 0.3 mg/dL	< 0.5 mL/kg/h for 6–12 h
2	2.0–2.9 times baseline	< 0.5 mL/kg/h for 12 or more h
3	3.0 times baseline or increase to $\geq$ 4.0 mg/dL or initiation of renal replacement therapy	Anuria for $\geq$ 12 h or < 0.3 mL/kg/h for $\geq$ 24 h

Adapted from Kidney Disease: Improving Global Outcomes Acute Kidney Injury Work Group. KDIGO clinical practice guideline for acute kidney injury. Kidney Inte Suppl.2012;2:1-138.

Box 2
Perioperative prevention and treatment of acute kidney injury

Perioperative Prevention and Treatment Strategies
    Monitor serum creatinine and urine output to detect and stage kidney injury
    In high-risk patients without hemorrhagic shock, use isotonic crystalloids rather than colloids
    for intravascular volume expansion
    Avoid nephrotoxic agents including radiocontrast, if possible
    Use vasopressors and fluids in high-risk patients with vasomotor shock
    Use perioperative protocol-based management of hemodynamics and oxygenation
    Maintain normoglycemia
    Avoid protein restriction to prevent or delay renal replacement therapy
    Target 20 kcal/kg/day to 30 kcal/kg/day enterally in patients with AKI
    Avoid diuretics except in volume overload

Adapted from Kidney Disease: Improving Global Outcomes Acute Kidney Injury Work Group.
KDIGO clinical practice guideline for acute kidney injury. Kidney Inte Suppl.2012;2:1-138.

---

of key supportive measures like volume management, maintenance of normotension, and avoiding nephrotoxic agents.[57] This bundle is designed to be applied in tandem with a determination of the etiology of disease when possible, for instance urinary tract obstruction or injury requiring intervention. The KDIGO guidelines have been evaluated in several randomized controlled trials and were found to decrease AKI occurrence even in high-risk surgical populations.[62,63]

Perioperative fluid management deserves special mention in prevention and mitigation of postsurgical AKI. Renal perfusion pressure is dependent in part upon adequate intravascular volume, yet volume overload leads to high renal venous pressure, increased renal interstitial edema, and consequent reduced renal blood flow. Both intravascular hypovolemia and fluid overload have been associated with an increased risk of decreased eGFR after surgery.[64] Accordingly, a large body of research has been devoted to determining the appropriate amount of fluid to mitigate the risk of postoperative AKI. The 2018 RELIEF trial was a robust pragmatic international trial that randomized 3000 patients undergoing major abdominal surgery to liberal or restrictive fluid therapy in the first 24 hours during and following surgery.[65] Patients in the liberal arm received a median of 6.1 L of fluid resuscitation with a median of 3.7 L in the restrictive arm. The restrictive arm had a higher rate of AKI (8.6% vs 5.0%, P<.001), need for renal replacement therapy, and surgical site infections, though long-term survival outcomes were similar across both arms. These findings provide evidence that a liberal (albeit modestly so) perioperative fluid repletion strategy is needed in order to maintain adequate renal perfusion, with recent consensus guidelines for AKI from the Acute Disease Quality Initiative recommending not using restrictive or zero-balance perioperative fluid regimens in major elective surgery.[64]

SUMMARY

Chronic liver and renal disease present a perioperative challenge, though risk prediction and methodical preoperative evaluation of cirrhosis and CKD can help to mitigate the risk of mortality and morbidity including postoperative AKI. The use of risk scores in cirrhosis has proven to be valuable in predicting postoperative outcomes, while preoperative renal risks are especially delineated by the presence and stage of CKD. The prevention and mitigation of postoperative AKI is paramount. In all cases, the implementation of guideline-based interventions can improve the postsurgical course of these complex patient populations.

CLINICS CARE POINTS

- Preoperative risk assessment for patients with chronic liver disease should focus on severity of liver disease, including the presence of cirrhosis and portal hypertension that may warrant preoperative optimization.
- The VOCAL-Penn risk score has superior accuracy compared with traditional perioperative risk prediction models in patients with cirrhosis and incorporates type and urgency of surgical procedure.
- CKD is the most potent risk factor for postoperative AKI and a strong predictor of adverse perioperative outcomes including mortality.
- Postoperative AKI can be classified via KDIGO definitions, and its prevention and management should include implementation of the KDIGO guideline bundle of care.
- Restrictive fluid therapy during and after major elective surgery is associated with a higher rate of postoperative AKI and should be avoided.

DISCLOSURES

The authors have nothing to disclose.

REFERENCES

1. Im GY, Lubezky N, Facciuto ME, et al. Surgery in patients with portal hypertension: a preoperative checklist and strategies for attenuating risk. Clin Liver Dis 2014;18(2):477–505.
2. HARVILLE DD, SUMMERSKILL WH. Surgery in acute hepatitis. Causes and effects. JAMA 1963;184:257–61.
3. Greenwood SM, Leffler CT, Minkowitz S. The increased mortality rate of open liver biopsy in alcoholic hepatitis. Surg Gynecol Obstet 1972;134(4):600–4.
4. Stravitz RT, Lee WM. Acute liver failure. Lancet 2019;394(10201):869–81.
5. Karvellas CJ, Bajaj JS, Kamath PS, et al. AASLD Practice guidance on Acute-on-chronic liver failure and the management of critically Ill patients with cirrhosis. Hepatology 2023. https://doi.org/10.1097/HEP.0000000000000671.
6. Rinella ME, Lazarus JV, Ratziu V, et al. A multisociety Delphi consensus statement on new fatty liver disease nomenclature. Hepatology 2023;78(6):1966–86.
7. Scaglione S, Kliethermes S, Cao G, et al. The epidemiology of cirrhosis in the united states: a population-based study. J Clin Gastroenterol 2015;49(8):690–6.
8. Estes C, Razavi H, Loomba R, et al. Modeling the epidemic of nonalcoholic fatty liver disease demonstrates an exponential increase in burden of disease. Hepatology 2018;67(1):123–33.
9. Tessiatore KM, Mahmud N. Trends in surgical volume and in-hospital mortality among United States cirrhosis hospitalizations. Ann Gastroenterol 2021;34(1):85–92.
10. Mahmud N, Fricker Z, Hubbard RA, et al. Risk prediction models for postoperative mortality in patients with cirrhosis. Hepatology 2021;73(1):204–18.
11. Newman KL, Johnson KM, Cornia PB, et al. Perioperative evaluation and management of patients with cirrhosis: risk assessment, surgical outcomes, and future directions. Clin Gastroenterol Hepatol 2020;18(11):2398–414.e3.
12. Teh SH, Nagorney DM, Stevens SR, et al. Risk factors for mortality after surgery in patients with cirrhosis. Gastroenterology 2007;132(4):1261–9.

13. Canillas L, Pelegrina A, Álvarez J, et al. Clinical guideline on perioperative management of patients with advanced chronic liver disease. Life 2023;13(1).

14. Johnson KM, Newman KL, Green PK, et al. Incidence and risk factors of postoperative mortality and morbidity after elective versus emergent abdominal surgery in a national sample of 8193 patients with cirrhosis. Ann Surg 2021;274(4): e345–54.

15. Gholson CF, Provenza JM, Bacon BR. Hepatologic considerations in patients with parenchymal liver disease undergoing surgery. Am J Gastroenterol 1990;85(5): 487–96.

16. Sato K, Kawamura T, Wakusawa R. Hepatic blood flow and function in elderly patients undergoing laparoscopic cholecystectomy. Anesth Analg 2000;90(5): 1198–202.

17. Intraobserver and interobserver variations in liver biopsy interpretation in patients with chronic hepatitis C. The French METAVIR Cooperative Study Group. Hepatology 1994;20(1):15–20.

18. Friedman SL. Mechanisms of hepatic fibrogenesis. Gastroenterology 2008; 134(6):1655–69.

19. Garcia-Tsao G, Abraldes JG, Berzigotti A, et al. Portal hypertensive bleeding in cirrhosis: Risk stratification, diagnosis, and management: 2016 practice guidance by the American Association for the study of liver diseases. Hepatology 2017;65(1):310–35.

20. Smith A, Baumgartner K, Bositis C. Cirrhosis: diagnosis and management. Am Fam Physician 2019;100(12):759–70.

21. Cusi K, Isaacs S, Barb D, et al. American Association of Clinical Endocrinology Clinical Practice Guideline for the Diagnosis and Management of Nonalcoholic Fatty Liver Disease in Primary Care and Endocrinology Clinical Settings: Co-Sponsored by the American Association for the Study of Liver Diseases (AASLD). Endocr Pract 2022;28(5):528–62.

22. Rinella ME, Neuschwander-Tetri BA, Siddiqui MS, et al. AASLD Practice Guidance on the clinical assessment and management of nonalcoholic fatty liver disease. Hepatology 2023;77(5):1797–835.

23. Talwalkar JA, Kurtz DM, Schoenleber SJ, et al. Ultrasound-based transient elastography for the detection of hepatic fibrosis: systematic review and meta-analysis. Clin Gastroenterol Hepatol 2007;5(10):1214–20.

24. Ozturk A, Olson MC, Samir AE, et al. Liver fibrosis assessment: MR and US elastography. Abdom Radiol (NY) 2022;47(9):3037–50.

25. Mahmud N, Kaplan DE, Taddei TH, et al. Frailty is a risk factor for postoperative mortality in patients with cirrhosis undergoing diverse major surgeries. Liver Transplant 2021;27(5):699–710.

26. Pinzani M, Rosselli M, Zuckermann M. Liver cirrhosis. Best Pract Res Clin Gastroenterol 2011;25(2):281–90.

27. Child CG, Turcotte JG. Surgery and portal hypertension. Major Probl Clin Surg 1964;1:1–85.

28. Mahmud N, Fricker Z, Panchal S, et al. External validation of the vocal-penn cirrhosis surgical risk score in 2 large, independent health systems. Liver Transplant 2021;27(7):961–70.

29. Patton H, Heimbach J, McCullough A. AGA clinical practice update on bariatric surgery in cirrhosis: expert review. Clin Gastroenterol Hepatol 2021;19(3):436–45.

30. Mosko JD, Nguyen GC. Increased perioperative mortality following bariatric surgery among patients with cirrhosis. Clin Gastroenterol Hepatol 2011;9(10):897–901.

31. Johnson KM, Newman KL, Berry K, et al. Risk factors for adverse outcomes in emergency versus nonemergency open umbilical hernia repair and opportunities for elective repair in a national cohort of patients with cirrhosis. Surgery 2022; 172(1):184–92.

32. Mahmud N, Goldberg DS, Abu-Gazala S, et al. Modeling optimal clinical thresholds for elective abdominal hernia repair in patients with cirrhosis. JAMA Netw Open 2022;5(9):e2231601.

33. Northup PG, Friedman LS, Kamath PS. AGA clinical practice update on surgical risk assessment and perioperative management in cirrhosis: expert review. Clin Gastroenterol Hepatol 2019;17(4):595–606.

34. Northup PG, Garcia-Pagan JC, Garcia-Tsao G, et al. Vascular liver disorders, portal vein thrombosis, and procedural bleeding in patients with liver disease: 2020 practice guidance by the american association for the study of liver diseases. Hepatology 2021;73(1):366–413.

35. Kaplan DE, Bosch J, Ripoll C, et al. AASLD practice guidance on risk stratification and management of portal hypertension and varices in cirrhosis. Hepatology 2023. https://doi.org/10.1097/HEP.0000000000000647.

36. Manzano-Nunez R, Jimenez-Masip A, Chica-Yanten J, et al. Unlocking the potential of TIPS placement as a bridge to elective and emergency surgery in cirrhotic patients: a meta-analysis and future directions for endovascular resuscitation in acute care surgery. World J Emerg Surg 2023;18(1):30.

37. Weeder PD, Porte RJ, Lisman T. Hemostasis in liver disease: implications of new concepts for perioperative management. Transfusion medicine reviewsJuly 2014;107–13.

38. Terrault N, Chen YC, Izumi N, et al. Avatrombopag before procedures reduces need for platelet transfusion in patients with chronic liver disease and thrombocytopenia. Gastroenterology 2018;155(3):705–18.

39. Tateishi R, Seike M, Kudo M, et al. A randomized controlled trial of lusutrombopag in Japanese patients with chronic liver disease undergoing radiofrequency ablation. J Gastroenterol 2019;54(2):171–81.

40. United Stated Renal Data System 2022 Annual Data Report. Available at: https://usrds-adr.niddk.nih.gov/2022. Accessed February 25, 2024.

41. Kidney Disease. KDIGO 2012 clinical practice guideline for the evaluation and management of chronic kidney disease. Kidney Inter Suppl 2013;3(1):1–136.

42. Chawla LS, Eggers PW, Star RA. Kimmel PL. Acute kidney injury and chronic kidney disease as interconnected syndromes. N Engl J Med 2014;371(1):58–66.

43. Zarbock A, Koyner JL, Hoste EAJ, et al. Update on perioperative acute kidney injury. Anesth Analg 2018;127(5):1236–45.

44. Grams ME, Sang Y, Coresh J, et al. Acute kidney injury after major surgery: a retrospective analysis of veterans health administration data. Am J Kidney Dis 2016;67(6):872–80.

45. Nadim MK, Forni LG, Bihorac A, et al. Cardiac and vascular surgery-associated acute kidney injury: The 20th International Consensus Conference of the ADQI (Acute Disease Quality Initiative) Group. J Am Heart Assoc 2018;7(11).

46. Wang C, Gao Y, Tian Y, et al. Prediction of acute kidney injury after cardiac surgery from preoperative N-terminal pro-B-type natriuretic peptide. Br J Anaesth 2021;127(6):862–70.

47. Hobson C, Lysak N, Huber M, et al. Epidemiology, outcomes, and management of acute kidney injury in the vascular surgery patient. J Vasc Surg 2018;68(3): 916–28.

48. Cabezuelo JB, Ramírez P, Ríos A, et al. Risk factors of acute renal failure after liver transplantation. Kidney Int 2006;69(6):1073–80.
49. Hedley AJ, Roberts MA, Hayward PA, et al. Impact of chronic kidney disease on patient outcome following cardiac surgery. Heart Lung Circ 2010;19(8):453–9.
50. Lin JC, Liang WM. Mortality and complications after hip fracture among elderly patients undergoing hemodialysis. BMC Nephrol 2015;16:100.
51. Gajdos C, Hawn MT, Kile D, et al. Risk of major nonemergent inpatient general surgical procedures in patients on long-term dialysis. JAMA Surg 2013;148(2): 137–43.
52. Tuot DS, Plantinga LC, Hsu CY, et al. Chronic kidney disease awareness among individuals with clinical markers of kidney dysfunction. Clin J Am Soc Nephrol 2011;6(8):1838–44.
53. Shlipak MG, Tummalapalli SL, Boulware LE, et al. The case for early identification and intervention of chronic kidney disease: conclusions from a Kidney Disease: Improving Global Outcomes (KDIGO) Controversies Conference. Kidney Int 2021;99(1):34–47.
54. Huen SC, Parikh CR. Predicting acute kidney injury after cardiac surgery: a systematic review. Ann Thorac Surg 2012;93(1):337–47.
55. Fielding-Singh V, Vanneman MW, Grogan T, et al. Association between preoperative hemodialysis timing and postoperative mortality in patients with end-stage kidney disease. JAMA 2022;328(18):1837–48.
56. Lameire N, Van Biesen W, Vanholder R. Acute renal failure. Lancet 2005 Jan 29-Feb 4 2005;365(9457):417–30.
57. Kidney Disease: Improving Global Outcomes Acute Kidney Injury Work Group. KDIGO clinical practice guideline for acute kidney injury. Kidney Int Suppl 2012;2:1–138.
58. Priyanka P, Zarbock A, Izawa J, et al. The impact of acute kidney injury by serum creatinine or urine output criteria on major adverse kidney events in cardiac surgery patients. J Thorac Cardiovasc Surg 2021;162(1):143–51.e7.
59. Sun LY, Wijeysundera DN, Tait GA, et al. Association of intraoperative hypotension with acute kidney injury after elective noncardiac surgery. Anesthesiology 2015; 123(3):515–23.
60. Hu J, Chen R, Liu S, et al. Global incidence and outcomes of adult patients with acute kidney injury after cardiac surgery: a systematic review and meta-analysis. J Cardiothorac Vasc Anesth 2016;30(1):82–9.
61. Cheungpasitporn W, Thongprayoon C, Kittanamongkolchai W, et al. Comparison of renal outcomes in off-pump versus on-pump coronary artery bypass grafting: A systematic review and meta-analysis of randomized controlled trials. Nephrology 2015;20(10):727–35.
62. Göcze I, Jauch D, Götz M, et al. Biomarker-guided Intervention to Prevent Acute Kidney Injury After Major Surgery: The Prospective Randomized BigpAK Study. Ann Surg 2018;267(6):1013–20.
63. Zarbock A, Küllmar M, Ostermann M, et al. Prevention of Cardiac Surgery-Associated Acute Kidney Injury by Implementing the KDIGO Guidelines in High-Risk Patients Identified by Biomarkers: The PrevAKI-Multicenter Randomized Controlled Trial. Anesth Analg 2021;133(2):292–302.
64. Prowle JR, Forni LG, Bell M, et al. Postoperative acute kidney injury in adult noncardiac surgery: joint consensus report of the Acute Disease Quality Initiative and PeriOperative Quality Initiative. Nat Rev Nephrol 2021;17(9):605–18.
65. Myles PS, Bellomo R, Corcoran T, et al. Restrictive versus Liberal Fluid Therapy for Major Abdominal Surgery. N Engl J Med 2018;378(24):2263–74.

Perioperative Medication Management

Preethi Patel, MD, Christopher Whinney, MD, SFHM*

KEYWORDS

- Perioperative • Medication • Cardiovascular • Anesthesia • Diabetes
- Polypharmacy • Complications

KEY POINTS

- Clinicians should take a complete medication history and reconcile medications preoperatively, including nonprescription medications and herbal regimens.
- Stop medications not essential for short-term quality of life and increase surgical risk, and continue essential medications that are controlling disease states that affect perioperative risk.
- Ensure medications that are stopped due to surgical risk concerns are resumed postoperatively to mitigate decompensation of chronic conditions and improve outcomes.

INTRODUCTION

At least 48.6% of the population of the United States has taken at least 1 prescription medication in the past 30 days and 12.5% of the population takes 5 or more prescriptions.[1] The most prescribed drugs are cardiovascular medications, analgesics, and vitamins. At least 50% of patients going to surgery are on some type of prescription medication.[2] Most of the medications that are taken prior to surgery are unrelated to the surgical procedure; polypharmacy is a predictor for postoperative complications, such as side effects and drug withdrawal.

Unfortunately, little evidence is available to inform decision-making regarding regulation of most classes of medications prior to surgery. It lies to the discretion of the treating physician, surgeon, or the primary care physician to make decisions about holding, continuing, or tapering medications before surgery. This gets more confusing with the advent of medications with unusual dosing regimens such as antidiabetic and antirheumatic medications, especially when determining timing of surgery after the last dose.[3]

GENERAL PRINCIPLES IN PERIOPERATIVE MEDICATION MANAGEMENT

Reliable medication reconciliation is the cornerstone of an effective medication plan in the perioperative period. A thorough medication history should be obtained. Potential

Department of Hospital Medicine, Cleveland Clinic Lerner College of Medicine, Integrated Hospital Care Institute, Cleveland Clinic, 9500 Euclid Avenue, M2 Annex, Cleveland, OH 44195, USA
* Corresponding author.
E-mail address: whinnec@ccf.org

Med Clin N Am 108 (2024) 1135–1153
https://doi.org/10.1016/j.mcna.2024.05.002
medical.theclinics.com
0025-7125/24/© 2024 Elsevier Inc. All rights reserved, including for text and data mining, AI training, and similar technologies.

sources of medication reconciliation include the patient, family members, the dispensing pharmacy, the primary care provider, the patient's dialysis center, the patient's home health nurse or aide, or the patient's postacute care facility in case the patient is unable to do so. Patients should be encouraged to bring their latest medication list or bottles to the preoperative clinic to have the correct information about dosing, scheduling, and compliance. This additional step is especially recommended for patients with memory and compliance issues and who use multiple pharmacies to fill their medications. All prescriptions and non-prescription medications such as over the counter medications, herbal medications, vitamins, and dietary supplements should be recorded. An accurate preoperative medication reconciliation will bestow an added benefit of setting the baseline for patients to resume medications after surgery either in the hospital or after discharge.

It is considered safe to continue medications that do not cause harm through the perioperative period. For example, medication that helps in managing underlying hypertension and hyperlipidemia is safe and should be continued. Medications that have a withdrawal potential when abruptly stopped should be continued or if deemed to be harmful to the patient tapered off. **Table 1** highlights common medication classes that can produce perioperative withdrawal.

Medications that increase perioperative complications such as bleeding, wound healing, postop infection, kidney injury, and hypoglycemia are normally withheld before surgery and resumed once the healing process starts usually within a few hours to a few weeks.

It is imperative to customize the perioperative medication plan to the surgery being performed and the anesthesia plan. For example, if the surgery is a low-risk procedure under local anesthesia, in a bloodless field, medications such as antiplatelet agents and anticoagulants can be safely continued.[4]

If the patient is expected or is at a risk to have a prolonged nothing by mouth status postoperatively, such as some colorectal or gastrointestinal (GI) surgeries, it is necessary to have a plan where in medications with withdrawal potential can be given through an alternative route or exchanged by a therapeutic equivalent that can be administered through a different route.

Critical medications such as antirejection or antiseizure medications in which therapeutic levels dictate the efficacy of the medications should not be stopped in the perioperative period due to the risk of rejection or seizure and should be closely monitored in the postoperative period.

The anesthesia plan and the postop pain management regimens should be formulated to avoid harmful drug interactions with the patient's existing medication regimen.

This review will touch on some of the most common medications encountered in the perioperative setting and examine the evidence behind each recommendation. The authors will defer discussion of endocrine medicines—insulins, non-insulin diabetes agents (except Sodium-glucose cotransporter-2 [SGLT-2] inhibitors), thyroid medications, and glucocorticoids to chapter 13 dedicated to Endocrine Care of the Surgical Patient.

Cardiovascular Medications

These medications are prescribed for hypertension, hyperlipidemia, coronary artery disease, stroke, congestive heart failure (CHF), and arrhythmias. Since these conditions still account for the greatest number of deaths in the United States, they tend to be widely prescribed and encountered, leading to a good body of literature regarding their use in the perioperative period. These medications affect vital

Table 1
Medications concerning for perioperative withdrawal risk

Medication Class	Examples	Symptoms	Management
Beta Blockers	Metoprolol, carvedilol, bisoprolol, atenolol, sotalol, propranolol	Tachycardia, hypertension	Continue orally (PO) dose as tolerated or intravenous (IV) metoprolol or esmolol if nil per os (NPO) status.
Alpha Blockers	Doxazosin, phenoxybenzamine, prazosin, terazosin	Tachycardia, hypertension	Continue PO dose as tolerated; or use IV phenoxybenzamine or clonidine patch.
Statins	Atorvastatin, rosuvastatin, simvastatin	Myocardial infarction or stroke risk with plaque destabilization	Continue if able to tolerate po (no parenteral option).
Steroids	Prednisone, prednisolone, methylprednisolone	Risk for adrenal insufficiency rare, dose and duration dependent; also dependent on presence of primary adrenal insufficiency (AI)vs treatment for non AI-related condition	Continue home daily dose in most cases; stress dose steroids if large surgical stressor.
Antidepressants	Selective serotonin reuptake inhibitors (SSRIs) (paroxetine, sertraline, fluoxetine); serotonin-norepinephrine reuptake inhibitors (SNRIs) (venlafaxine, desvenlafaxine, duloxetine)	Sweating, dizziness, flu-like symptoms, chills, fatigue, tremors, paresthesias	Continue if able to tolerate po (no parenteral option currently available in the United States).
Opioids	Morphine, fentanyl, hydromorphone, oxycodone, hydrocodone	Abdominal cramps, diarrhea, nausea, vomiting, shivering, tachycardia, anxiety, agitation mydriasis, yawning	Continue at least 25% of the home dose, topical fentanyl or parenteral infusions if unable to tolerate PO route.
Benzodiazepines	Alprazolam, lorazepam, clonazepam, diazepam	Sweating, tachycardia, nausea, visual changes, tremor, confusion, restlessness; rarely seizures, psychosis	Continue oral or intravenous dosing at least 25%–50% of dose; taper off preoperatively over 3–6 months if time permits.

parameters such as heart rate, blood pressure, and blood flow; hence, it is essential to examine the impact of these medications on the patient in the preoperative setting, adjust the dosing if necessary, and give time to achieve a steady state preoperatively before the patient is optimized for surgery.

Although the optimal intraoperative blood pressure or heart rates for best surgical outcomes are still up for debate, avoiding extremes is always a wise strategy in the immediate preoperative setting. Several retrospective studies and metanalysis had shown an association between intraoperative hypotension and adverse postoperative events such as acute kidney injury (AKI). Most end-organ damage reported in these studies occurred with mean arterial pressures (MAP) lower than 65 mm Hg and with prolonged exposure.[5,6] However, a recent prospective study examining strategies at mitigating intraoperative hypotension or hypertension by medication adjustment preoperatively has not shown any differences in cardiovascular outcomes in patients whose intraoperative MAP were controlled between 60 and 79 mm Hg versus 80 mm Hg and above (**Table 2**).[7]

Beta blockers

Beta blocking medications are commonly used for many cardiovascular conditions. They have a class 1 recommendation from the American College of Cardiology (ACC)/American Heart Association (AHA) for compensated heart failure, angina,

Table 2
Consensus recommendations for the preoperative management of cardiac medications

Medication Class	Hold/Continue on Day of Surgery	Additional Considerations
Alpha- Adrenoceptor blockers	Continue	Ensure adequate hydration due to risk of hypotension with prolonged fasting.
Angiotensin-converting enzyme inhibitors	Continue	Consider holding if concern for intraoperative hypotension or acute kidney injury.
Angiotensin II receptor blockers	Continue	Consider holding if concern for intraoperative hypotension or acute kidney injury.
Angiotensin receptor blocker-neprilysin inhibitors	Hold	Consider cardiology input if given for severe congestive heart failure with reduced ejection fraction.
Beta-adrenoceptor inhibitors	Continue	Risk of withdrawal if held.
Calcium-channel blockers	Continue	
Centrally acting sympatholytic medications	Continue	Risk of rebound hypertension if held.
Direct-acting vasodilators	Continue	
Loop diuretics	Hold	May continue with low-risk procedures under local anesthesia or sedation or at risk for volume overload.
Thiazide diuretics	Continue	
Potassium-sparing diuretics	Continue or hold	Based on fluid status assessement.
Digoxin	Continue	Check levels once in the postop period.
SGLT-2 inhibitors	Hold for 3 d	Check metabolites in the postop period.

Sunil K. Sahai et al., Preoperative Management of Cardiovascular Medications: A Society for Perioperative Assessment and Quality Improvement (SPAQI) Consensus Statement, Mayo Clinic Proceedings, 97 (9), 2022, 1734-1751, https://doi.org/10.1016/j.mayocp.2022.03.039.

coronary artery disease, hypertension, and some arrythmias. They also have Food and Drug Administration (FDA) approval for migraine prophylaxis, hyperthyroidism, portal hypertension, essential tremor, and other conditions.

This class of medication has been extensively studied in the preoperative period due to their ability to modify the chronotropic and inotropic effects of catecholamines on the beta receptors leading to improvement in the supply demand balance of cardiac perfusion.[8]

It has been shown that initiating a betablocker before surgery on high-risk patients has a beneficial effect on postop cardiac complications such as myocardial infarction and ischemia.[9,10] However, a randomized controlled trial (RCT) published in 2008 showed that the benefits achieved by beta blocker initiation were offset by increased risk of hypotension, bradycardia, stroke, and death.[11] A systematic review undertaken for the ACC/AHA guidelines for preoperative betablocker also came to a similar conclusion. There are not enough data currently to recommend initiation of beta blockers to reduce postop cardiac complications in all patients. In patients who have an indication for use of a beta blocker, starting this medication prior to surgery should be accompanied by close monitoring of their heart rate, blood pressure, and general tolerance.[12,13]

The timing of initiation of betablocker before surgery for other indications is not clear yet but in patients who were started on a betablocker 60 days prior to surgery seemed to have similar risk of stroke than the betablocker-naive patients.[14] There is currently no consensus about a preoperative safe period to start betablockers. However, if a betablocker is started for indications mentioned earlier, the authors recommend initiating at least 7 days prior to surgery to assess for tolerance and steady state.

In patients already on betablockers, there is evidence that stopping it before surgery may lead to withdrawal symptoms of angina or congestive heart failure (CHF) exacerbation[15] Hence, in patients taking betablockers, it is recommended to continue them throughout the perioperative period. Heart rate and blood pressure monitoring in the intraoperative and postoperative period is recommended; however, incidence of intraoperative hypotension seems to be low in patients on chronic betablocker therapy.[16]

Alpha-adrenergic blockers

Alpha blockers are medications that are prescribed for benign prostatic hypertrophy (BPH), essential hypertension, and pheochromocytoma. They act by blocking the effect of sympathomimetics and catecholamines on postsynaptic alpha receptors on vascular smooth muscle cells leading to vasodilation and hypotension.

There are 3 types of alpha blockers in the market currently. The non-selective alpha blockers such as phenoxybenzamine and phentolamine are FDA approved for management of pheochromocytoma in the preoperative and intraoperative period to prevent hypertensive crises.[17] The selective alpha 1 blockers are FDA approved for BPH and essential hypertension. These medications include prazosin, terazosin, doxazosin, etc. The ALLHAT trial noted an increased risk of adverse cardiac events with the use of doxazosin and now these medications are used as fourth-line or fifth-line agents for hypertension management as part of a multidrug approach.[18] There is a high incidence of orthostatic hypotension and risk of falls and hence these medications are given at bedtime. These medications are recommended to continue in the perioperative period.

One consideration in the use of these medications is the higher risk of intraoperative floppy iris syndrome and vision failure in patients getting cataract surgery due to their mechanism of action. The risk does not seem to be mitigated by stopping these medications in the preoperative setting but intraoperative measures undertaken by the ophthalmologists may be helpful in preventing this complication.[19]

Angiotensin-converting enzyme inhibitors and angiotensin receptor blockers
These medications are FDA recommended as first-line therapy for hypertension in diabetic patients, proteinuria in kidney disease, heart failure with reduced ejection fraction less than 40%, and after myocardial infarction. They act by inhibiting the renin angiotensin aldosterone system and decreasing the effects of angiotensin II which is a potent vasoconstrictor. They also block the effect of angiotensin II on the adrenal cortex and pituitary leading to reduced aldosterone and antidiuretic hormone production.

The use of these medications just before surgery has been a highly debated topic in anesthesiology for years. Case reports of intractable intraoperative hypotension have been published since the 1990s and confirmed by small observational studies.[20,21]

However, more recent published literature has yielded conflicting results leading to different recommendations from different societies. In 2014, the ACC/AHA recommended that it is reasonable to continue these medications in the preoperative period due to large studies that did not show any increased incidence in mortality, renal failure, or cardiac complications due to hypotension from these agents. However, more studies since then have noted a trend toward higher risk of postoperative kidney injury and cardiac complications with the use of these medications[22,23] Since then, the Canadian Cardiovascular Society guidelines have recommended withholding angiotensin-converting enzyme inhibitors (ACEI)/angiotensin receptor blockers (ARB) for 24 hours prior to surgery[24] while the European Society of Cardiology guidelines recommend withholding for 24 hours if the indication is for hypertension and continuing it if given for heart failure.[25] Other societies such as the Society for Perioperative Assessment and Quality Improvement (SPAQI) and Perioperative Quality Initiative have set out similar recommendations.[26] Most recently, the SPACE trial found that stopping renin-angiotensin system inhibitors before non-cardiac surgery did not reduce myocardial injury, and increased the risk of clinically significant acute hypertension.[27] Ongoing randomized controlled trials that are currently being conducted should hopefully shed more light on this question; the authors recommend continuing these agents in most patients, but it is reasonable to hold these prior to surgery if concerns for hemodynamic instability, large blood loss or fluid shifts, or postoperative AKI.[28–30]

Calcium channel blockers
The calcium channel blockers (CCBs) are classified into 2 distinct kinds: dihydropyridines and non-dihydropyridines. These medications bind to the long L-type calcium channels and block the inward movement of calcium in the myocardium and peripheral vasculature. The dihydropyridines such as nifedipine and amlodipine primarily act in the peripheral blood vessels leading to vasodilation and hypotension. The non-dihydropyridines such as verapamil and diltiazem act on the myocardium leading to inhibitory chronotropic and inotropic effects. The CCBs are FDA approved for treatment of arrythmias, hypertension, coronary spasm, and Raynaud's phenomena among others.

These medications are well tolerated in the perioperative period and there are data suggesting that they may be beneficial in patients going for cardiac and vascular surgery particularly in preventing postop arrythmias.[31,32] It is recommended to be continued in the perioperative setting without interruptions.

Diuretics
Diuretics and diuretic-type medications are a group of several different classes of medications that help in excreting water from the body thereby helping in restoring the fluid balance. Most diuretics work by inhibiting the renal tubular sodium channels

thereby affecting the fluid and electrolyte balance in the body. The different classes of medications in this group work in different parts of the renal tubule. Osmotic diuretics such as mannitol, and diuretic-type medications such as sodium-glucose cotrans-porter-2 (SGLT-2) inhibitors increase the intraluminal osmolarity thereby drawing free water into the collecting tubule while the newer aquaretic agents such as the vap-tans block vasopressin receptors and only affect free water excretion.[33]

The loop diuretics which act on the thick ascending Loop of Henle are some of the most efficacious ones in this group. They are FDA approved for acute decompensated heart failure and ascites in liver cirrhosis. The addition of aldosterone receptor blockers such as spironolactone is recommended for chronic left ventricular dysfunction with ejection fraction less than 35%. Thiazide diuretics, which act on distal convoluted tubular is one of the first-line agents for essential hypertension. Other agents such as carbonic anhydrase inhibitors are used for open angle glaucoma.

The controversy surrounding these agents is due to their effect on intravascular volume status and electrolyte balance in a surgical patient who is going to be nil per os on the day of surgery and hypothetical risk of AKI due to their mechanism of action. The concern for hypotension due to volume depletion in patients on loop diuretics was studied in an RCT of 193 patients which showed no difference in patients who took the medication on the morning of surgery versus those who were not on it.[34] There was a trend toward AKI in patients who were on chronic diuretics in an observational cohort study done in the VA population with postop kidney injury.[35] However, most of the recommendations for diuretic management come from expert consensus and guidance. SPAQI and the Perioperative Quality Initiative recommend continuing thiazide and aldosterone receptor blockers on the day of surgery but to hold the loop diuretics.

In the postoperative setting, especially in cardiac surgery patients, fluid management with diuretics is one way to mitigate the fluid retention that occurs with cardiopulmonary bypass. However, aquaretics such as tolvaptans are showing a benefit in reducing the incidence of AKI and electrolyte imbalances in that population.[36]

Other antihypertensive medications

Clonidine acts by blocking the central sympathetic outflow thereby reducing the symptoms of sympathetic stimulation such as hypertension, anxiety, and tachycardia. Due to these sympatholytic properties, clonidine was studied as a potential medication in reducing perioperative myocardial ischemia in the POISE-2 trial. The trial showed no benefit when given to clonidine-naïve patients, but increased the risk of intraoperative and non-fatal cardiac arrest.[37]

Clonidine has a large withdrawal effect and, if taken chronically, should be continued through surgery uninterrupted due to risk of hypertension and tachycardia on the day of surgery.

Hydralazine is a direct vasodilator and is used as a third-line or fourth-line agent in the treatment of hypertension. It causes reflex tachycardia and is usually used in conjunction with a betablocker. There are no data to guide the use of this medication in the perioperative setting, but expert opinion recommends continuing the medication through the surgical episode.

Congestive heart failure medications

Angiotensin receptor-neprolysin inhibitor. Sacrubitril/Valsartan is the only medication that is approved so far for this group of new drugs developed for the treatment of heart failure. It is now approved for use in patients with heart failure both reduced and preserved ejection fraction according to the ACC/AHA guidelines on heart failure management based on the favorable data from the PARADGIM- HF study that compared angiotensin receptor-neprolysin inhibitor (ARNI) with enalapril.[37]

Physiologic effects of heart failure lead to the release of natriuretic hormones as a compensatory mechanism to promote natriuresis, diuresis, and vasodilation. This leads to reduced blood pressure, sympathetic tone, and aldosterone levels which are all beneficial effects of these hormones. The enzyme neprolysin metabolizes the natriuretic hormones, and sacubitril works by inhibiting this enzyme. Neprolysin also breaks down angiotensin II and bradykinin and inhibiting this increases the levels of both these hormones as well. Hence, it is used in conjunction with an ARB to block the angiotensin II effect. Because ACEI also causes an increase in bradykinin levels, the risk of angioedema is elevated. ACC/AHA recommends stopping ACEI at least 3 days before an ARNI is started.

There is no current literature or studies that give us guidance as to how this medication affects physiology during surgery; hence, expert statements and consensus recommend holding this medication 24 hours prior to surgery similar to an ACEI or ARB and restarting it within 48 hours after surgery or when patient is able to resume per os (PO) intake.

Sodium-glucose cotransporter-2 inhibitors. SGLT-2 inhibitors are anti-diabetic medications that act by preventing the reabsorption of glucose from the proximal convoluted tubules leading to a diuretic effect as noted earlier. They have shown cardiorenal protective effect and now are FDA approved for treatment of CHF in both diabetic and non-diabetic patients.[37] Use of these medications is associated with an increased risk of urinary tract infection and, diabetic and euglycemic ketoacidosis (eDKA) presumably due to glucagon stimulation and lipolysis in times of stress such as surgery or fasting.[38] Recent data suggest that all patients on SGLT-2 inhibitors are at risk for postoperative eDKA and the risk is reduced with longer hold times prior to surgery. [39]

It is recommended to hold these medications at least 3 days prior to surgery and minor procedures that require patients to fast. All patients postoperatively should have laboratory parameters monitored for development of eDKA.

Digoxin. Digoxin is one of the oldest medications used for congestive heart failure and supraventricular tachycardia. It has a narrow therapeutic window and levels are monitored occasionally. It is generally safe and the authors recommend continuing this medication in the perioperative setting and discontinuation might precipitate tachycardia and heart failure.[26]

Ivabradine. Ivabradine is selective sinus node inhibitor and was shown to improve composite cardiac outcomes when used in concert with a betablocker. ACC/AHA now recommends it for New York Heart Association (NYHA) class II and III patients already on goal directed medical therapy with an elevated heart rate. Ivabradine is fairly new and no guidelines are present to inform its management in the perioperative setting. However, it was shown to reduce intraoperative tachycardia in a single-center study.[40]

If continued, it is recommended to closely monitor patients for bradycardia.[41]

Opioids and pain medications
Patients on chronic opioid therapy present a challenge in the postoperative period, as pain control is often suboptimal due to higher postoperative analgesic requirements, opioid-induced hyperalgesia, and the risk of drug withdrawal.[42,43] Opioids should be continued as close to preoperative doses as possible, with attention to

adverse effects of opioids including respiratory depression and sedation especially with concurrent anesthesia. At least 50% of the preoperative opioid dose is required to prevent withdrawal. Ideally, clinicians should continue the preoperative opioid formulation in the postoperative period; however, it is reasonable to rotate opioids at equipotent doses to address uncontrolled pain. Multimodal analgesia planning including nonopioid and nonpharmacologic approaches can help reduce postoperative opioid requirements.[44] Consultation with Pain Medicine may be considered in complicated cases.

Patients with substance use disorders may present for surgery on therapeutic opioid agonists (eg, methadone), opioid antagonists (eg, naltrexone), or combination agonist and antagonist therapy (eg buprenorphine and naltrexone). These regimens complicate pain management strategies, but careful planning can mitigate uncontrolled pain in these patients.[45] Methadone generally should be continued preoperatively as well as postoperatively once the patient is tolerating oral intake. Naltrexone will cause resistance to the analgesic effect of opioids for 4 to 5 days after an oral dose, but increased opioid sensitivity may manifest after this time. If minimal pain is expected after surgery, continuation of naltrexone with the use of multimodal analgesia is appropriate. If moderate to severe pain is anticipated requiring opioid therapy, stop oral naltrexone 48 to 72 hours before surgery, and use both opioid and nonopioid analgesics.[46,47] Patients receiving intramuscular naltrexone should be scheduled for surgery 28 days or more after the last administered dose.

Buprenorphine management is more challenging, as one must balance the risk of withdrawal with discontinuation, versus the risk of poor control and high-dosage agonist requirements with continuation. In most cases, this can be continued, but published algorithms can help navigate this challenge based on home doses and anticipated levels of postoperative pain.[47,48]

Nonsteroidal anti-inflammatory agents (NSAIDs) are commonly used analgesics that inhibit cyclooxygenase (COX) enzymes and interfere with prostaglandin synthesis, thus decreasing systemic inflammatory responses including pain and fever. The 2 isoforms of these enzymes, COX-1 (which affects gastric cytoprotection and platelet aggregation) and COX-2 (more specific to cytokine induction and inflammation), dictate management of these medications. NSAIDs inhibiting COX-1 (ibuprofen, naproxen, and others) should be held in advance of surgery due to bleeding risk concerns. Recommendations for duration of holding preoperatively are variable based on half-life, but best practice guidelines suggest 7 days before surgery.[49] COX-2 inhibitors (celecoxib) can be continued preoperatively and on the day of surgery, and in some cases are encouraged as a strategy for reduction in postoperative opioid usage.[44]

Headache agents. Ergotamine and related agents specifically treat migraine headaches and activate serotonin receptors in intracranial blood vessels leading to vasoconstriction. Due to the risk of serotonin syndrome and hypertensive crisis, these agents should be held at least 2 days prior to elective surgery.[44,50]

Butalbital is a barbiturate that is commonly used for vascular or tension headaches in combination with acetaminophen, aspirin, and caffeine. It primarily affects gamma-aminobutyric acid receptors and can lead to central nervous system and respiratory depression, and may have an additive effect with anesthetics. This should be held on the day of surgery if not taking chronically. If used chronically, patient should take to avoid withdrawal, and if possible weaned over the prior 2 weeks if patients are using these agents chronically.[44]

Serotonin 5HT 1 B/1D receptor agonists, better known as "triptans," are used specifically for migraine treatment. Theoretic concerns exist for serotonin syndrome, mostly in conjunction with selective serotonin reuptake inhibitors (SSRIs) and seroto-nin norepinephrine reuptake inhibitors (SNRIs), as well as monoamine oxidase A (MAO-A) inhibition. These agents can affect drug metabolism via the cytochrome P450 pathways. Consensus recommendations are to hold these agents on the day of surgery.[44,51]

Immunosuppressive agents

Immunosuppression is used for preventing rejection of organ transplantation as well as for various autoimmune rheumatologic and GI conditions. The decision for continuing these medications through surgery is nuanced and should be made with the prescribing clinician. The caveat is that the surgical procedure severity and the risk of infection must be balanced with the risks of disease relapse and transplant or-gan rejection. In most cases, these agents should be continued through the surgical episode, with the exception of cyclophosphamide, which should be held for 4 weeks prior to elective surgery, due to risk of infection, and cardiac and bone marrow toxicity.[52] In cases of less severe systemic lupus erythematosis (SLE), medications such as mycophenolate and azathioprine can be held for 7 days preoperatively; if SLE is severe, these can be continued through surgery.[53] GI immunomodulators are used for inflammatory bowel disease or organ transplants, and data are limited to small single-center studies. Purine analogs such as 6-mercaptopurine and azathio-prine, as well as methotrexate, do not increase postoperative complications and are safe to continue.[54]

Tumor necrosis factor (TNF) inhibitors (infliximab, adalimumab, golimumab, and certolizumab) are used for both GI and inflammatory arthritic conditions, and they are known to increase the risk of infection and malignancy in general, but perioperative literature on these agents historically has been conflicting.[55] The Prospective Cohort of Ulcerative Colitis and Crohn's Disease Patients Undergoing Surgery to Identify Risk Factors for Post-Operative Infection (PUCCINI) trial published in 2022 found no asso-ciation between preoperative TNFi use and postoperative infectious or wound healing complications.[56] Thus, it is likely safe to continue these agents in the absence of active infection, although discussion with treating surgeons and gastroenterologists is still reasonable; the American College of Rheumatology (ACR)/Association of Hip and Knee Surgeons (AAHKS) guidelines for arthroplasty patients suggest holding these agents for a full-dose cycle.[53] Other monoclonal agents should be held for 1 dosing interval before surgery; the Janus kinase inhibitor tofactinib should be held for 7 days prior to surgery, as it has a black box warning for risk of thrombosis.[44] Appro-priate venous thromboembolism (VTE) prophylaxis should be provided for these pa-tients if surgery is required within this 7-day window (**Table 3**).

Psychiatric medications

There is an increasing use of psychotropic agents in patients undergoing elective noncardiac surgeries. Evidence-based guidelines for management of psychotropic medications are limited as data are primarily derived from case reports and expert opinion, with few RCTs. One must consider the potential for side effects and interac-tion with anesthetic agents balanced with the risk of withdrawal with abruptly stopping these agents, leading to decompensation of their psychiatric condition. Most of these agents should be continued through the perioperative setting. However, there are selected issues with some of these agents.[57]

Tricyclic antidepressants act to inhibit uptake of norepinephrine and serotonin. These agents have anticholinergic, antihistaminic, and alpha-1 receptor antagonism. They also prolong the QT corrected for heart rate (QTc) interval and lower seizure

Table 3
Immunosuppressive agents

Medication Class	Hold/Continue on Day of Surgery	Special Considerations
Corticosteroids	Continue	Risk for adrenal insufficiency rare, dose and duration dependent; also dependent on presence of primary AI vs treatment for non AI- related condition; usual daily dose is required in most cases.
Purine Analogues. 6-Mercaptopurine azathioprine	Continue	
Methotrexate	Continue	
Tumor Necrosis Factor Inhibitors (infliximab, adalimumab, golimumab, certolizumab)	Hold for at least 1 dosing interval before surgery (ie, if taken every 4 wk, schedule surgery 5 wk after the last dose)	PUCCINI trial does not suggest increased risk of infection with continuation in inflammatory bowel disease surgery; unclear if this extrapolates to other surgical types; consult with the prescribing clinician and surgeon to discuss the relevant risks and benefits of therapy interruption.
Monoclonal Antibodies (ustekinumab, vedolizumab, natalizumab)	Hold for at least 1 dosing interval before surgery	Consult with the prescribing clinician and surgeon to discuss the relevant risks and benefits of therapy interruption.
Tofacitinib	Hold for 7 d before surgery	

threshold. There is concern about arrhythmias in this patient population conjunction with certain anesthetics or sympathomimetic agents; literature to support this is very limited. It is recommended to continue these agents through surgery unless there is a substantial risk of arrhythmias, in which case these can be tapered between 7 and 14 days prior to surgery.[57]

Selective serotonin reuptake inhibitors are commonly used agents for depression and anxiety. These agents may increase risk of bleeding and need for transfusion due to their effects on platelet aggregation. This is primarily noted in combination with NSAID use.[58] The literature on this association is inconsistent, noted especially in hip and knee arthroplasties and breast surgeries.[59,60] However, stopping these agents could lead to exacerbation of mood disorders and a withdrawal syndrome. These generally can be continued unless there is a substantial risk of bleeding or a higher risk surgery from bleeding consequences such as neurosurgery. These agents should be tapered several weeks prior to surgery and consideration of an alternate antidepressant regimen in this circumstance. It is also recommended to avoid non-steroidal or antiplatelet agents in the perioperative setting when patients are on SSRIs.

Monoamine oxidase inhibitors (MAOIs) are less commonly utilized today but are used in refractory mood disorders. Nonselective MAOIs lead to accumulation of biogenic amines in the central and autonomic nervous system. The use of sympathomimetic agents like ephedrine can lead to severe hypertensive crisis. In addition, serotonin syndrome in conjunction with dextromethorphan and pyridine as well as inhibition of hepatic microsomal environment enzymes involved in opioid metabolism can lead to accumulation of free opioids and increased sedation and respiratory depression. MAO-safe techniques are reported and in general avoidance of meperidine and dextromethorphan, as well as use of direct-acting sympathomimetics is recommended.[57,61]

Antipsychotics are generally safe and should be continued through surgery unless known QT interval prolongation or clinical arrhythmias are present.[62,63] They do have some interactions with cytochrome P450 2D6 (CYP-2D6) and cytochrome P450 3A4 (CYP3A4) drug metabolism and can interact with other drugs used in the perioperative period, including agents like midazolam and ketamine. If patients cannot take in oral medication, parenteral forms of atypical antipsychotics are available, as well as oral dissolvable formulations of agents such as olanzapine and risperidone.

Benzodiazepines are generally safe to continue although withdrawal symptoms may manifest if they are stopped abruptly. They are commonly used in the perioperative period to reduce anxiety. It should be noted that increased tolerance to perioperative anesthetic and sedative agents may be observed in patients on chronic benzodiazepine therapy **(Table 4)**.[57]

Table 4
Psychiatric medications

Medication Class	Hold/Continue on Day of Surgery	Special Considerations
SSRIs SNRIs	Continue Continue	Risk for discontinuation syndrome, hyponatremia due to syndrome of inappropriate ADH (SIADH), some bleeding risk increase with nonsteroidal inflammatory drugs (NSAIDs); serotonin syndrome with other serotonergic drugs; Extrapyrimal symptoms and neuroleptic malignant syndrome (NMS) with metoclopramide.
Tricyclic antidepressants	Continue	Hypertension with indirect sympathomimetics, anticholinergic effect, cytochrome P450 2D6 (CYP-2D6) metabolism; withdrawal syndrome; QT corrected for heart rate (QTc) prolongation; EPS with metoclopramide, serotonin syndrome with other serotonergic drugs.
Tetracyclic antidepressants	Continue	Mirtazapine serotonin syndrome with other serotonergic drugs; QTc prolongation; CNS depression with benzodiazepines; hyponatremia, bleeding risk with warfarin
Monoamine Oxidase Inhibitors (MAO)	Continue with MAO Safe anesthesia, or stop 2 wk before surgery	Risk for hypertensive crisis with indirect sympathomimetics (ephedrine) (ABSOLUTE contraindication). Risk of serotonin syndrome with serotoninergic opiates (meperidine, methadone, tramadol); tyramine-free diet preoperatively; direct sympathomimetics are the agents of choice for hypotension treatment.
Dupropion	Continue	Decreases seizure threshold, dose adjust for impaired renal and hepatic function; inhibits CYP-2D6.

Gastrointestinal medications

Proton pump inhibitors are commonly used agents for gastroesophageal reflux disease, peptic ulcer disease, and other indications. They block gastric acid production by inhibiting the hydrogen potassium ATPase pump on the parietal cell membrane. These agents are generally safe to continue through surgery. There are more recent concerns about hypomagnesemia and arrhythmogenic potential, interactions with CYP 450 metabolism drugs, and diminished antiplatelet deflation effectiveness of clopidogrel. PPIs are also associated with pneumonia in hospitalized patients. Literature does not support that these will reduce the risk of aspiration pneumonitis from intubation and mechanical ventilation; however, it is still considered safe to continue these agents.[48]

H2 receptor antagonists are also used for gastric acid suppression. Potential complications with these agents include concerns for postoperative delirium, QT interval prolongation in cognition with other medications, and possible alteration of gastric colonization leading to increased risk for nosocomial pneumonia. However, these complications are rare and these agents are considered safe in the perioperative setting.

Particulate antacid formulations such as aluminum hydroxide, calcium carbonate, or sucralfate are also commonly used. The American Society of Anesthesiologists strongly recommends discontinuing these on the morning of surgery, especially the particulate antacids listed earlier, due to a higher risk and severity of aspiration injury. Sodium citrate and magnesium trisilicate are nonparticulate antacids and may be safer to use from an aspiration standpoint on the day of surgery.[58]

5HT3 antagonists are commonly used agents for nausea and vomiting management period. It is recommended to be cautious with these agents especially when using concurrently with medications that prolong the QT interval or have serotonergic properties.

Dopamine agonists such as promethazine, prochlorperazine, droperidol, and metoclopramide are safe to use up to and including the morning of surgery unless there are also concerns with QT prolongation and risk for extrapyramidal side effects.[48]

Vitamins are generally safe to take except for the concern for increasing bleeding risk with vitamin E. Most other over the counter supplements that are not FDA approved may have multiple ingredients that are not specifically evaluated. Consensus guidelines suggest most of these should be held approximately 2 weeks prior to elective surgery. If this is not possible, or patients continue to take these up to the day of surgery, it becomes necessary to have a conversation with the surgeon, anesthesiologist, and treating clinicians, and the patient regarding the risk benefit of the procedure in terms of bleeding, arrhythmias, sedation, and other potential complications.[60,61]

Parkinson's disease

Parkinson's disease medications have a complex pharmacodynamic and side effect profile that requires consideration of risks and benefits of continuation versus discontinuation. These are typically dopaminergic agonists which can lead to delirium and orthostatic hypotension. However, withdrawal of these agents can lead to breakthrough parkinsonian symptoms as well as orthostatic hypotension and dysautonomia, with increased risk of aspiration and gastric dysmotility. Consensus guidelines suggest that all these agents be continued on the morning of surgery, including carbidopa/levodopa, dopamine agonists such as pramipexole and ropinirole, monoamine oxidase B inhibitors, catechol-O-methyl transferase (COMT) inhibitors, and Amantadine. However, it is reasonable to check electrocardiogram (EKG) for QTc interval measurement, as well as serum creatinine, electrolytes, and liver function testing if these have not been done for the ongoing management of the patient's Parkinsons' medications.[62]

RESUMING MEDICATIONS AFTER SURGERY

There is evidence that failure to resume cardiovascular medications that were held before surgery leads to harms such as heart failure exacerbation, hypertension, and even mortality.[63,64] Hence, it is imperative that once patients can resume a diet, most of their home medications should be reinitiated. As noted previously, a reliable medication reconciliation in the preoperative setting and on admission to the hospital can serve as a baseline for drug dosing and schedules.

High-risk medications such as anticoagulants or antiplatelet medication should be resumed after discussion with the surgical team ensuring hemostasis has been achieved. If there is prolonged interruption of an anticoagulant or antiplatelet, it is important to have an alternative strategy based on the indication. Once the medication is resumed, close monitoring of the blood counts should be undertaken.

It is common for medications to be withheld due to development of AKI postoperatively. In such a case, a clear channel of communication should be established with the patient's outpatient provider to ensure that the patient has a follow-up appointment with labs within a week of discharge if the patient is discharged prior to the complete resolution of AKI.

Medications started in the hospital for a temporary postoperative condition such as delirium and postoperative atrial fibrillation should be tapered or stopped before discharge or at least have a postoperative plan that can be executed once patient is discharged.

Insulin dose adjustments are quite common in the hospital due to nil per os (NPO) status, lack of appetite, and fewer food choices. This is also a high-risk medication and any changes should be communicated to the patient's outpatient provider.

Leveraging technology and the electronic health record for seamless transitions of care and improved communication, educating patients and providers regarding their medication changes, and ensuring an accurate medication reconciliation are some ways in which we can mitigate the risk of dropped medications in the postoperative setting.[65]

CLINICS CARE POINTS

- Take a complete medication history including over the counter medications, herbal agents, vitamins and dietary supplements.
- Contact the patient's pharmacy if they are unable to provide a clear history.
- Continue medications with the potential for withdrawal syndromes and keep existing medical conditions stable, if they do not impact the surgical milleu.
- Stop medications that affect surgical or anesthetic outcomes including bleeding risk, wound healing, postoperative infection risk, and kidney or liver dysfunction.
- Do not prescribe beta blockers solely for perioperative cardiovascular risk reduction; continue beta blockers in patients already on them.
- If patients have indications for beta blockade outside of the surgical condition, start them at least 7 days before surgery to assess for hemodynamic tolerance.
- Stop SGLT-2 inhibitors 3-4 days prior to elective surgery to mitigate the risk of euglycemic DKA.

- In most low to intermediate risk surgeries in pateints on corticosteroids, stress dose steroids are not required; continuing the patient's home dose of corticosteroid is adequate.
- Realize that resuming medications postoperatively is essential to maintain stability of medical conditions; discuss with the surgical teams regarding the timing of resuming high risk medications such as anticoagulants, antiplatelet agents, and insulins.

DISCLOSURE

Dr P. Patel has no disclosures of interest. Dr C. Whinney receives compensation from UpToDate as a coauthor on the topic, "Perioperative Medication Management"

REFERENCES

1. Available at: www.cdc.gov/nchs/fastats/drug-use-therapeutic.htm. Accessed June 3, 2024.
2. Kennedy JM, van Rij AM, Spears GF, et al. Polypharmacy in a general surgical unit and consequences of drug withdrawal. Br J Clin Pharmacol 2000;49(4): 353–62.
3. Goodman SM, Springer B, Guyatt G, et al. 2017 American College of Rheumatology/American Association of Hip and Knee Surgeons guideline for the perioperative management of antirheumatic medication in patients with rheumatic diseases undergoing elective total hip or total knee arthroplasty. Arthritis Care Res 2017. https://doi.org/10.1002/acr.23274.
4. Sweitzer B, Rajan N, Schell D, et al. Preoperative care for cataract surgery: the society for ambulatory anesthesia position statement. Anesth Analg 2021;133(6): 1431–6.
5. Wesselink EM, Kappen TH, Torn HM, et al. Intraoperative hypotension and the risk of postoperative adverse outcomes: a systematic review. Br J Anaesth 2018;121:706–21.
6. Gregory A, Stapelfeldt WH, Khanna AK, et al. Intraoperative hypotension is associated with adverse clinical outcomes after noncardiac surgery. Anesth Analg 2021;132(6):1654–65.
7. Marcucci M, Painter TW, Conen D, et al. Hypotension-avoidance versus hypertension-avoidance strategies in noncardiac surgery : an international randomized controlled trial. Ann Intern Med 2023;176(5):605–14.
8. Devereaux PJ, Goldman L, Cook DJ, et al. Perioperative cardiac events in patients undergoing noncardiac surgery: a review of the magnitude of the problem, the pathophysiology of the events and methods to estimate and communicate risk. CMAJ (Can Med Assoc J) 2005;173:627–34.
9. Mangano DT, Layug EL, Wallace A, et al. Effect of atenolol on mortality and cardiovascular morbidity after noncardiac surgery. multicenter study of perioperative ischemia research group. N Engl J Med 1996;335:1713–20.
10. Lindenauer PK, Pekow P, Wang K, et al. Perioperative beta-blocker therapy and mortality after major noncardiac surgery. N Engl J Med 2005;353:349–61.
11. Devereaux PJ, Yang H, Yusuf S, et al, POISE Study Group. Effects of extended-release metoprolol succinate in patients undergoing non-cardiac surgery (POISE trial): A andomized controlled trial. Lancet 2008;371:1839–47.
12. Wijeysundera DN, Duncan D, Nkonde Price C, et al. Perioperative beta blockade in noncardiac surgery: A systematic review for the 2014 ACC/AHA guideline on perioperative cardiovascular evaluation and management of patients undergoing

noncardiac surgery: a report of the american college of cardiology/american heart association task force on practice guidelines. J Am Coll Cardiol 2014;64: 2406–25.

13. Alegria S, Costa J, Vaz-Carneiro A, et al. Perioperative beta-blockers for preventing surgery-related mortality and morbidity. Rev Port Cardiol (Engl Ed) 2019; 38(10):691–4.

14. McKenzie NL, Parker Ward R, Nagele P, et al. Preoperative β-blocker therapy and stroke or major adverse cardiac events in major abdominal surgery: a retrospective cohort study. Anesthesiology 2023;138:42–54.

15. Wallace AW, Au S, Cason BA. Association of the pattern of use of perioperative b-blockade and postoperative mortality. Anesthesiology 2010;113(4):794–805.

16. Mol KHJM, Liem VGB, van Lier F, et al. Intraoperative hypotension in noncardiac surgery patients with chronic beta-blocker therapy: A matched cohort analysis. J Clin Anesth 2023;89:111143.

17. Hiremat S, Ruscika M. Alpha-blocker use and the risk of hypotension and hypotension-related clinical events in women of advanced age. Hypertension 2019;74:645–51.

18. Christou CD, Tsinopoulos I, Ziakas N, et al. Intraoperative floppy iris syndrome: updated perspectives. Clin Ophthalmol 2020;14:463–71.

19. Powell CG, Unsworth J, McVey FK. Severe hypotension associated with angiotensin-converting enzyme inhibition in anaesthesia. Anaesth Intensive Care 1998;26:107–9.

20. Rosenman DJ, McDonald FS, Ebbert JO, et al. Clinical consequences of withholding versus administering renin-angiotensin-aldosterone system antagonists in the preoperative period. J Hosp Med 2008;3:319–25.

21. Roshanov PS, Rochwerg B, Patel A, et al. Withholding versus continuing angiotensin-converting enzyme inhibitors or angiotensin II receptor blockers before noncardiac surgery: an analysis of the Vascular events In noncardiac Surgery patients cOhort andomized prospective cohort. Anesthesiology 2017;126: 16–27.

22. Hollmann C, Fernandes NL, Biccard BM. A systematic review of outcomes associated with withholding or continuing angiotensin-converting enzyme inhibitors and angiotensin receptor blockers before noncardiac surgery. Anesth Analg 2018;127:678–87.

23. Duceppe E, Parlow J, MacDonald P, et al. Canadian Cardiovascular Society guidelines on perioperative cardiac risk assessment and management for patients who undergo noncardiac surgery. Can J Cardiol 2017;33:17–32.

24. Kristensen SD, Knuuti J, Saraste A, et al. 2014 ESC/ESA guidelines on non-cardiac surgery: cardiovascular assessment and management: the joint task force on non-cardiac surgery: cardiovascular assessment and management of the European Society of Cardiology (ESC) and the European Society of Anaesthesiology (ESA). Eur Heart J 2014;35:2383–431.

25. Sanders RD, Hughes F, Shaw A, et al. Perioperative Quality Initiative-3 Workgroup; POQI chairs; Physiology group; Preoperative blood pressure group; Intraoperative blood pressure group; Postoperative blood pressure group. Perioperative Quality Initiative consensus statement on preoperative blood pressure, risk and outcomes for elective surgery. Br J Anaesth 2019;122:552–62.

26. Sahai SK, Balonov K, Bentov N, et al. Preoperative Management of Cardiovascular Medications: A Society for Perioperative Assessment and Quality Improvement (SPAQI) Consensus Statement. Mayo Clin Proc 2022;97(9):1734–51.

27. Ackland GL, Patel A, Abbott TEF, et al. Discontinuation vs. continuation of renin-angiotensin system inhibition before non-cardiac surgery: the SPACE trial. Eur Heart J 2024;45(13):1146–55.
28. Legrand M, Futier E, Leone M, et al. Impact of renin-angiotensin system inhibitors continuation versus discontinuation on outcome after major surgery: protocol of a multicenter randomized, controlled trial (STOP-or-NOT trial). Trials 2019;20:160.
29. Yang YF, Zhu YJ, Long YQ, et al. Withholding vs. continuing angiotensin-converting enzyme inhibitors or angiotensin receptor blockers before non-cardiac surgery in older patients: study protocol for a multicenter randomized controlled trial. Front Med (Lausanne) 2021;8:654700.
30. Misra S, Parida S, Sahajanandan R, et al. ACE investigators. The effect of continuing versus withholding angiotensin-converting enzyme inhibitors/angiotensin II receptor blockers on mortality and major adverse cardiovascular events in hypertensive patients undergoing elective non-cardiac surgery: study protocol for a multi-centric open-label andomized controlled trial. Trials 2022;23(1):670.
31. Wijeysundera DN, Beattie WS, Rao V, et al. Calcium antagonists reduce cardiovascular complications after cardiac surgery: a meta-analysis. J Am Coll Cardiol 2003;41(9):1496–505.
32. Qvavadze T, Lurie F, Russell T. Association of beta blockers and calcium channel blockers with arrhythmia after carotid intervention. J Vasc Surg 2023;77(4):21S.
33. Arumugham V.B., Shahin M.H., Therapeutic Uses of Diuretic Agents. 2023. In: StatPearls [Internet]. Treasure Island (FL): StatPearls Publishing; 2024. Available at: https://pubmed.ncbi.nlm.nih.gov/32491770/. Accessed June 6, 2024.
34. Khan NA, Campbell NR, Frost SD, et al. Risk of intraoperative hypotension with loop diuretics: a randomized controlled trial. Am J Med 2010;123(11):1059, e1-8.
35. Grams ME, Sang Y, Coresh J, et al. Acute kidney injury after major surgery: a retrospective analysis of veterans health administration data. Am J Kidney Dis 2016;67(6):872–80.
36. Nishi H. Advent of New perioperative care for fluid management after cardiovascular surgery: A review of current evidence. J Cardiol 2020;75(6):606–13.
37. Devereaux PJ, Sessler DI, Leslie K, et al. Clonidine in patients undergoing noncardiac surgery. N Engl J Med 2014;370:1504–13.
38. Heidenreich PA, Bozkurt B, Aguilar D, et al. 2022 AHA/ACC/HFSA guideline for the management of heart failure: a report of the american college of cardiology/american heart association joint committee on clinical practice guidelines. Circulation 2022;145(18):e895–1032.
39. Peters AL, Buschur EO, Buse JB, et al. Euglycemic diabetic ketoacidosis: a potential complication of treatment with sodium–glucose cotransporter 2 inhibition. Diabetes Care 2015;38(9):1687–90.
40. Steinhorn B, Wiener-Kronish J. Dose-dependent relationship between SGLT2 inhibitor hold time and risk for postoperative anion gap acidosis: a single-centre retrospective analysis. Br J Anaesth 2023;131(4):682e686.
41. Banerjee A, Mishra S. Use of preoperative single dose ivabradine for perioperative hemodynamic stabilization during non-cardiac elective surgery under general anesthesia: a pilot study. J Clin Med Res 2021;13:343–54.
42. Correll D.J., Pain Management. In: Cohn S.L., editor. *Decision Making in Perioperative Medicine: Clinical Pearls*. McGraw Hill; New York, NY, 2021. Available at: https://accessmedicine.mhmedical.com/content.aspx?bookid=3023&sectionid=254145045. Accessed June 07, 2024.
43. Goel A, Azargive S, Weissman JS, et al. Perioperative pain and addiction interdisciplinary network (PAIN) clinical practice advisory or perioperative management

of buprenorphine: results of a modified Delphi process. Br J Anaesth 2019; 123(2):e333–42.

44. Russell LA, Craig C, Flores EK, et al. Preoperative management of medications for rheumatologic and HIV diseases: society for perioperative assessment and quality improvement (spaqi) consensus statement. Mayo Clin Proc 2022 Aug; 97(8):1551–71. PMID: 35933139.

45. Jiang M, Deng H, Chen X, et al. The efficacy and safety of selective COX-2 inhibitors for postoperative pain management in patients after total knee/hip arthroplasty: a meta-analysis. J Orthop Surg Res 2020;15(1):39.

46. Walkembach J, Brüss M, Urban BW, et al. Interactions of metoclopramide and ergotamine with human 5-HT3A receptors and human 5-HT reuptake carriers [published correction appears in Br J Pharmacol. 2005;146(8):1156]. Br J Pharmacol 2005;146(4):543–52.

47. Orlova Y, Rizzoli P, Loder E. Association of coprescription of triptan antimigraine drugs and selective serotonin reuptake inhibitor or selective norepinephrine reuptake inhibitor antidepressants with serotonin syndrome. JAMA Neurol 2018;75(5): 566–72.

48. Russell LA, Craig C, Flores EK, et al. Preoperative Management of Medications for Rheumatologic and HIV Diseases: Society for Perioperative Assessment and Quality Improvement (SPAQI) Consensus Statement. Mayo Clin Proc 2022 Aug;97(8):1551–71. PMID: 35933139.

49. Pfeifer KJ, Selzer A, Whinney CM, et al. Preoperative Management of Gastrointestinal and Pulmonary Medications: Society for Perioperative Assessment and Quality Improvement (SPAQI) Consensus Statement. Mayo Clin Proc 2021 Dec; 96(12):3158–77. PMID: 34736777.

50. Mowlah RK, Soldera J. Risk and management of post-operative infectious complications in inflammatory bowel disease: A systematic review. World J Gastrointest Surg 2023;15(11):2579–95.

51. Cohen BL, Fleshner P, Kane SV, et al. Prospective Cohort Study to Investigate the Safety of Preoperative Tumor Necrosis Factor Inhibitor Exposure in Patients With Inflammatory Bowel Disease Undergoing Intra-abdominal Surgery. Gastroenterology 2022;163(1):204–21.

52. Oprea AD, Keshock MC'O, Glasser AY, et al. Preoperative Management of Medications for Psychiatric Diseases: Society for Perioperative Assessment and Quality Improvement Consensus Statement. Mayo Clin Proc 2022;97(2):397–416.

53. Roose SP, Rutherford BR. Selective serotonin reuptake inhibitors and operative bleeding risk: a review of the literature. J Clin Psychopharmacol 2016;36(6):704–9.

54. Belay ES, Penrose CT, Ryan SP, et al. Perioperative selective serotonin reuptake inhibitor use is associated with an increased risk of transfusion in total hip and knee arthroplasty. J Arthroplasty 2019;34(12):2898–902.

55. Gärtner R, Cronin-Fenton D, Hundborg HH, et al. Use of selective serotonin reuptake inhibitors and risk of re-operation due to post-surgical bleeding in breast cancer patients: a Danish population-based cohort study. BMC Surg 2010;10:3.

56. Ebrahim ZY, O'Hara J, Borden L, et al. Monoamine oxidase inhibitors and elective surgery. Cleve Clin J Med 1993;60(2):129–30.

57. Kudoh A, Katagai H, Takase H, et al. Effect of preoperative discontinuation of antipsychotics in schizophrenic patients on outcome during and after anaesthesia. Eur J Anaesthesiol 2004;21(5):414–6.

58. Kudoh A. Perioperative management for chronic schizophrenic patients. Anesth Analg 2005;101(6):1867–72.

59. Practice guidelines for preoperative fasting and the use of pharmacologic agents to reduce the risk of pulmonary aspiration: application to healthy patients undergoing elective procedures: an updated report by the American Society of Anesthesiologists Task Force on Preoperative Fasting and the Use of Pharmacologic Agents to Reduce the Risk of Pulmonary Aspiration. Anesthesiology 2017; 126(3):376–93.

60. Ang-Lee MK, Moss J, Yuan CS. Herbal medicines and perioperative care. JAMA 2001;286(2):208–16.

61. Cummings KC, Keshock M, Ganesh R, et al. Preoperative management of surgical patients using dietary supplements: society for perioperative assessment and quality improvement (SPAQI) consensus statement. Mayo Clin Proc 2021;96(5): 1342–55.

62. Oprea AD, Keshock MC'O, Glasser AY, et al. Preoperative management of medications for neurologic diseases: society for perioperative assessment and quality improvement consensus statement. Mayo Clin Proc 2022;97(2):375–96.

63. Lee SM, Takemoto S, Wallace AW. Association between withholding angiotensin receptor blockers in the early postoperative period and 30-day mortality: A cohort study of the veterans affairs healthcare system. Anesthesiology Open Access 2015;123(2):2–8.

64. Mudumbai SC, Takemoto S, Cason BA, et al. Thirty-day mortality risk associated with the postoperative nonresumption of angiotensin-converting enzyme inhibitors: a retrospective study of the Veterans Affairs Healthcare System. J Hosp Med 2014;9:289–96.

65. Available at: https://www.ismp.org/resources/temporarily-holding-medication-orders-safely-order-prevent-patient-harm. Accessed June 3, 2024.

The Patient with Hip Fracture

Michael D. Rudy, MD*, Paul J. Grant, MD

KEYWORDS

- Hip fracture • Perioperative management • Timing of surgery
- Venous thromboembolism prophylaxis

KEY POINTS

- Hip fractures are a common cause of morbidity and mortality particularly among those of advanced age.
- Surgical intervention is warranted for the vast majority of patients sustaining hip fracture and should be completed within a day of sustaining injury unless there are acute medical concerns that would preclude safely taking the patient to surgery.
- Patients with hip fracture are at high risk for venous thromboembolism. Pharmacologic prophylaxis while hospitalized and up to 35 days after surgery is essential.
- Early postoperative interventions including early mobilization and physical therapy can improve the functional outcomes of patients with hip fracture.

INTRODUCTION

Hip fractures refer to any fracture of the proximal femur from the femoral head to 5 cm below the lesser trochanter.[1] Hip fractures account for more than 300,000 annual hospital admissions in the United States at an estimated cost of US$10 to 15 billion annually.[1–4]

The lifetime prevalence of hip fractures is estimated at 5% to 10% in men and 15% to 20% in women although there is significant geographic variability. The risk of hip fracture increases exponentially with age, and globally, hip fractures are projected to nearly double in incidence by the year 2050.[2,4–6] Hip fractures are associated with high, but declining mortality rates. Present estimates of in-hospital, 30 day, and 1 year mortality rates after hip fracture are 2.5%, 5% to 10%, and 20% to 25%, respectively.[1,4,7–10] Less than half of surviving patients will have returned to their baseline function at 1 year after sustaining a hip fracture.[11]

Division of Hospital Medicine, Department of Internal Medicine, University of Michigan Medical School, Ann Arbor, MI, USA
* Corresponding author. 1500 East Medical Center Drive, SPC 5257, Ann Arbor, MI 48109.
E-mail address: mikerudy@med.umich.edu

Med Clin N Am 108 (2024) 1155–1169
https://doi.org/10.1016/j.mcna.2024.04.004   medical.theclinics.com

RISK FACTORS FOR HIP FRACTURE

The majority of hip fractures in older adults result from falls from a standing height. Known risk factors for hip fractures and falls resulting in such are shown in **Table 1**.[9,12-15]

DIAGNOSIS OF HIP FRACTURE

Hip fracture should be clinically suspected in patients presenting with a history of trauma including ground level fall with concomitant pain, swelling or ecchymosis in the area of the hip or upper leg, difficulty with weight-bearing, or a change in mobility. Broader symptoms including vague knee, buttock, or groin pain in the absence of trauma may signal a pathologic fracture. Leg external rotation and shortening may be evident in the setting of displaced fractures.

Diagnosis of hip fracture is usually based on plain radiography that has a sensitivity exceeding 90%, although rates of occult hip fracture may be as high as 40% in those with high clinical suspicion but normal radiographs.[16,17] In these cases, the preferred next diagnostic imaging options are summarized in **Table 2**. Bone scans (which can be falsely normal up to 3 days after fracture) are generally not indicated for radiograph-normal suspected hip fracture.[17]

CATEGORIZATION OF HIP FRACTURES

Hip fractures are anatomically categorized as intracapsular (including the femoral head and neck) or extracapsular (trochanteric, intertrochanteric, and subtrochanteric), and functionally characterized as stable (nondisplaced or impacted) or unstable (displaced).[1,9] Femoral neck fractures and intertrochanteric fractures are most commonly encountered in clinical practice, particularly in older adults sustaining falls.

SURGICAL MANAGEMENT OF HIP FRACTURE

Orthopedic surgical consultation should be obtained in all patients diagnosed with hip fracture. Extensive discussion of the surgical treatment of hip fracture is beyond the scope of this article; however, a general understanding of surgical considerations may be helpful for nonorthopedic providers. An overview of hip fracture anatomy and surgical repair types are shown in **Fig. 1**.

In general, nondisplaced femoral neck fractures are repaired by internal fixation with screws.[1,18,19] Internal fixation is also usually the treatment of choice for younger patients (ie, <50 years old) with higher impact trauma resulting in displaced femoral

Table 1 Risk factors for hip fractures	
Female sex	Excessive alcohol use
Advanced age	Chronic systemic corticosteroid exposure
Low body mass index/malnutrition	Personal history of fragility fracture
Osteoporosis	Factors that increase fall risk: • Physical inactivity • Dementia • Visual impairment • Use of medications/drugs that increase the risk of falls[a]

[a] Well-described medication classes include benzodiazepines, opiates, and antidepressants.

Table 2
American College of Radiology preferred imaging modalities for radiograph-normal suspected hip fractures

Modality	Advantages	Disadvantages
Computed tomography (CT) pelvis and hips without intravenous contrast	Quick, widely available and generally well tolerated	Only ~80–90% sensitive for radiograph-normal fractures
MRI pelvis and affected hip without intravenous contrast	Near 100% sensitivity/specificity	Slower and more expensive than CT; may be more challenging for patient to complete study

From: Ross AB, Lee KS, Chang EY, et al. American College of Radiology ACR Appropriateness Criteria: Acute Hip Pain-Suspected Fracture. 2018. Online: https://acsearch.acr.org/docs/3082587/ Narrative.

neck fractures as there is benefit to maintaining native bone and joint anatomy, and hip prostheses may not offer sufficient durability for these patients. Displaced femoral neck fractures in older adults are usually treated with either total hip arthroplasty (THA; replacement of the femoral head and acetabulum with surgical prosthesis) or hemiarthroplasty (replacement of the femoral head only). Although arthroplasties are associated with greater operative time, blood loss, risk of infection, and hip dislocation compared to internal fixation, they are associated with lower risk of reoperation and better functional outcomes, and thus remain the surgical treatment of choice for older patients with displaced femoral neck fracture.[18,20,21] The choice between THA and hemiarthroplasty for displaced femoral neck fracture in older adults remains

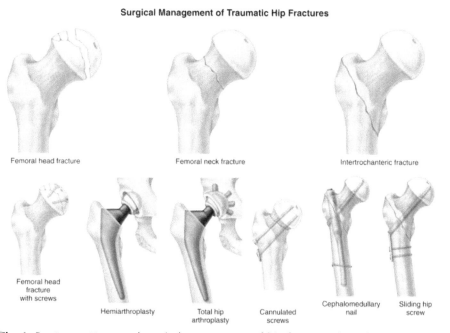

Fig. 1. Fracture patterns and surgical management of hip fractures. (Brandon S. Huggins, Michael S. Sridhar, Chapter 124 Traumatic Hip Fractures. In ed. Miller, M. D., Hart, J., & MacKnight, J. M. (2019). Essential orthopaedics, 2nd edition, Elsevier.)

controversial, but the American Academy of Orthopedic Surgeons (AAOS) and National Institute of Clinical Excellence (NICE; UK) both currently favor THA for higher functioning/independently ambulating older adults who are candidates for the higher surgical risk associated with THA.[18,22]

Extracapsular fractures are also usually treated surgically. Stable intertrochanteric fractures may by treated with intramedullary nails or a sliding hip screw with the latter representing a shorter, less bloody, and more cost-effective option.[1,18,23] Unstable intertrochanteric and subtrochanteric fractures are preferably treated with intramedullary nails owing to better functional outcomes and lower rates of malunion, reoperation, and potentially, a mortality benefit.[18,24,25]

The AAOS has an interactive online tool to help guide surgical management in older adults based on fracture type, baseline mobility/functional status, and pre-existing arthritis.[26]

NONOPERATIVE MANAGEMENT OPTIONS

The vast majority of patients presenting with hip fracture benefit from surgical intervention. Consideration for nonoperative management is generally limited to patients who are nonambulatory at baseline with minimal pain, sustain nondisplaced fractures, or have advanced medical comorbidities with limited life expectancy including advanced dementia.[27–29] In general, outcomes following hip repair in patients with advanced medical comorbidities including frailty and dementia are poor, but nonoperative outcomes are worse. A retrospective cohort study of over 3000 patients with advanced dementia demonstrated mortality rates of 35% and 62% at 6 months and 24 months after hip fracture, respectively, with much higher mortality rates among those managed nonoperatively.[27] The recently published FRAIL-HIP study, evaluated frail, institutionalized adults aged 70 years or older presenting with proximal femur fractures.[30] Patients (or their proxies) who opted for surgery had a higher risk of adverse events including infection (urinary tract, pneumonia), delirium, and longer hospital admissions. However, patients undergoing surgery were more likely to regain mobility and had much lower mortality rates at 30 days (25% vs 81%) and 6 months (48% vs 94%). Notably, both patients and their proxies had similarly positive attitudes toward their treatment decisions highlighting the importance of shared decision-making.[30] Several other studies have demonstrated that nonoperative management of hip fractures more than doubles the risk of 1 year mortality, even when accounting for underlying medical comorbidities.[31–33]

In considering hip fracture surgery in patients with significant comorbidities or limited life expectancy, shared decision-making is paramount when weighing the upfront risk of surgical intervention (perioperative complications, surgical pain, and delirium) with the downstream benefits of better long-term pain control, mobility, and increased life expectancy.[27–30]

TIMING OF HIP FRACTURE SURGERY

When elected, surgical treatment of hip fracture should proceed expeditiously absent any acute medical concerns (see later discussion). A number of studies have sought to address the optimal timing of hip fracture repair. "Early" surgery (variably defined as <24, <48, or <72 hours) was associated with significantly reduced mortality and in-hospital complications of pneumonia and pressure sores in a systematic review and meta-analysis of over 13,000 patients.[34] A population-based retrospective cohort study comprising over 70 hospitals and 40,000 patients with hip fracture in Ontario, Canada, found an inflection point at 24 hours at which longer times for surgical repair was associated with an increase in mortality and medical complications including pulmonary embolism, myocardial infarction, and pneumonia.[35] These findings persisted when propensity-score matching was performed accounting for baseline comorbidities, fracture pattern, and surgery type performed. Several other studies controlling for major comorbidities, which may result in delayed surgery, have not shown the same mortality benefit but have shown lower risk of complications including pressure ulcers, urinary tract infections, pulmonary complications, less postoperative pain, and reduced hospital length of stay.[36–39]

The HIP ATTACK trial of nearly 3000 patients in 17 countries randomized patients to "accelerated surgery" (median surgery 6 hours from presentation) versus "standard-care" (median surgery 24 hours from presentation).[40] There were no differences in mortality or a composite of major medical complications at 90 days. Patients undergoing accelerated surgery were quicker to mobilize and had a shorter hospital length of stay by about 1 day. There was also a modest reduction in delirium in those undergoing accelerated surgery.[40]

The 2021 AAOS hip fracture guidelines recommend surgery within 24 to 48 hours of admission.[18] The 2023 NICE guidelines recommend performing surgery "on the day of, or the day after, admission."[22]

EVALUATING FOR SURGICAL DELAY

Because of the time-critical nature of hip fracture surgery, the decision to delay surgery for further medical evaluation or optimization should not be taken lightly. Active severe medical problems may necessitate delaying surgery as proceeding without appropriate intervention may result in unacceptable perioperative risks (**Table 3**). Once these issues are adequately addressed, surgery should proceed as soon as possible.[18,22]

COMANAGEMENT

A multidisciplinary care model for treating patients with hip fracture is beneficial given the time-sensitive nature of surgery requiring rapid evaluation of often older and medically comorbid patients. Many hospitals have established successful pathways where patients presenting with hip fracture are rapidly evaluated by both medical physicians and orthopedic surgeons. Service models include patient admission to either a medical service with orthopedic surgery consulting, an orthopedic service with a medicine provider consulting, or a comanagement model where both medical and orthopedic

Table 3	
Medical conditions that may warrant delaying hip fracture surgery	
Acute coronary syndrome	Acutely decompensated heart failure
Severe/symptomatic valvular disease (eg, aortic stenosis)	Active malignant cardiac arrhythmias
Severe pulmonary hypertension (especially with right ventricular dysfunction)	Pneumonia or decompensated pulmonary disease (eg, acute exacerbation of chronic obstructive pulmonary disease or asthma)
Sepsis or shock	Severe coagulopathy or anemia
Diabetic ketoacidosis or hyperosmolar hyperglycemic state	Life-threatening electrolyte or metabolic derangements (eg, severe hypokalemia or hyperkalemia, and severe acidemia)

providers dually provide primary in-hospital care for the patient with delineated roles.[41]

Most recent studies have shown significant benefit from medical comanagement for patients with hip fracture including reduced postoperative complications (ie, delirium, infections, and transfer to the intensive care unit), decreased time to surgery, and reduced hospital length of stay.[42–44] Functional outcomes and cost of care may also be improved by comanagement care models.[42,45,46] The data supporting a potential mortality reduction with hip fracture comanagement are less certain.[18,47–49] As a result of these benefits, the AAOS has a "strong" (highest) recommendation for interdisciplinary care programs for the treatment of older adult with hip fractures.[18]

MEDICATION CONSIDERATIONS FOR HIP FRACTURE SURGERY
Antiplatelet Agents

Given the expediency with which hip fracture surgery should be performed, recent intake of blood thinning agents, which might delay less urgent surgeries, may be of particular concern. The use of aspirin and/or clopidogrel is not clearly associated with an increased risk of mortality or bleeding with hip fracture surgery performed within 48 hours, and delaying surgery due to antiplatelet exposure is associated with harm.[50–53] The AAOS recommends "not delaying hip fracture surgery for patients on aspirin and/or clopidogrel."[54] While other $P2Y_{12}$ inhibitors (ie, prasugrel, ticagrelor, and cangrelor) lack robust data with regard to timing of hip fracture surgery, they should be treated similar to clopidogrel as postponing hip fracture surgery for these medications would place patients beyond the recommended surgical timeframe.[55]

Vitamin K Antagonists

Consensus guidelines for delaying hip fracture surgery in the setting of anticoagulation are lacking, and there is significant variability in practice patterns among orthopedic surgeons.[56] In general, the target international normalized ratio (INR) for patients receiving vitamin K antagonists (VKA, ie, warfarin) in whom anticoagulation must be interrupted for elective surgery is less than 1.5.[55,57,58] If acute INR lowering is deemed necessary, prothrombin complex concentrate (PCC), when available, is preferred over fresh frozen plasma (FFP) due to more rapid INR correction, better hemostasis, lower transfusion volumes, and lower risk of adverse transfusion reactions.[59] Early administration of vitamin K (which provides slower, but more durable INR lowering than FFP or PCC) is often used in conjunction with blood products as part of a VKA reversal protocol and has shown to be effective in avoiding unnecessary and potentially harmful delays in hip fracture surgery.[60–62]

Direct Oral Anticoagulants

The direct oral anticoagulants (DOACs; ie, rivaroxaban, apixaban, edoxaban, and dabigatran) are rarely monitored by laboratory testing. Although DOACs are typically held for 1 to 2 days preoperatively for elective procedures (longer for neuraxial anesthesia and in certain clinical circumstances with elevated bleeding risk), guidelines for DOAC management in the setting of hip fracture are lacking.[55,63] For example, the 2022 American College of Chest Physicians Guidelines pertain specifically to elective surgery/procedures. They acknowledge that while preoperative laboratory testing for patients receiving DOACs before urgent (including hip fracture) surgery may be considered, routine coagulation testing (eg, INR and activated partial thromboplastin time) may not reliably exclude residual anticoagulant effects of DOACs and that more specific tests (eg, DOAC-calibrated antifactor Xa levels) may not be readily available and of are of uncertain clinical utility.[55]

A recently published systematic review and meta-analysis found only a handful of studies comparing patients prescribed DOACs who underwent timely hip fracture repair (mean time ~30 hours) with non-DOAC-treated controls. They found no difference in bleeding or mortality, but higher frequency of blood transfusions for DOAC-treated patients, which appears to be partly driven by an included study where patients receiving DOACs presented with lower average hemoglobin levels compared with the nonanticoagulated cohort.[64] Another systematic review and meta-analysis of patients prescribed DOACs prior to hip fracture surgery did not show a difference with respect to mortality or transfusion requirements whether a time-reversal strategy (surgery >36 hours from presentation) was employed or early surgery (surgery within 36 hours of presentation) was performed.[65] The delay in taking patients to surgery in the setting of recent DOAC use has been posited as a potential culprit for increased mortality.[65,66] Regarding active reversal of DOACs, only the monoclonal antibody idarucizumab is Food and Drug Administration (FDA) approved for reversal of dabigatran in urgent/emergent surgery.[67] Coagulation factor Xa (recombinant), inactivated-zhzo is not FDA-approved for preoperative anticoagulation reversal of the factor Xa inhibitors apixaban and rivaroxaban and may increase thrombosis risk.[68] Although not FDA-approved for this indication, PCCs are effective in reversing factor Xa inhibitors and can be considered prior to urgent hip fracture surgery.[69,70]

Anesthesia Considerations

Although decisions regarding the optimal choice of anesthesia is beyond the scope of this study, recent data have provided a better understanding of the potential differences of general versus neuraxial anesthesia for patients undergoing hip fracture repair. Two recent randomized controlled trials compared general to neuraxial (spinal and epidural) anesthesia in patients undergoing hip fracture repair and found no differences in mortality and hospital length of stay.[71,72] Furthermore, no difference was observed in the incidence of postoperative delirium, a condition that was thought to be more associated with exposure to general anesthesia. Given the patient-specific complexities that require careful consideration when choosing anesthesia, the final decision should always be determined by the anesthesiologist.

Venous Thromboembolism Prophylaxis

Venous thromboembolism (VTE) is a well-known complication of surgery, and patients with hip fracture are among those with the highest risk for VTE. Despite this risk, consensus guidelines are lacking regarding the optimal approach to VTE prophylaxis in patients with hip fracture.

The various pharmacologic agents available for VTE prophylaxis for patients with hip fracture are listed in **Table 4** with key recommendations from major societal guidelines.[18,73–75] Low-molecular weight heparin (LMWH) has the most robust data supporting its use in the hip fracture population and tends to be the favored option in professional society guidelines. However, with the surge in popularity of DOACs for many clinical indications over the past several years, there has been a noticeable shift away from injectable anticoagulants in favor of these oral options. This also appears to be true of aspirin, an agent that has become widely accepted for VTE prophylaxis after total hip and total knee arthroplasty. Furthermore, given the lack of strong recommendations from national guidelines, some providers will switch from an injectable drug while hospitalized (ie, enoxaparin) to an oral option upon hospital discharge (ie, aspirin or a DOAC). Although not FDA-approved, this strategy would seem to be a valid

Table 4
Pharmacologic venous thromboembolism prophylaxis options for the patient with hip fracture

Drug	Dose and Route of Administration	FDA Approval for Hip Fracture	Comments/Guideline Recommendations from the ACCP,[73] ASH,[74] NICE,[75] and AAOS[18,a]
LMWH (ie, enoxaparin)	40 mg sc once daily or 30 mg sc bid (do not give within 12 h presurgery or postsurgery)	Yes	• Drug cost and patient discomfort may be a limitation • ACCP 2012 guidelines: preferred agent • ASH 2019 guidelines: preferred agent with no preference over low-dose unfractionated heparin (LDUH; ASH does not comment on aspirin, VKA, fondaparinux, or DOACs) • NICE 2018 guidelines: preferred agent (along with fondaparinux)
Fondaparinux	2.5 mg sc once daily (first dose 6–8 h postoperatively)	Yes	• Drug cost and patient discomfort may be a limitation • NICE 2018 guidelines: preferred agent (along with LMWH)
LDUH	5000 units sc 3 times a day	Yes	• Can be used in the hospital setting but not recommended for home use given the multiple daily injections
VKA (ie, warfarin)	Dosed orally for goal INR 2–3	Yes	• Achieving and maintaining a therapeutic INR within 30–35 d can be challenging • Requires frequent INR testing to ensure therapeutic dosing • Multiple drug–drug and drug–food interactions exist
Aspirin	Doses vary, but typically 81–162 mg po once daily	No	• Increasingly used, possibly lower efficacy and lower bleeding risk than alternatives
DOACs	Apixaban 2.5 mg po bid Rivaroxaban 10 mg po once daily Dabigatran 220 mg po once daily	No	• Increasingly used despite limited data in hip fracture patients • Avoid dabigatran if creatinine clearance is <30 mL/min • ACCP 2012 guidelines: can be considered for patients who decline injections

Abbreviations: AAOS, American Academy of Orthopedic Surgeons; ACCP, American College of Chest Physicians; ASH, American Society of Hematology; FDA, US Food and Drug Administration; INR, international normalized ratio; NICE, National Institute of Clinical Excellence (UK); po, per os (by mouth); sc, subcutaneous.
a AAOS 2021 guidelines state there is insufficient evidence to recommend a specific agent (but mention aspirin, VKA, LMWH, and DOACs as considerations).

approach as studies (including a recent systematic review and meta-analysis) have shown DOACs do have equivalent efficacy and bleeding risk compared to LMWH in patients with hip fracture.[76]

Despite limited evidence, mechanical VTE prophylaxis is routinely administered in the hospital setting in addition to drug therapy. The duration of pharmacologic VTE prophylaxis is generally recommended for at least 1 month but preferably up to 35 days.

POSTOPERATIVE CARE AND CONSIDERATIONS
Physical Therapy

Although the ultimate goal of hip fracture surgery is to have the patient return to their prefracture level of function, this is achieved in less than half of patients.[11] Physical therapy initiated early in the postoperative period is paramount in order to maximize physical recovery. Clinical practice guidelines from the American Physical Therapy Association[77] recommend the following for older adults with hip fracture:

- Treatment in a multidisciplinary team that includes physical therapy and early mobilization.
- Daily inpatient physical therapy after hip fracture surgery with duration as tolerated.
- Assisted transfers out of bed and ambulation as soon as possible after surgery and continued at least daily thereafter (unless contraindicated by a medical or surgical reason)
- Additional therapies for several weeks/months after hospital discharge. These therapies should include strength, balance, functional, and gait training to address physical limitations and fall risk.

Pressure Ulcers

Pressure ulcers can lead to increased risk of infection, pain, and prolonged hospitalization. The incidence of pressure ulcers in patients with hip fracture ranges from 10% to 40%.[78] Factors that have been associated with an increased risk of pressure ulcers in hip fracture patients include[79,80]

- Longer wait times before surgery
- Intensive care unit stay
- Longer length of surgery
- General anesthesia
- Age greater than 80 years
- Length of time a urinary catheter was used
- Length of time pain was present

Frequent patient repositioning has been shown to reduce the risk of developing pressure ulcers in patients with hip fracture.[80]

Osteoporosis

Patients who sustain a low-energy hip fracture (ie, a fall from standing height) have osteoporosis.[81] The risk of hip fracture recurrence is high but can be reduced with effective treatment of the underlying osteoporosis. While calcium and vitamin D supplementation seem reasonable, specific amounts of recommended intake for patients with a fragility hip fracture are largely unknown. However, all patients with osteoporosis are advised to participate in regular weight-bearing activities and receive pharmacologic treatment.

Bisphosphonate therapy remains the mainstay of osteoporosis treatment and has been shown to improve outcomes in hip fracture patients in clinical trials. The landmark HORIZON trial was a randomized placebo-controlled trial of over 2100 patients with a low-trauma hip fracture.[82] Patients randomized to a once yearly infusion of zoledronic acid within 90 days of hip fracture repair had a 35% reduction in fracture recurrence and a 28% reduction in all-cause mortality at a median 1.9 year follow-up.

Despite ample data showing significant benefit from initiating early osteoporosis therapy in patients with hip fracture, treatment rates have been poor. A cohort study of over 97,000 patients with a fragility hip fracture demonstrated osteoporosis treatment rates decline from only 9.8% in 2004 to an abysmal 3.3% in 2015.[83] This illustrates the importance of inpatient providers (ie, orthopedic surgeons, hospitalists) to take steps ensuring their patients with hip fracture receive this important and evidence-based care. Solutions may include (1) clear communication with the patient's primary care provider to initiate osteoporosis treatment; (2) starting bisphosphonate therapy in the hospital or provide a prescription upon discharge; and (3) clearly documenting the diagnosis of osteoporosis in the patient's medical record. Many health systems have developed metabolic bone programs and/or clinics to ensure patients receive timely outpatient follow-up and treatment of fragility fractures.

DISCUSSION AND SUMMARY

Hip fractures are a frequent and increasing cause of hospitalizations in the elderly and are associated with significant morbidity including perioperative medical complications, reduced functional status, and significantly reduced life expectancy. Mortality rates have improved over time but remain high. Prompt diagnosis of hip fracture through clinical evaluation and imaging is imperative. Early surgical intervention (ideally within a day) is warranted in the vast majority of hip fractures to address pain, improve mobility, and reduce mortality. Surgical approach depends on fracture type, age, and baseline functioning. Delaying surgery for extensive preoperative testing or treatment is rarely necessary unless active severe medical problems are present. Shared decision-making on whether to proceed with surgery is particularly important for patients with life-limiting medical comorbidities, severe frailty, or advanced dementia. Anticoagulant use prior to hip fracture surgery may need to be addressed to reduce bleeding risk. Either general or neuraxial anesthesia can reasonably be utilized for hip fracture surgery with the ultimate decision at the discretion of the anesthesiologist. Important postoperative considerations for patients undergoing hip fracture surgery include appropriate VTE prophylaxis, early physical therapy interventions to improve mobility and functional status, and subsequent treatment of osteoporosis, which has been shown to reduce the risk of recurrent fractures and mortality.

CLINICS CARE POINTS

- Hip fractures, defined as fractures from the femoral head to 5 cm below the lesser trochanter are a major cause of morbidity in the elderly, with improving but still high associated mortality rates up to 20% to 25% at 1 year

- Diagnosis of hip fractures with urgent orthopedic consultation and early surgical intervention (ideally within a day) is associated with better outcomes compared to delayed surgery or nonoperative management

- Surgical delay should be limited to situations where active severe medical conditions make proceeding to surgery unsafe at that time

- Shared decision-making between providers and patients or their surrogates is particularly important in patients who are at high-risk for surgery or have significantly limited life expectancy due medical comorbidities, frailty, or advanced dementia

- The utilization of multidisciplinary treatment teams (surgical and medical) with surgical and medical providers is associated with reduced perioperative complications, time to surgery, and hospital length of stay

- Postoperative care for patients sustaining hip fracture should include VTE prophylaxis (though preferred chemoprophylactic agents vary by guideline), early physical therapy and subsequent treatment of osteoporosis

DISCLOSURE

The authors have nothing to disclose.

REFERENCES

1. Bhandari M, Swiontkowski M. Management of Acute Hip Fracture. N Engl J Med 2017;377:2053–62.
2. GBD 2019 Fracture Collaborators. Global, regional, and national burden of bone fractures in 204 countries and territories, 1990–2019: a systematic analysis from the Global Burden of Disease Study 2019. Lancet Health Long 2021;2(9):e580–92.
3. Williams SA, Chastek B, Sundquist K, et al. Economic burden of osteoporotic fractures in US managed care enrollees. Am J Manag Care 2020;26(5):e142–9.
4. Remily EA, Mohamed NS, Wilkie WA, et al. Hip fracture trends in america between 2009 and 2016. Geriatr Ortho Surg Rehab 2020;11:1–10.
5. Harvey N, Dennison E, Cooper C. Osteoporosis: impact on health and outcomes. Nat Rev Rheumatol 2010;6:99–105.
6. Sing C-W, Lin T-C, Bartholomew S, et al. Global epidemiology of hip fractures: secular trends in incidence rate, post-fracture treatment, and all-cause mortality. J Bone Min Res 2023;38(8):1064–75.
7. Tsang C, Bolton C, Burgon V, et al. Predicting 30 day mortality after hip fracture: evaluation of the national hip fracture database case-mix adjustment model. Bone Joint Res 2017;5(9):550–6.
8. Downey C, Kelly M, Quinlan JF. Changing trends in the mortality rate at 1-year post hip fracture - a systematic review. World J Orthop 2019;10(3):166–75.
9. Zuckerman JD. Hip fracture. N Engl J Med 1996;334:1519–25.
10. Leibson CL, Tosteson ANA, Gabriel SE, et al. Mortality, disability, and nursing home use for persons with and without hip fracture: a population-based study. J Am Geriatr Soc 2002;50:1644–50.
11. Dyer SM, Crotty M, Fairhall N, et al. A critical review of the long-term disability outcomes following hip fracture. BMC Geriatr 2016;16(1):158.
12. Thorell K, Ranstad K, Midlöv P, et al. Is use of fall risk-increasing drugs in an elderly population associated with an increased risk of hip fracture, after adjustment for multimorbidity level: a cohort study. BMC Geriatr 2014;4(14):131.
13. Johnston YA, Bergen G, Bauer M, et al. Implementation of the stopping elderly accidents, deaths, and injuries initiative in primary care: an outcome evaluation. Gerontol 2019;59(6):1182–91.
14. Waade RG, Molden E, Martinsen MI, et al. Psychotropics and weak opioid analgesics in plasma samples of older hip fracture patients – detection frequencies and consistency with drug records. Br J Clin Pharmacol 2017;83(6):1397–404.

15. Felson DT, Anderson JJ, Hannan MT, et al. Impaired vision and hip fracture. The Framingham Study. J Am Geriatr Soc 1989;37(6):495–500.

16. Haj-Mirzaian A, Eng J, Khorsani R, et al. Use of advanced imaging for radiographically occult hip fracture in elderly patients: a systematic review and meta-analysis. Radiology 2020;296(3):521–31.

17. Ross AB, Lee KS, Chang EY, et al. American college of radiology ACR appropriateness criteria: acute hip pain-suspected fracture. 2018. Available at: https://acsearch.acr.org/docs/3082587/Narrative.

18. American Academy of Orthopaedic Surgeons. Management of hip fractures in older adults: evidence-based clinical practice guideline. 2021. Available at: https://www.aaos.org/hipfxcpg.

19. Hoshino CM, O'Toole RV. Fixed angle devices versus multiple cancellous screws: what does the evidence tell us? Injury 2015;46(3):474–7.

20. Chammout GK, Mukka SS, Carlsson T, et al. Total hip replacement versus open reduction and internal fixation of displaced femoral neck fractures: a randomized long-term follow-up study. J Bone Joint Surg Am 2012;94(21):1921–8.

21. Bhandari M, Devereaux PJ, Swiontkowski MF, et al. Internal fixation compared with arthroplasty for displaced fractures of the femoral neck. A meta-analysis. J Bone Joint Surg Am 2003;85(9):1673–81.

22. National Institute for Health and Care Excellence (NICE). National clinical guideline centre. the management of hip fracture in adults. NICE Clinical Guidelines 2023;124. Available at: https://www.nice.org.uk/guidance/cg124/evidence/full-guideline-pdf-183081997.

23. Ahrengart L, Törnkvist H, Fornander P, et al. A randomized study of the compression hip screw and Gamma nail in 426 fractures. Clin Orthop Relat Res 2002;401: 209–22.

24. Parker MJ, Bowers TR, Pryor GA. Sliding hip screw versus the Targon PF nail in the treatment of trochanteric fractures of the hip: a randomised trial of 600 fractures. J Bone Joint Surg Br 2012;94(3):391–7.

25. Grønhaug KML, Dybvik E, Matre K, et al. Intramedullary nail versus sliding hip screw for stable and unstable trochanteric and subtrochanteric fractures : 17,341 patients from the Norwegian Hip Fracture Register. Bone Joint Lett J 2022; 104-B(2):274–82.

26. American Academy of Orthopedic Surgeons. Hip fracture in older adults: acute treatment. AAOS Appropriate Use Criteria 2023. Available at: https://www.orthoguidelines.org/go/auc/auc.cfm?auc_id=224954.

27. Berry SD, Rothbaum RR, Kiel DP, et al. Association and clinical outcomes with surgical repair of hip fracture vs nonsurgical management in nursing home residents with advanced dementia. JAMA Intern Med 2018;178(6):774–80.

28. Sullivan NM, Blake LE, George M, et al. Palliative care in the hip fracture patient. Geriatr Orthop Surg Rehabil 2019;10:1–7.

29. Ko FC, Morrison RS. Hip fracture: a trigger for palliative care in vulnerable older adults. JAMA Intern Med 2014;174(8):1281–2.

30. Loggers SAI, Willems HC, Van Balen R, et al. Evaluation of quality of life after nonoperative or operative management of proximal femoral fractures in frail institutionalized patients: the FRAIL-HIP study. JAMA Surg 2022;157(5):424–34.

31. van de Ree CLP, De Jongh MAC, Peeters CMM, et al. Hip fractures in elderly people: surgery or no surgery? a systematic review and meta-analysis. Geriatr Orthop Surg Rehabil 2017;8(3):173–80.

32. Shin ED, Sandhu KP, Wiseley BR, et al. Mortality rates after nonoperative geriatric hip fracture treatment: a matched cohort analysis. J Orthop Trauma 2023;37(5): 237–42.
33. Chlebeck JD, Birch CE, Blankstein M, et al. Nonoperative geriatric hip fracture treatment is associated with increased mortality: a matched cohort study. J Orthop Trauma 2019;33(7):346–50.
34. Simunovic N, Devereaux PJ, Sprague S, et al. Effect of early surgery after hip fracture on mortality and complications: systematic review and meta-analysis. Can Med Assoc J 2010;182(15):1609–16.
35. Pincus D, Ravi B, Wasserstein D, et al. Association between wait time and 30-day mortality in adults undergoing hip fracture surgery. JAMA 2017;318(20):1994–2003.
36. Fu MC, Boddapati V, Gausden EB, et al. Surgery for a fracture of the hip within 24 hours of admission is independently associated with reduced short-term postoperative complications. Bone Joint Lett J 2017; Sep;99-B(9):1216–22.
37. Vidán MT, Sánchez E, Gracia Y, et al. Causes and effects of surgical delay in patients with hip fracture: a cohort study. Ann Intern Med 2011;155(4):226–33.
38. Grimes JP, Gregory PM, Noveck H, et al. The effects of time-to-surgery on mortality and morbidity in patients following hip fracture. Am J Med 2002;112(9): 702–9.
39. Orosz GM, Magaziner J, Hannan EL, et al. Association of timing of surgery for hip fracture and patient outcomes. JAMA 2004;291(14):1738–43.
40. ATTACK Investigators HIP. Accelerated surgery versus standard care in hip fracture (HIP ATTACK): an international, randomised, controlled trial. Lancet 2020; 395(10225):698–708.
41. Sharma G, Kuo Y-F, Freeman J, et al. Comanagement of hospitalized surgical patients by medicine physicians in the United States. Arch Intern Med 2010;170(4): 363–8.
42. Rohatgi N, Weng Y, Kittle J, et al. Merits of surgical comanagement of patients with hip fracture by dedicated orthopaedic hospitalists. J Am Acad Orthop Surg Glob Res Rev 2021;5(3):e2000231.
43. Roy A, Heckman MG, Roy V. Associations between the hospitalist model of care and quality-of-care-related outcomes in patients undergoing hip fracture surgery. Mayo Clin Proc 2006;81(1):28–31.
44. Swart E, Kates S, McGee S, et al. The case for comanagement and care pathways for osteoporotic patients with a hip fracture. J Bone Joint Surg Am 2018; 100(15):1343–50.
45. Prestmo A, Hagen G, Sletvold O, et al. Comprehensive geriatric care for patients with hip fractures: a prospective, randomised, controlled trial. Lancet 2015; 385(9978):1623–33.
46. Swart E, Vasudeva BS, Makhni EC, et al. Dedicated perioperative hip fracture comanagement programs are cost-effective in high-volume centers: An economic analysis. Clin Orthop Relat Res 2016 Jan;474(1):222–3.
47. Maxwell BG, Mirza A. Medical comanagement of hip fracture patients is not associated with superior perioperative outcomes: a propensity score-matched retrospective cohort analysis of the national surgical quality improvement project. J Hosp Med 2020;15(8):468–74.
48. Batsis JA, Phy MP, Melton LJ, et al. Effects of a hospitalist care model on mortality of elderly patients with hip fractures. J Hosp Med 2007;2(4):219–25.
49. Mazzarello S, McIsaac DI, Montroy J, et al. Postoperative shared-care for patients undergoing non-cardiac surgery: a systematic review and meta-analysis. Can J Anaesth 2019;66(9):1095–105.

50. Hossain FS, Rambani R, Ribee H, et al. Is discontinuation of clopidogrel necessary for intracapsular hip fracture surgery? Analysis of 102 hemiarthroplasties. J Orthop Traumatol 2013;14(3):171–7.

51. Chechik O, Amar E, Khashan M, et al. In support of early surgery for hip fractures sustained by elderly patients taking clopidogrel: a retrospective study. Drugs Aging 2012;29(1):63–8.

52. Mattesi L, Noailles T, Rosencher N, et al. Discontinuation of plavix® (clopidogrel) for hip fracture surgery. A systematic review of the literature. Orthop Traumatol Surg Res 2016;102(8):1097–101.

53. Lu W, Yon DK, Lee SW, et al. Safety of early surgery in hip fracture patients taking clopidogrel and/or aspirin: a systematic review and meta-analysis. J Arthroplasty 2023;S0883:5403.

54. Brox WT, Roberts KC, Taksali S, et al. The American academy of orthopaedic surgeons evidence-based guideline on management of hip fractures in the elderly. J Bone Joint Surg Am 2015;97(14):1196–9.

55. Douketis JD, Spyropoulos AC, Murad MH, et al. Perioperative management of antithrombotic therapy: an american college of chest physicians clinical practice guideline. Chest 2022;162(5):e207–43.

56. White NJ, Reitzel SL, Doyle-Baker D, et al. Management of patients with hip fracture receiving anticoagulation: What are we doing in Canada? Can J Surg 2021; 64(5):E510–5.

57. Hornor MA, Duane TM, Ehlers AP, et al. American college of surgeons' guidelines for the perioperative management of antithrombotic medication. J Am Coll Surg 2018;227(5):521–36.

58. Spyropoulos AC, Douketis JD. How I treat anticoagulated patients undergoing an elective procedure or surgery. Blood 2012;120(15):2954–62.

59. Chai-Adisaksopha C, Hillis C, Siegal DM, et al. Prothrombin complex concentrates versus fresh frozen plasma for warfarin reversal. A systematic review and meta-analysis. Thromb Haemostasis 2016;116(5):879–90.

60. Moores TS, Beaven A, Cattell AE, et al. Preoperative warfarin reversal for early hip fracture surgery. J Orthop Surg 2015;23(1):33–6.

61. Ahmed I, Khan MA, Nayak V, et al. An evidence-based warfarin management protocol reduces surgical delay in hip fracture patients. J Orthop Traumatol 2014; 15(1):21–7.

62. You D, Xu Y, Krzyzaniak H, et al. Safety of expedited-surgery protocols in anticoagulant-treated patients with hip fracture: a systematic review and meta-analysis. Can J Surg 2023;66(2):E170–80.

63. Douketis JD, Spyropoulos AC, Kaatz S, et al. Perioperative bridging anticoagulation in patients with atrial fibrillation. N Engl J Med 2015;373(9):823–33.

64. Schuetze K, Eickhoff A, Dehner C, et al. Impact of oral anticoagulation on proximal femur fractures treated within 24 h - A retrospective chart review. Injury 2019; 50(11):2040–4.

65. Alcock HMF, Nayar SK, Moppett IK. Reversal of direct oral anticoagulants in adult hip fracture patients. A systematic review and meta-analysis. Injury 2021;52(11): 3206–16.

66. You D, Xu Y, Ponich B, et al. Effect of oral anticoagulant use on surgical delay and mortality in hip fracture. Bone Joint Lett J 2021;103-B(2):222–33.

67. Praxbind® (idaricizumab). Package insert. Boehringer-Ingelheim; 2021. Available at: https://www.accessdata.fda.gov/drugsatfda_docs/label/2015/761025 lbl.pdf.

68. ANDEXXA® (coagulation factor Xa (recombinant), inactivated-zhzo), 2023, Astra-Zeneca. Available at: https://www.fda.gov/media/113279/download?attachment.
69. Majeed A, Ågren A, Holmström M, et al. Management of rivaroxaban- or apixaban-associated major bleeding with prothrombin complex concentrates: a cohort study. Blood 2017;130(15):1706–12.
70. Song Y, Wang Z, Perlstein I, et al. Reversal of apixaban anticoagulation by four-factor prothrombin complex concentrates in healthy subjects: a randomized three-period crossover study. J Thromb Haemostasis 2017;15(11):2125–37.
71. Neuman MD, Feng R, Carson JL, et al. Spinal anesthesia or general anesthesia for hip surgery in older adults. N Engl J Med 2021;385(22):2025–35.
72. Li T, Li J, Yuan L, et al. Effect of regional vs general anesthesia on incidence of postoperative delirium in older patients undergoing hip fracture surgery: the RAGA randomized trial. JAMA 2022;327(1):50–8.
73. Falck-Ytter Y, Francis CW, Johanson NA, et al. Prevention of VTE in orthopedic surgery patients. antithrombotic therapy and prevention of thrombosis, 9th ed. american college of chest physicians evidence-based clinical practice guidelines. Chest 2012;141(2):e278S–325S.
74. Anderson DR, Morgano GP, Bennett C, et al. American Society of Hematology 2019 guidelines for management of venous thromboembolism: prevention of venous thromboembolism in surgical hospitalized patients. Blood Adv 2019; 3(23):3898–944.
75. National Institute for Health Care and Clinical Excellence. Venous thromboembolism in over 16s: reducing the risk of hospital-acquired deep vein thrombosis or pulmonary embolism. NICE Guideline 2019. Available at: https://www.nice.org.uk/guidance/ng89.
76. Nederpelt CH, Bijman Q, Krijnen P, et al. Equivalence of DOACs and LMWH for thromboprophylaxis after hip fracture surgery: systemic review and meta-analysis. Injury 2022;53(3):1169–76.
77. McDonough CM, Harris-Hayes M, Kristensen MT, et al. Physical therapy management of older adults with hip fracture: clinical practice guidelines linked to the international classification of functioning, disability and health from the academy of orthopaedic physical therapy and the academy of geriatric physical therapy of the american physical therapy association. J Orthop Sports Phys Ther 2021; 51(2):CPG1–81.
78. Beaupre LA, Jones CA, Saunders LD, et al. Best practices for elderly hip fracture patients. A systematic overview of the evidence. J Gen Intern Med 2005;20(11): 1009–25.
79. Baumgarten M, Margolis D, Berlin JA, et al. Risk factors for pressure ulcers among elderly hip fracture patients. Wound Repair Regen 2003;11(2):96–103.
80. Chiari P, Forni C, Guberti M, et al. Predictive factors for pressure ulcers in an older adult population hospitalized for hip fractures: a prognostic cohort study. PLoS One 2017;12(1):e0169909.
81. Siris ES, Adler R, Bilezikian J, et al. The clinical diagnosis of osteoporosis: a position statement from the National Bone Health Alliance Working Group. Osteoporos Int 2014;25(5):1439–43.
82. Lyles KW, Colon-Emeric CS, Magaziner JS, et al. Zoledronic acid in reducing clinical fracture and mortality after hip fracture. N Engl J Med 2007;357(18): 1799–809.
83. Desai RJ, Mahesri M, Abdia Y, et al. Association of osteoporosis medication use after hip fracture with prevention of subsequent nonvertebral fractures: an instrumental variable analysis. JAMA Netw Open 2018;1(3):e180826.

Approach to Patients with Cancer Going to Surgery

Win M. Aung, MD, DM, MBA, FRCP[a],*, Sunil K. Sahai, MD, SFHM[b,1]

KEYWORDS

- Preoperative evaluation • Perioperative medicine • Cancer • Surgery
- Chemotherapy • Radiation therapy • Anesthesia

KEY POINTS

- Physical deconditioning of patients with cancer is multifactorial cardiac, pulmonary disease, and/or the cancer itself.
- Oncology surgical procedures are time sensitive. Preoperative care in a multidisciplinary approach to optimize the patient's medical, functional, emotional, and nutritional optimization is essential for the best possible outcome. Timing of surgery should be balanced with patients' optimization.
- Neoadjuvant chemotherapy and radiation therapy has an impact on multiple organ systems. Regular monitoring, targeted testing, and supportive care, and medical optimization toward recovery are the goals.
- Goal-directed medical therapy is indicated for chronic medical conditions.

INTRODUCTION

The journey of an oncology patient undergoing surgery begins with meticulous preoperative care. This phase is critical for assessing and optimizing the patient's overall health, managing comorbidities, and tailoring surgical plans to maximize success while minimizing complications. Curative radical surgery or palliative symptomatic relief procedures need timely medical optimization to improve outcomes. In addition to pre-existing medical conditions, nutrition, functional status, and effects of concurrent neoadjuvant chemotherapy, radiation therapy, and immunotherapy should be considered. This article will focus specifically on the care of preoperative patients with cancer. Routine preoperative care of noncardiac surgery is described elsewhere.[1,2]

[a] Department of Medicine, University of Florida School of Medicine, UF Health, 653 West 8th Street, Jacksonville, FL 32209, USA; [b] Division of General Internal Medicine, Department of Medicine, The University of Texas Medical Branch, 4.174 John Sealy Annex, 301 University Boulevard, Galveston, TX 77550, USA
[1] Present address. 4523 Royal Bend Lane, Sugar Land, TX 77479.
* Corresponding author. UF Health, Faculty Clinic #3036; 653 West 8th Street, Jacksonville, FL 32209.
E-mail address: win.aung@jax.ufl.edu

Med Clin N Am 108 (2024) 1171–1183
https://doi.org/10.1016/j.mcna.2024.04.006   medical.theclinics.com
0025-7125/24/© 2024 Elsevier Inc. All rights reserved.

MULTIDISCIPLINARY ASSESSMENT

Oncology surgical procedures are typically time sensitive, and some of the patients' concurrent changes in clinical status after neoadjuvant therapy can be optimized. Patients with cancer face unique physiologic challenges in the perioperative period that impact their physical fitness for surgery. From side effects from treatment to medical comorbidities to cancer disease symptoms, patients with cancer are at risk for physical deconditioning[3] (**Fig. 1**). Anticipatory and supportive care rather than unnecessary testing to verify the functional decline could delay time-sensitive surgery. The preoperative assessment of oncology patients necessitates a collaborative effort involving surgeons, medical oncologists, radiation oncologists, anesthesiologists, psychotherapists, nutritionists, primary care physicians, hospitalists, and physical therapists. An analysis by Soones and colleagues showed that preoperative internal medicine consultation for patients with cancer was associated with a reduction in 30 day postoperative mortality.[4] Palliative care assessment and goals of care, including nonsurgical options, should be discussed, especially if the disease burden is increased. This multidisciplinary approach ensures a comprehensive understanding of the patient's cancer history, treatment course, current status, and wishes. The team should address patients' concerns, expectations, risk–benefit trade-offs, and effective communication with simple language to fit the patient's health literacy. Integrating these perspectives allows for a tailored preoperative plan that addresses the cancer and the patient's overall health.

Cardiovascular System

Oncology patients often present with cardiovascular challenges due to the effects of cancer and previous treatments. The debility of an oncology patient leading to poor exercise tolerance should not be attributed to pre-existing cardiac disease alone. In addition to pre-existing cardiovascular disease, poor functional status may be due

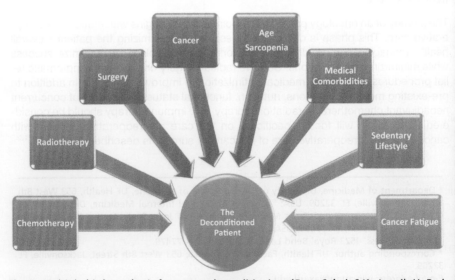

Fig. 1. Multiple hit hypothesis for cancer deconditioning. (*From* Sahai, S.K., Ismail, H. Perioperative Implications of Neoadjuvant Therapies and Optimization Strategies for Cancer Surgery. *Curr Anesthesiol Rep* 5, 305–317 (2015). https://doi.org/10.1007/s40140-015-0121-x with permission.)

to physical deconditioning from the cancer itself. In addition, the perioperative clinician should be aware of side effects from treatment that may compromise cardiac function. Common chemotherapeutic agents affecting cardiac function are summarized in **Table 1** Side effects of chemotherapeutic agents include left ventricular systolic dysfunction, endothelial damage, systemic hypertension, vasospastic and thromboembolic ischemic myocardial injury, arrhythmias, and QT interval (QT) prolongation.[5] Anthracycline agents such as doxorubicin, daunorubicin, epirubicin, and mitoxantrone are well documented to cause direct and nonreversible myocardial injury. Myocardial toxicity can be observed within 1 to 3 days after administration of chemotherapy, manifested as pericarditis or myocarditis[6] or late-onset heart failure as restrictive or dilated cardiomyopathy after 1 year.[7] Pyrimidine analogs such as 5-fluorouracil and capecitabine may cause coronary spastic-induced ischemia.[8] Alkylating agents such as cyclophosphamide may cause myocarditis.[9] There are reports of corrected QT (QTc) prolongation after the use of conventional chemotherapy, such as arsenic trioxide, vadimezan, and capecitabine, in up to 20% of patients. However, there is no report of fetal arrhythmia.[10] Cisplatin, primarily used for gastric cancer, has a significant number of both venous (62.7%) and arterial (15.6%) thrombosis.[11] Microtubule inhibitors such as paclitaxel, docetaxel, and cabazitaxel can be cardiotoxic in up to 2.3% to 8% of patients, causing bradycardia and autonomic dysfunction.[11] The degree of damage and reversibility depends on anthracyclines versus nonanthracyclines, the presence or absence of risk factors (pre-existing heart disease, hypertension, and extreme age), cumulative dose, and combination chemotherapy.[3]

Perioperative cardiac risk assessment should be evidence based and follow a structured pathway (**Fig. 2**). Proper cardiac risk stratification, regular monitoring of electrocardiogram (ECG), troponin, and pro-B-type natriuretic peptide, scheduled noninvasive cardiac monitoring such as limited echocardiogram to assess left ventricular function, concurrent use of cardioprotective agents such as dexrazoxane and angiotensin-converting enzyme inhibitors (ACEIs) are recommended to optimize the patient preoperatively. A retrospective cohort study of over 35,000 newly diagnosed patients with esophageal and gastric cancer using ACEI/angiotensin receptor blockers (ARBs) was associated with significantly lower mortality.[12] Along with cardiac protection, the additional effects of inhibiting tumor angiogenesis and proliferation may also be beneficial.

Pulmonary System

Radiation-induced pneumonitis is common (33.3%) in patients who received radiation either by conventional or stereotactic approach.[13] Pulmonary complications after chemotherapy are often challenging to clinicians due to the probability of multifactorial components such as typical and atypical (fungal, *Pneumocystis jirovecii*, mycobacterial) pneumonia, pulmonary thromboembolism, metastasis, and direct lung injury from chemotherapy. Chemotherapy-induced lung injury can be acute, such as pneumonitis, diffuse alveolar hemorrhage, nonspecific interstitial pneumonia, capillary leak syndrome (acute respiratory distress syndrome [ARDS]), and cryptogenic organizing pneumonia. Late effects of treatment may manifest as pulmonary fibrosis and/or pulmonary hypertension. A careful clinical assessment along with computed tomography (CT) imaging will help to differentiate among the common radio pathologic patterns.[14] Pulmonary function tests should not be a routine preoperative evaluation for noncardiac surgery (NCS) and should be reserved for patients scheduled for lung resection.[15] Chemotherapeutic agents affecting pulmonary function are summarized in **Table 2**. Bleomycin-induced lung injury is usually dose-dependent and can occur in 6% to 10% of patients.[16] Most acute lung injuries are self-limited and nonfatal; however,

Table 1
Common chemotherapeutic agents affecting cardiac function

Therapeutic Class	Agent	Effect
Anthracyclines	Daunorubicin, doxorubicin, epirubicin, idarubicin, valrubicin, and mitoxantrone	Direct myocardial injury
Pyrimidine analog	5-Fluorouracil and capecitabine	Coronary spasm/ischemia
Alkylating agents	Cyclophosphamide	Myocarditis
Antiangiogenic	Combretastatin and vadimezan	QT prolongation
Antimetabolites	Capecitabine	—
Other	Arsenic trioxide	—
Platinum	Cisplatin	Thrombosis
Angiogenesis inhibitors	Bevacizumab, sunitinib, and sorafenib	Arterial hypertension
Taxanes	Paclitaxel and docetaxel	Bradyarrhythmia Autonomic dysfunction

diffuse alveolar hemorrhage, pulmonary hemorrhage, and ARDS can be life threatening. Limited oxygen supplementation during surgery,[17] titrated usage of intravenous hydration to avoid fluid overload, and judicious use of preoperative lung expansion maneuvers have been proposed to enhance pulmonary outcomes.

Renal System

Patients with malignancy are at risk for sepsis, tumor lysis, and poor par oral (PO) intake that may affect kidney function. Along with the use of nephrotoxic chemotherapeutic agents, pre-existing chronic kidney disease and diabetes lead to the development of worsening renal function. Hypercalcemia was observed in 20% to 30% of malignancies and may have a compounded effect on kidney injury.[18] The highest risk of renal injury occurs in patients with renal cancer, multiple myeloma, leukemia, and posthematopoietic stem cell transplant.[19] Common chemotherapeutic agents affecting renal function are summarized in **Table 3**. Bevacizumab and other angiogenesis inhibitors may cause renal injury by thrombotic microangiopathy (TMA) along with concomitant accelerated hypertension. A pyrimidine analog, gemcitabine, infrequently causes TMA.[20] Interferon (IFN) alpha is used to treat patients with chronic myeloid leukemia, often associated with minimal change and focal segmental glomerulosclerosis.[18]

Management of patients with chemotherapy-induced acute kidney injury (AKI) is primarily supportive of careful monitoring of strict intake output and fluid management. Monitoring electrolytes and daily assessment of hydration, along with bedside inferior vena cava assessment, can be useful. Low magnesium level is associated with AKI in critically ill patients, and prophylactic magnesium infusion in major cancer surgery perioperatively may improve estimated glomerular filtration rate (eGFR) after surgery.[21]

Gastrointestinal System

Nausea and vomiting associated with chemotherapy is a well-known side effect. It can be observed in up to 60% to 80% of patients.[22] Treatment is primarily anticipated and

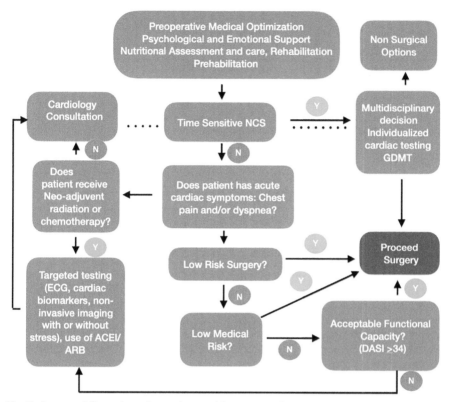

Fig. 2. Proposed flow sheet for patients with cancer going to surgery. ACEI, Angiotensin converting enzyme inhibitor; ARB, angiotensin receptor blocker; DASI, Duke Activity Status Index; ECG, electrocardiogram; GDMT, Goal-directed medical therapy, NCS, noncardiac surgery.

supportive care. Pre-emptively treatment with dexamethasone, 5-HT3 receptor antagonists such as ondansetron, palonosetron, and olanzapine added in the early days of chemotherapy (days 2–4) achieved effective relief of symptoms in 79% of patients.[23]

Table 2
Common chemotherapeutic agents affecting pulmonary function

Therapeutic Class	Agent	Effect
Folate antagonist	Methotrexate	Eosinophilic pneumonia Hypersensitivity pneumonitis Pulmonary edema, pleural effusion
Nitrogen mustards	Cyclophosphamide	Pulmonary hemorrhage (high dose) Pulmonary fibrosis
Antibiotic	Bleomycin	Eosinophilic pneumonia Cryptogenic organizing pneumonia Diffuse alveolar hemorrhage Pulmonary fibrosis
Angiogenesis inhibitor	Bevacizumab	Diffuse alveolar hemorrhage
Taxanes	Paclitaxel, docetaxel	Interstitial infiltrates

Table 3
Common chemotherapeutic agents affecting renal function

Therapeutic Class	Agent	Effect
Angiogenesis inhibitor	Bevacizumab, axitinib, sorafenib, and sunitinib	TMA
Pyridine analog	Gemcitabine	—
Immunomodulator	INFs	Glomerulopathies
Bisphosphonates	Pamidronate and zoledronate	—
Folate antagonist	Methotrexate	Crystalline-induced AKI
Platinum containing compound	Cisplatin and carboplatin	Interstitial nephritis
Alkylating agent	Ifosfamide	—
Anthracycline	Adriamycin	—
Anaplastic lymphoma kinase inhibitor	Crizotinib	—

Diarrhea is another common gastrointestinal (GI) side effect of chemotherapy, especially with regimens including 5-fluorouracil and irinotecan.[24] Immune checkpoint inhibitors (ICIs) are also associated with diarrhea in 19% to 50% of the patients.[25] The use of loperamide in mild diarrhea and somatostatin analog, octreotide, in severe diarrhea is generally recommended along with intravenous (IV) hydration therapy. The use of budesonide, probiotics, or antibiotic therapy for chemotherapy-induced diarrhea has not been proven beneficial.[26]

Chemotherapy-induced neutropenia occasionally leads to bacterial overgrowth and invasion of the cecal wall, leading to typhlitis.[27] The patient experienced right lower quadrant abdominal pain with fever, and a CT scan showed localized cecal wall thickening with fat strands with or without abscess formation. Bowel rest, IV fluids, and broad-spectrum antibiotics are the standards of care, and surgical consultation is recommended. Colonoscopy is contraindicated.

Immunotherapy-induced hepatitis occurs between 5% and 10% of the patient. [28] Incidence can be higher in patients receiving combination immunotherapy. Diagnosis is made after the exclusion of other possible etiologies. Treatment is usually supportive care for mild cases, and high-dose corticosteroids are needed for grade 3 to 4 hepatitis.[29] Immunotherapy should be discontinued permanently in those circumstances.

Hematological System

Anemia is common in patients with cancer, and supportive nutritional care along with oral iron and vitamin supplements before surgery is a standard of care. In contrast to popular belief, parenteral iron therapy was neither associated with a timely rise of hemoglobin before surgery nor reduced the likelihood of blood transfusion in patients with iron deficiency anemia.[30]

Patients with leukopenia have traditionally been considered as poor surgical candidates. However, a retrospective cohort study using National Surgical Quality Improvement Program (NSQIP) data based on the 4369 patients who received chemotherapy before surgery including 20.2% who had leukopenia is not associated with increased mortality or morbidity.[31] Usual neutropenic precautions should be exercised.

Thrombocytopenia is a frequent finding in patients with cancer, either due to the disease process or secondary to chemotherapeutic agents. Platelet counts over 50,000/μL are considered adequate for most surgical procedures. Platelet transfusion is the mainstay therapy for severe chemotherapy-induced thrombocytopenia. Prophylactic antifibrinolytic therapy, such as tranexamic acid, does not influence the bleeding outcome.[32] The role of epsilon-aminocaproic acid, the other antifibrinolytic agent, versus prophylactic platelet transfusion to prevent bleeding in patients with hematological malignancies (the PROBLEMA trial) is still ongoing.[33] Changes in anticoagulation and antiplatelet management is recommended when platelets are less than 50,000/μL.[34]

Targeted Therapies

In the last several years, the introduction of molecular targeted immunotherapy as a treatment of cancer has transformed cancer care. ICIs/blockers leverage the body's immune system to attack cancerous cells. Monoclonal antibodies and other targeted agents may have side effects with perioperative implications, mostly in terms of an immune-related adverse effect (IRAE). IRAEs are a consequence of immunomodulation by these agents and usually manifest as inflammation and autoimmune reactions. In general, adverse effects are temporally related to the last dose administered. If IRAEs are suspected, consultation with the treating oncologist is recommended. Treatment of severe effects usually requires high-dose steroids and supervision by the treating oncologist.

Patients who receive chimeric antigen receptor T (CAR-T) cell immunotherapy are at risk for cytokine release syndrome and other neurotoxicities in the immediate treatment period[35] (**Fig. 3**[36]). Since CAR-T treatments are usually confined to comprehensive cancer centers, they have the expertise to address these adverse effects. The perioperative clinician should be aware of the late effects of cytokine release syndrome, including neurotoxicity, steroid-induced myopathy (deconditioning), and cardiovascular complications (cardiomyopathy and dysrhythmias) and investigate as needed.

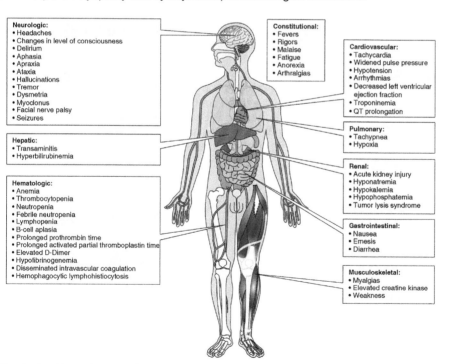

Fig. 3. Cytokine release syndrome.

NUTRITIONAL ASSESSMENT AND SUPPORT

Malnutrition is a common concern in oncology patients, ranging from 10% to 85% of patients,[37] impacting both treatment response and surgical outcomes. Wasting of muscle mass (sarcopenia) was associated with an increased risk of complications after GI tumor resection.[38] Nutritional assessment and support are integral to preoperative care, involving strategies such as dietary counseling, enteral or parenteral nutrition, and vitamin supplementation. Enteral nutrition is the preferred mode of therapy, and parenteral nutrition should be reserved for patients with poor GI tolerance. European Society of Clinical Nutrition and Metabolism (ESPEN) recommends taking 800 mL of carbohydrate drinks the night before surgery and 400 mL 2 hours before surgery instead of traditional overnight fasting. It does not increase the risk of aspiration, reduces preoperative discomfort and anxiety, and reduces the length of stay (LOS).[39] ESPEN also recommends early resumption of oral clear liquid intake, demonstrating no increased risk of impaired healing on the anastomosis, rather than enhancing postoperative recovery and improving infection rate. Parenteral nutrition should be reserved for patients who do not tolerate oral or enteral feeds for 7 days. Optimizing nutritional status reduces the risk of postoperative complications and supports the body's healing ability. Nutritional therapy support with greater than 25 kcal/kg (ideal body weight) per day for at least 10 days is recommended for patients with malnutrition (weight loss >10%–15% in 6 months, body mass index < 18.5 kg/m^2, Subjective Global Assessment grade C, nutritional risk screening >5, and serum albumin <30 g/L).[40]

Functional Status

Patient function status declined generally in patients with malignancy. Physical deconditioning of patients with cancer is multifactorial. In addition to a catabolic state, premorbid medical conditions, concurrent radiation, chemotherapy, pain associated with malignancy, and depression may all contribute to progressive functional decline (see **Fig. 1**). Several risk stratification methods are available to access the quantitative functional status. Metabolic equivalents less than 4 are an established landmark as poor functional capacity. Duke Activity Status Index (DASI) less than 34 is associated with poor cardiac outcome.[41] A cardiopulmonary exercise test (CPET) is an easily accessible office-based test and can guide prehabilitation.[42] The Eastern Cooperative Oncology Group and Palliative Performance Scale questionnaire have subjective assessments. The incremental shuttle walk test uses the cutoff distance of 250 m to predict postoperative morbidity, and the 6 minute walk test provides objective value when CPET is not readily available.[43]

Psychological and Emotional Support

The psychological and emotional well-being of oncology patients is paramount in the preoperative phase. As many as 40% of patients with cancer experience significant emotional and social stress during treatment.[44] Patients have a certain level of anxiety in general. However, preoperative anxiety and depression are associated with poor presurgical health status, postoperative pain, and functional recovery.[45] Psychosocial assessments, counseling, and support groups can help alleviate anxiety, depression, and fears associated with surgery. Integrating mental health services into preoperative care enhances patient resilience, coping mechanisms, and overall satisfaction with their care.

Prehabilitation Programs

Structured prehabilitation programs, encompassing physical exercise, nutritional guidance, and psychological support, have demonstrated benefits in improving functional capacity and reducing postoperative complications. Engaging in an active physical activity program before surgery improves overall clinical outcomes. Integrating prehabilitation into the preoperative care pathway prepares patients for surgery, enhancing their physical and mental resilience. Aerobic exercise combined with inspiratory muscle training is safe and effective in improving functional status, tolerating surgery, and adjuvant therapy,[46] and reducing the length of hospital stay.

Postoperative Care

Enhanced Recovery After Surgery guidelines are available and tailored to specific surgical procedures.[47] Cancer surgery-specific enhanced recovery protocols have shown to improve outcomes.[48–50] The goals of postoperative care are to decrease metabolic and inflammatory stress, obtain adequate pain control, start early enteral feeding, early removal of drainage tube, early mobilization, shorten hospital LOS, and to hasten the return to normal function. Adequate pain control is crucial to promote mobilization. Opioid medication should be minimized, especially in elderly patients and those with poor renal and hepatic clearance. Acetaminophen, cyclooxygenase 2 (COX2) inhibitors, in combination with gabapentinoids has shown significant pain relief.[51] ESPEN provided a strong consensus about initiating PO clear liquid within an hour after surgery.[39] Introducing clear fluid in postoperative day, one does not cause impairment of GI anastomosis healing[52] and leads to significantly reduced LOS.[53] Pharmacologic anxiolytics such as benzodiazepine should be avoided. The American Society of Clinical Oncology recommends pharmacologic thromboprophylaxis for up to 4 weeks in patients undergoing major abdominal surgery in patients with malignancy.[54]

CLINICS CARE POINTS

- Oncology surgical procedures are time sensitive. Preoperative care is a multidisciplinary approach to optimize the patient's medical, functional, emotional, and nutritional optimization is essential for the best possible outcome. The timing of surgery should be balanced with patients' optimization.

- Physical deconditioning of patients with cancer is multifactorial.

- Neoadjuvant chemotherapy and radiation therapy have an impact on multisystems. Regular monitoring, targeted testing, supportive care, and medical optimization toward recovery are the goals.

- Use of ACEI/ARBs showed added benefit in the overall survival of patients with concurrent cardiovascular pathology.

- Careful clinical evaluation along with CT imaging will help to differentiate common pulmonary pathology in oncology patients.

- Adequate hydration, adjusting the rate of chemotherapy, and correction of magnesium level enhance eGFR after surgery.

- Neutropenic patients may proceed with standard precautions.

- Limiting nothing par oral (NPO) time and encouraging early oral intake enhances postoperative recovery.

SUMMARY

The preoperative care of oncology patients is a dynamic and complex process that requires a holistic and individualized approach. Collaboration among health care professionals, optimization of cardiovascular and pulmonary function, nutritional support, psychological well-being, and the integration of prehabilitation programs are essential components of a successful preoperative care strategy. By addressing the unique needs of oncology patients before surgery, health care providers can contribute significantly to improved surgical outcomes and enhanced quality of life for these individuals.

REFERENCES

1. Fleisher LA, Fleischmann KE, Auerbach AD, et al, American College of Cardiology, American Heart Association. 2014 ACC/AHA guideline on perioperative cardiovascular evaluation and management of patients undergoing noncardiac surgery: a report of the American College of Cardiology/American Heart Association Task Force on practice guidelines. J Am Coll Cardiol 2014;64(22):e77.

2. Halvorsen S, Mehilli J, Cassese S, et al. 2022 ESC Guidelines on cardiovascular assessment and management of patients undergoing non-cardiac surgery. Eur Heart J 2022;43(39). https://doi.org/10.1093/eurheartj/ehac270.

3. Sahai SK, Ismail H. Perioperative implications of neoadjuvant therapies and optimization strategies for cancer surgery. Current Anesthesiology Reports 2015; 5(3):305–17.

4. Soones TN, Guo A, Foreman JT, et al. Preoperative internal medicine evaluation is associated with a reduction in 30-day postoperative mortality risk in patients with cancer. Perioperative Care and Operating Room Management 2022;26:100240.

5. Magnano LC, Martínez Cibrian N, Andrade González X, et al. Cardiac complications of chemotherapy: role of prevention. Curr Treat Options Cardiovasc Med 2014;16(6). https://doi.org/10.1007/s11936-014-0312-7.

6. Hagberg CA, Nates JL, Riedel BP, et al. Perioperative care of the cancer patient E-book. 1st edition. UK: Elsevier Health Sciences; 2022. p. 46–55.

7. Wilkinson EL, Sidaway JE, Cross MJ. Cardiotoxic drugs Herceptin and doxorubicin inhibit cardiac microvascular endothelial cell barrier formation, resulting in increased drug permeability. Biology Open 2016;5(10):1362–70.

8. Suter TM, Ewer MS. Cancer drugs and the heart: importance and management. Eur Heart J 2013;34(15):1102–11.

9. Dhesi S, Chu MP, Blevins G, et al. Cyclophosphamide-Induced Cardiomyopathy. Journal of Investigative Medicine High Impact Case Reports 2013;1(1). 232470961348034.

10. Porta-Sánchez A, Gilbert C, Spears D, et al. Incidence, diagnosis, and management of qt prolongation induced by cancer therapies: a systematic review. J Am Heart Assoc 2017;6(12). https://doi.org/10.1161/jaha.117.007724.

11. Storozynsky E. Multimodality assessment and treatment of chemotherapy-induced cardiotoxicity. Future Cardiol 2015;11(4):421–4.

12. Li PC, Huang RY, Yang YC, et al. Prognostic impact of angiotensin-converting enzyme inhibitors and angiotensin receptors blockers in esophageal or gastric cancer patients with hypertension - a real-world study. BMC Cancer 2022;22:430.

13. Cousin F, Desir C, Ben Mustapha S, et al. Incidence, risk factors, and CT characteristics of radiation recall pneumonitis induced by immune checkpoint inhibitor in lung cancer. Radiother Oncol 2021;157:47–55.

14. Dhamija E, Meena P, Ramalingam V, et al. Chemotherapy-induced pulmonary complications in cancer: Significance of clinicoradiological correlation. Indian J Radiol Imag 2020;30(01):20–6.

15. Brunelli A, Kim AW, Berger KI, et al. Physiologic evaluation of the patient with lung cancer being considered for resectional surgery: Diagnosis and management of

lung cancer, 3rd ed: American College of Chest Physicians evidence-based clinical practice guidelines. Chest 2013 May;143(5 Suppl):e166S–90S. Erratum in: Chest. 2014 Feb;145(2):437.

16. Keijzer A, Kuenen B. Fatal pulmonary toxicity in testis cancer with bleomycin-containing chemotherapy. J Clin Oncol 2007;25(23):3543–4.

17. Goldiner PL, Schweizer O. The hazards of anesthesia and surgery in bleomycin-treated patients. PubMed 1979;6(1):121–4.

18. Rosner MH, Dalkin AC. Onco-nephrology: the pathophysiology and treatment of malignancy-associated hypercalcemia. Clin J Am Soc Nephrol 2012;7(10): 1722–9.

19. Salahudeen AK, Doshi SM, Pawar T, et al. Incidence rate, clinical correlates, and outcomes of AKI in patients admitted to a comprehensive cancer center. Clin J Am Soc Nephrol 2013;8:347–54.

20. Perazella MA. Onco-nephrology: renal toxicities of chemotherapeutic agents. Clin J Am Soc Nephrol 2012;7(10):1713–21.

21. Oh TK, Oh AY, Ryu JH, et al. Retrospective analysis of the association between intraoperative magnesium sulfate infusion and postoperative acute kidney injury after major laparoscopic abdominal surgery. Sci Rep 2019;9(1).

22. Natale JJ. Overview of the prevention and management of CINV. Am J Manag Care 2018;24(18 Suppl):S391–7.

23. Hashimoto H, Abe M, Tokuyama O, et al. Olanzapine 5 mg plus standard antiemetic therapy for the prevention of chemotherapy-induced nausea and vomiting (J-FORCE): a multicentre, randomised, double-blind, placebo-controlled, phase 3 trial. Lancet Oncol 2020;21(2):242–9. Erratum in: Lancet Oncol. 2020 Feb;21(2): e70.

24. Stein A, Voigt W, Jordan K. Chemotherapy-induced diarrhea: pathophysiology, frequency and guideline-based management. Ther Adv Med Oncol 2010;2(1): 51–63.

25. Gupta A, De Felice KM, Loftus EV Jr, et al. Systematic review: colitis associated with anti-CTLA-4 therapy. Aliment Pharmacol Ther 2015;42(4):406–17.

26. Wei D, Heus P, van de Wetering FT, et al. Probiotics for the prevention or treatment of chemotherapy- or radiotherapy-related diarrhoea in people with cancer. Cochrane Database Syst Rev 2018;8(8):CD008831.

27. Andreyev HJ, Davidson SE, Gillespie C, et al, British Society of Gastroenterology, Association of Colo-Proctology of Great Britain and Ireland, Association of Upper Gastrointestinal Surgeons, Faculty of Clinical Oncology Section of the Royal College of Radiologists. Association of Colo-Proctology of Great Britain and Ireland; Association of Upper Gastrointestinal Surgeons; Faculty of Clinical Oncology Section of the Royal College of Radiologists. Practice guidance on the management of acute and chronic gastrointestinal problems arising as a result of treatment for cancer. Gut 2012;61(2):179–92.

28. Larkin J, Chiarion-Sileni V, Gonzalez R, et al. Combined Nivolumab and Ipilimumab or Monotherapy in Untreated Melanoma. N Engl J Med 2015;373(1):23–34 . Erratum in: N Engl J Med. 2018 Nov 29;379(22):2185.

29. Eigentler TK, Hassel JC, Berking C, et al. Diagnosis, monitoring and management of immune-related adverse drug reactions of anti-PD-1 antibody therapy. Cancer Treat Rev 2016;45:7–18.

30. Ploug M, Kroijer R, Qvist N, et al. Preoperative intravenous iron treatment in colorectal cancer: experience from clinical practice. J Surg Res 2022;277:37–43.

31. Grant HM, Davis LL, Garb J, et al. Preoperative leukopenia does not affect outcomes in cancer patients undergoing elective and emergent abdominal surgery: A brief report. Am J Surg 2020;220(1):132–4.

32. Amar D, Grant FM, Zhang H, et al. Antifibrinolytic therapy and perioperative blood loss in cancer patients undergoing major orthopedic surgery. Anesthesiology 2003;98:337–42.

33. NCT02074436 Prevention of bleeding in hematological malignancies with antifibrinolytic (epsilon aminocaproic acid). Available at: https://clinicaltrials.gov/ct2/show/NCT02074436. [Accessed 18 February 2024].

34. Leader A, Hofstetter L, Spectre G. Challenges and advances in managing thrombocytopenic cancer patients. J Clin Med 2021;10(6):1169.

35. Zhang Y, Qin D, Shou AC, et al. Exploring CAR-T cell therapy side effects: mechanisms and management strategies. J Clin Med 2023;12(19):6124.

36. Brudno Jennifer N, Kochenderfer James N. Toxicities of chimeric antigen receptor T cells: recognition and management. Blood 2016;127(26):3321–30.

37. Brajcich BC, Stigall K, Walsh DS, et al. Preoperative nutritional optimization of the oncology patient: a scoping review. J Am Coll Surg 2022;234(3):384–94.

38. Simonsen C, de Heer P, Bjerre ED, et al. Sarcopenia and postoperative complication risk in gastrointestinal surgical oncology: a meta-analysis. Ann Surg 2018 Jul;268(1):58–69.

39. Weimann A, Braga M, Carli F, et al. ESPEN practical guideline: clinical nutrition in surgery. Clin Nutr 2021;40(7):4745–61.

40. Fukuda Y, Yamamoto K, Hirao M, et al. Prevalence of malnutrition among gastric cancer patients undergoing gastrectomy and optimal preoperative nutritional support for preventing surgical site infections. Ann Surg Oncol 2015;22(S3):778–85.

41. Wijeysundera DN, Pearse RM, Shulman MA, et al, METS study investigators. Assessment of functional capacity before major non-cardiac surgery: an international, prospective cohort study. Lancet 2018;391(10140):2631–40.

42. West M, Jack S, Grocott MP. Perioperative cardiopulmonary exercise testing in the elderly. Best Pract Res Clin Anaesthesiol 2011;25(3):427–37.

43. Sinclair RC, Batterham AM, Davies S, et al. Validity of the 6 min walk test in predicting the anaerobic threshold before major non-cardiac surgery. Br J Anaesth 2012 Jan;108(1):30–5.

44. Pranjic N, Bajraktarevic A, Ramic E. Distress and ptsd in patients with cancer: cohort study case. Mater Sociomed 2016;28(1):12–6.

45. Rosenberger PH, Jokl P, Ickovics J. Psychosocial factors and surgical outcomes: an evidence-based literature review. J Am Acad Orthop Surg 2006;14(7):397–405.

46. Cesario A, Dall'Armi V, Cusumano G, et al. Post-operative pulmonary rehabilitation after lung resection for NSCLC: A follow-up study. Lung Cancer 2009;66(2):268–9.

47. Guidelines. ERAS® Society. Available at: :https://erassociety.org/guidelines/ Enhanced Recovery After Surgery (ERAS) Guidelines 2019 Assessed January 22, 2024.

48. Sánchez-Pérez B, Ramia JM. Does enhanced recovery after surgery programs improve clinical outcomes in liver cancer surgery? World J Gastrointest Oncol 2024;16(2):255–8.

49. Pagano E, Pellegrino L, Robella M, et al, ERAS-colorectal Piemonte group. Implementation of an enhanced recovery after surgery protocol for colorectal cancer in

a regional hospital network supported by audit and feedback: a stepped wedge, cluster randomized trial. BMJ Qual Saf 2024;bmjqs(2023):016594.

50. Grilo N, Crettenand F, Bohner P, et al. Impact of Enhanced Recovery after Surgery® Protocol Compliance on Length of Stay, Bowel Recovery and Complications after Radical Cystectomy. Diagnostics (Basel) 2024;14(3):264.

51. Hurley RW, Cohen SP, Williams KA, et al. The analgesic effects of perioperative gabapentin on postoperative pain: a meta-analysis. Reg Anesth Pain Med 2006 May-Jun;31(3):237–47.

52. Feo CV, Romanini B, Sortini D, et al. Early oral feeding after colorectal resection: a randomized controlled study. ANZ J Surg 2004;74(5):298–301.

53. Barlow R, Price P, Reid TD, et al. Prospective multicentre randomized controlled trial of early enteral nutrition for patients undergoing major upper gastrointestinal surgical resection. Clin Nutr 2011;30(5):560–6.

54. Lyman GH, Khorana AA, Falanga A, et al. American society of clinical oncology guideline: recommendations for venous thromboembolism prophylaxis and treatment in patients with cancer. J Clin Oncol 2007;25(34):5490–505.

Endocrine Care for the Surgical Patient

Diabetes Mellitus, Thyroid and Adrenal Conditions

Carlos E. Mendez, MD[a],*, Jason F. Shiffermiller, MD, MPH[b],
Alejandra Razzeto, MD[c], Zeina Hannoush, MD[c]

KEYWORDS

- Perioperative management • Endocrine • Thyroid • Hypothyroidism
- Hyperthyroidism • Diabetes mellitus • Hyperglycemia • Adrenal

KEY POINTS

- Patients with hyperglycemia, thyroid dysfunction, and adrenal insufficiency face increased perioperative risk, which may be mitigated by appropriate management.
- Hyperglycemia has been associated with increased perioperative morbidity and mortality in patients with and without diabetes.
- Hemoglobin A1c may not be reliable in certain populations; fructosamine and continuous glucose monitoring are emerging alternatives.

DIABETES AND HYPERGLYCEMIA

Hyperglycemia, defined for hospitalized patients as a serum glucose greater than 140 mg/dL,[1] occurs in approximately 40% of patients undergoing noncardiac surgery and in up to 80% of patients undergoing cardiac surgery. Approximately one-third of patients with postoperative hyperglycemia have no previous history of diabetes,[2,3] and a glycosylated hemoglobin (HbA1c) can help differentiate undiagnosed diabetes (HbA1c ≥ 6.5%) from new or stress hyperglycemia (HbA1c of < 6.5%).[4,5] Hyperglycemia has been associated with increased perioperative morbidity and mortality in patients with and without diabetes. Patients undergoing cardiac surgery with poor glycemic control have significantly higher risk of overall complications, including

[a] Division of General Internal Medicine, Medical College of Wisconsin, 8701 West Watertown Plank Road, Milwaukee, WI 53226, USA; [b] Division of Hospital Medicine, Department of Internal Medicine, University of Nebraska Medical Center, 986435 Nebraska Medical Center, Omaha, NE 68198-6435, USA; [c] Division of Endocrinology, Diabetes and Metabolism, Department of Internal Medicine, University of Miami, Miller School of Medicine, FL 33136, USA
* Corresponding author.
E-mail address: cmendez@mcw.edu

Med Clin N Am 108 (2024) 1185–1200
https://doi.org/10.1016/j.mcna.2024.04.007
0025-7125/24/Published by Elsevier Inc.
medical.theclinics.com

deep sternal wound infections and death.[6,7] In general surgical patients, a postoperative glucose greater than 140 mg/dL has been identified as one of the strongest predictors for surgical-site infections.[8] Overall, the detrimental effects of hyperglycemia in the perioperative period have been seen in multiple surgical populations, including the orthopedic, neurosurgical, vascular, colorectal, and oncologic among others (**Table 1**).

In patients without diabetes, the presence of hyperglycemia has unexpectedly been found to be much more deleterious than in those with a previous diabetes diagnosis. In hospitalized patients, the association between new hyperglycemia and higher in-hospital mortality has been well recognized.[9] Similarly, patients presenting with acute coronary syndromes with hyperglycemia, but without diabetes, have a significantly higher risk for congestive heart failure, cardiogenic shock, and death, than those without hyperglycemia, or with hyperglycemia but a previous diagnosis of diabetes.[10,11] In the surgical population, this paradox has also been observed in patients undergoing both cardiac and noncardiac surgeries.[12–14] Adequate management of hyperglycemia through the use of intravenous insulin protocols for cardiac surgical patients or subcutaneous basal-bolus insulin regimens for noncardiac surgical patients has shown to significantly decrease risk of perioperative complications.[6,15,16] Thus, the proper identification of high-risk surgical candidates becomes increasingly important to facilitate timely detection and management of hyperglycemia and avoid or decrease risks of poor outcomes during the perioperative period.

PREOPERATIVE EVALUATION
HbA1c

The HbA1c test has been conventionally used to evaluate the quality of glycemic control in the preoperative period. The American Diabetes Association recommends a target HbA1c lower than 8% before elective surgeries whenever possible.[21] However, the evidence linking preoperative HbA1c levels with postoperative complications has been inconsistent.[22–27] It is not clear why HbA1c fails to perform well as a preoperative risk stratification tool, but it may be partly due to the inherent properties of the test. HbA1c is correlated with average glucose over the preceding 60 to 90 days,[28] but provides limited information on more recent glucose control. It also provides no information on hypoglycemia or glycemic variability, which are independent risk factors for morbidity and mortality in the surgical population.[1,22,23,29] Additionally, a variety of medical conditions can impact erythrocyte lifespan and falsely raise or lower the HbA1c levels.[24]

Alternate Measures of Preoperative Glycemic Control

Given the limitations to the use of HbA1c, alternate methods for assessing preoperative glycemic control have been emerging. Fructosamine, a measure of nonenzymatic glycation of circulating proteins, provides an approximation of average glucose over the preceding 2 to 3 weeks.[25] An elevated fructosamine (>293 μmol/L) before surgery has been associated with a markedly increased risk of prosthetic joint infection in patients undergoing total knee and hip arthroplasty. Unlike fructosamine, HbA1c failed to show a significant association with complications.[26,27] In patients with diabetes who are preparing for surgery, particularly those in whom a recent change in glycemic control is suspected, preoperative fructosamine measurement may be of benefit.

Another tool in the preoperative setting is continuous glucose monitors (CGMs). Recent estimates are that as many as 13% of patients with type 2 diabetes (DM2) in the community have used a CGM.[28] These devices can be particularly valuable

Author	Population	Study Design	Sample Size	Outcomes	Significance
Furnary et al,[6] 2003	Cardiac (CABG)	Observational	5,534	Increased DSWI, LOS, costs, and death	$P<.05$
McGirt et al,[17] 2006	Vascular (CEA)	Observational	1,201	Increased stroke, MI, and death	$P<.05$
Chrastil et al,[18] 2015	Orthopedic (total joint)	Observational	13,272	Increased periprosthetic joint infection	$P<.05$
Mohan et al,[19] 2015	Colorectal	Observational	5,145	SSI, sepsis, death	$P<.05$
Frisch et al,[20] 2010	Noncardiac (general, neurosurgery, oncology, orthopedic, vascular, thoracic, urology, otolaryngology and gynecology)	Observational	3,184	Increased infections, renal failure, MI, and mortality	$P<.05$

Table 1
Adverse effects of postoperative hyperglycemia across surgical populations

Abbreviations: CABG, coronary artery bypass graft surgery; CEA, carotid endarterectomy; DSWI, deep sternal wound infections; LOS, length of stay; MI, myocardial infarction; SSI, surgical site infections.

during the preoperative evaluation because the quality of recent glycemic control can be quickly assessed by reviewing key metrics from either a recent report or directly from the user's reader device or smartphone. A time in range greater than 70%, time below range less than 4%, and a coefficient of variation (%CV) of less than 36% are considered optimal goals for most patients with diabetes.[30]

Preoperative Medication Management

Noninsulin diabetes medications

The preoperative management of noninsulin diabetes medications is crucial for ensuring patient safety during surgery (**Table 2**). Among noninsulin medications, metformin continues to be the most widely used agent for the management of DM2 in the United States.[31] Due to the concern that surgery in patients taking metformin may precipitate lactic acidosis, current recommendations from expert bodies are to hold metformin on the day of surgery for patients with preserved renal function with longer interruptions being discouraged.[21,32] Nevertheless, metformin should be avoided in conditions predisposing to lactic acidosis, such as acute kidney injury, decompensated heart failure, hypoxemia, alcoholism, cirrhosis, contrast dye exposure, sepsis, and shock.[33]

Sodium–glucose cotransporter 2 (SGLT-2) inhibitors present unique challenges in the perioperative setting. Due to their potential for increased risk of urogenital infections, acute kidney injury, dehydration, hypotension, and euglycemic diabetic ketoacidosis (DKA), the Food and Drug Administration (FDA) recommends discontinuing canagliflozin, dapagliflozin, and empagliflozin at least 3 days before scheduled surgery, and ertugliflozin at least 4 days prior.[34] Euglycemic DKA is particularly dangerous as it can be precipitated by surgery and may go unrecognized by clinicians.

Table 2
Summary of recommendations for the preoperative management of non-insulin diabetes medications

Medication Class	Agents	Day(s) Before Surgery	Morning of Surgery
Alpha-glucosidase inhibitors	Acarbose, Miglitol	Continue	Hold
Biguanides	Metformin	Continue	Hold
DPP-4 inhibitors	Vildagliptin, sitagliptin, saxagliptin, linagliptin, alogliptin	Continue	Hold
GLP-1 agonists	Liraglutide, lixisenatide, semaglutide*, dulaglutide*, tirzepatide*	Continue daily agents Hold weekly agents 1 wk prior*	Hold
Insulin secretogogues (sulfonylureas, glinides)	Glipizide, glyburide, glimepiride repaglinide, nateglinide	Continue	Hold
SGLT-2 inhibitors	Dapagliflozin, canagliflozin, empagliflozin, ertugliflozin*	Hold 3–4* days prior	Hold
Thiazolidinediones	Pioglitazone	Continue	Hold

Glucagon-like peptide-1 (GLP-1) agonists, increasingly used for the management of DM2 and obesity, enhance insulin production in a glucose-dependent manner while decreasing glucagon activity.[35] Additionally, they suppress appetite and slow gastric emptying, resulting in increased satiety and reduced postprandial hyperglycemia.[36,37] A small number of perioperative studies have shown the efficacy of GLP-1 in achieving glycemic control during surgery without significant complications.[38,39] However, case reports and retrospective evidence in patients undergoing esophagogastroduodenoscopy have raised concern for pulmonary aspiration risk in patients taking GLP-1 agonists.[40–42] Due to the concern for aspiration, consensus guidance from the American Society of Anesthesiologists advises that weekly GLP-1 agonists should be held 1 week prior to surgery and daily agents should be held on the day of surgery.[43] Given this recommendation, and until more evidence is available, it seems reasonable to consider holding these agents before surgery.

Insulin secretogogues, including sulfonylureas and glinides, stimulate endogenous insulin secretion and carry an increased risk of hypoglycemia, especially in older patients and those with impaired renal function.[44] The recommendation is to withhold these medications on the morning of surgery.[21,32] It is also recommended that thiazolidinediones and alpha-gucosidase inhibitors be held on the morning of surgery.[1,45] Although they would not be expected to cause hypoglycemia, there are concerns for potential side effects from these agents and a lack of evidence for their perioperative benefit.[45,46] Similarly, due to mixed and limited evidence of benefit from dipeptidyl-peptidase-4 inhibitors in preventing postoperative hyperglycemia, recommending their continued use on the day of surgery is not generally warranted for most patients.[32]

Insulin therapy

For patients presenting for surgery on insulin, an appropriate perioperative insulin regimen is critical to maintaining glycemic control while minimizing hyperglycemia

Table 3
Summary of recommendations for the preoperative management of insulin therapy

Insulin Type	Agents	Day(s) Before Surgery	Morning of Surgery
Long-acting	Glargine, detemir, degludec	Continue, consider a 25% reduction the night prior	Continue, consider a 25% reduction
Intermediate-acting	NPH	Continue, consider a 25% reduction the night prior	Decrease dose by 50%
Short-/rapid-acting	Regular, aspart, lispro, glulisine	Continue	Hold, may use for treatment of hyperglycemia per a protocol
Premixed	Human NPH/regular 70/30; insulin lispro protamine/ lispro 75/25	Continue	Consider a 50% reduction (glucose >120 mg/dL), or hold if glucose ≤120 mg/dL
Insulin U-500		Continue	Consider a 50% reduction (glucose >120 mg/dL), or hold if glucose ≤120 mg/dL

and hypoglycemia (**Table 3**). The different insulin preparations, including long-acting (eg, glargine, detemir, degludec), intermediate-acting (NPH insulin), short-acting, and rapid-acting insulin (eg, regular, aspart, lispro, glulisine), require specific dose adjustments based on their time of onset, peaks, and duration. Long-acting insulin should generally be continued both before and on the day of surgery, with a potential 20% to 25% dose reduction on the evening before or morning of surgery, especially for patients prone to hypoglycemia.[21] Intermediate-acting insulin, specifically NPH insulin, may be continued before surgery and on the day of surgery, but with a 50% dose reduction on the morning of surgery, and possibly a 25% reduction the evening before, particularly for patients at risk of hypoglycemia.[32] Short-acting and rapid-acting insulin, such as regular human insulin and analogues, should be held on the day of surgery when the patient is fasting. However, they can be used on the day of surgery if necessary for correcting hyperglycemia following institutional protocols for administration. Premixed insulin preparations combining intermediate and short rapid-acting insulin (eg, 70/30) or concentrated insulin (U-500) should generally be continued the day before surgery, but their use on the morning of surgery should be based on the patient's blood sugar measurement, with adjustments as needed. For instance, a reduction of 50% of the morning dose for glucose levels over 120 mg/dL and completely holding the dose for glucose levels under 120 mg/dL has been recommended.[47]

Intraoperative and Postoperative Glycemic Control

Achieving target glucose levels while avoiding hyperglycemia, hypoglycemia, and glycemic variability is the ultimate goal during the intraoperative and postoperative periods. In general, insulin therapy is the most validated and recommended strategy for treating hyperglycemia in surgical patients during and after surgery.[21,44]

Determining the appropriate insulin regimen and dosing to be used will vary depending on factors such as required inpatient level of care (critically ill vs noncritically ill), outpatient regimen, quality of glycemic control prior to admission, current glucose levels, and nutritional status.[47] For inpatient management of hyperglycemia in noncritical care settings, a glycemic goal of 100 to 180 mg/dL is recommended, while for most critically ill individuals, a goal of 140 to 180 mg/dL is recommended as stricter goals may not improve outcomes and are associated with more hypoglycemia.[21,48] For the majority of patients undergoing noncardiac general surgery, basal insulin plus pre-meal short-acting or rapid-acting insulin (basal-bolus) is recommended as this therapy has been associated with improved glycemic outcomes and lower rates of perioperative complications compared to sliding scale correction insulin alone without basal insulin dosing.[16] For patients with type 1 diabetes or those with insulin-requiring DM2 undergoing prolonged procedures such as cardiac surgeries requiring intensive care, continuous intravenous insulin infusion using validated written or computerized protocols is the recommended approach for achieving specific glycemic goals and avoiding hypoglycemia.[49]

Continuous Glucose Monitoring and Insulin Pumps

An increasing number of patients use continuous glucose monitoring devices and insulin pumps. Integration of these technologies has allowed the recent adoption of automated insulin delivery devices (AIDs).[50] Although several reports have advocated for the safe and effective use of insulin pumps and AIDs in the perioperative period, it is imperative that the decision to continue to use these devices during and after surgery is made in consensus with the patient, as well as the surgical and anesthesia teams. Health care providers must be familiar with the basic functioning of these devices. Consultation with an endocrinologist is warranted in the management of these patients.[51,52] In general, for prolonged procedures where patients will require intensive care and are not expected to resume oral intake in the early postoperative period, transition to intravenous insulin infusion as per protocol is recommended.[45] Conversely, for procedures of short or moderate duration, after which patients are expected to regain consciousness and resume oral intake in a short period of time, continuing the use of the AID/CGM would be considered appropriate.[46] **Fig. 1** shows the recommended approach to patients wearing insulin pumps presenting to surgery.[53]

THYROID DISORDERS
Preoperative Screening

Thyroid disorders, both hypothyroidism and hyperthyroidism, can significantly impact perioperative risk. Preoperative thyroid stimulating hormone (TSH) measurement is not routinely indicated but should be performed when symptoms or signs suggestive of thyroid disease are present and in all patients with known thyroid disease. If performed within the previous 3 months, repeat testing is not necessary in patients taking a stable dose of medication with documented euthyroidism.[54] It should be noted that, due to the long half-life of free thyroxine (T4), it may take a month to reach an euthyroid state after dose adjustments. Delaying procedures until this is achieved might not always be possible.

Hypothyroidism Clinical Manifestations

Untreated hypothyroidism poses increased risks during surgery, with the severity of thyroid dysfunction dictating the likelihood and type of complications. While a multitude of organ systems can be affected, the greatest concern is for precipitation of

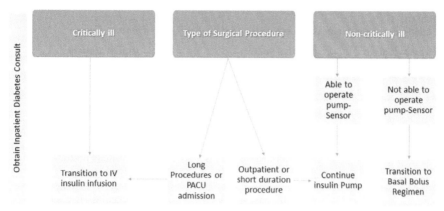

Fig. 1. Perioperative management of insulin pumps. (Mendez, C.E., Umpierrez, G.E. Management of Type 1 Diabetes in the Hospital Setting. Curr Diab Rep 17, 98 (2017). https://doi.org/10.1007/s11892-017-0919-7.)

myxedema coma, a life-threatening condition characterized by coma, hypothermia, and cardiorespiratory collapse. Additionally, cardiovascular complications are common, including reduced cardiac output, hypotension, myocardial infarction, bradycardia, irregular heartbeat, and prolonged QT interval. Respiratory complications are also a concern, including hypoventilation. Other concerns include difficult intubation, increased sensitivity to anesthesia, constipation, and delayed wound healing.[55–57]

Management of Hypothyroidism

Thyroid hormone replacement with oral levothyroxine is the standard of care and main treatment for patients with hypothyroidism. Levothyroxine can be started at a dose of 1.6 mcg/kg/day after complete thyroidectomy or radioactive iodine ablation. Lower doses should be used in patients with thyroid reserve. Thyroid function tests should be monitored 5 to 6 weeks after treatment changes, and further dose adjustments should be made based on the results.

The risk for postsurgical complications in the uncontrolled hypothyroid patient needs to be balanced with the urgency of the procedure. We divide the management according to 3 levels of severity of hypothyroidism: *mild*: patients with subclinical hypothyroidism (elevated TSH with normal free T4 levels); *moderate*: patients with elevated TSH, low free T4 without the features of severe hypothyroidism; and *severe*: patients with myxedema coma, severe symptoms of hypothyroidism like altered mentation, pericardial effusion, heart failure, or free T4 less than 0.5 ng/dL.[54]

Table 4 summarizes the perioperative management recommendations in patients with hypothyroidism based on the severity of thyroid dysfunction and the urgency of surgery.

In stable hypothyroid patients on chronic oral LT4 replacement undergoing surgery, thyroid hormone may be safely withheld for up to several days, if not eating. Intravenous or intramuscular administration should be considered if enteral resumption is not achieved within 5 to 7 days.[58]

Hyperthyroidism Clinical Manifestations

Patients with hyperthyroidism are at increased risk of perioperative complications. Hyperthyroidism can affect various organ systems, but cardiovascular complications are

Table 4		
Perioperative management recommendations in patients with hypothyroidism		
Hypothyroidism	**Elective Surgery**	**Urgent Surgery**
Mild	Proceed with surgery Start/adjust levothyroxine treatment as above	Proceed with surgery Start/adjust levothyroxine treatment as above
Moderate	• Start/adjust levothyroxine treatment as above • Postpone surgery until the euthyroid state is restored	Proceed with surgery Start/adjust levothyroxine treatment as above • Close monitoring for possible postoperative complications
Severe	• Start/adjust levothyroxine treatment as above. • Delay surgery until the euthyroid state is restored	• Treat as soon as the diagnosis is made with intravenous (IV) levothyroxine, loading dose of 200–300 mg followed by 50–100 mg daily. Consider IV liothyronine if there is a concern for precipitating myxedema coma • In patients needing heart revascularization, starting treatment may not be beneficial • If concerns for concomitant adrenal insufficiency, give corticosteroid prior to thyroid hormone • Close monitoring for possible postoperative complications

the primary concern, including arrhythmias, high output heart failure, and acute coronary events. The catabolic state associated with severe hyperthyroidism contributes to a cascade of complications including electrolyte imbalances, myopathy, respiratory weakness, anorexia with malnutrition, and hyperthermia leading to dehydration. Thyroid storm is a rare but potentially fatal complication that can be precipitated by surgery or anesthesia and can culminate in cardiovascular collapse and death.[59]

Management of Hyperthyroidism

Oral thionamides, such as methimazole and propylthiouracil, inhibit the thyroid peroxidase enzyme and decrease thyroid hormone synthesis by follicular cells. These agents are the standard of care and main treatment for patients with primary hyperthyroidism due to Graves' disease and toxic multinodular goiter. non-steroidal anti-inflammatory drugs (NSAIDs) and/or corticosteroids can be beneficial in the management of some patients with thyroiditis, which is characterized by the release of presynthetized thyroid hormone from thyroid follicles. Thyroiditis can be caused by viral infections, radiation, medication, or other factors acutely damaging follicular thyroid cells. Patients presenting with hyperthyroidism, regardless of the etiology, can benefit from the addition of beta-blockers to help manage their symptoms. Certain

Table 5
Perioperative management recommendations in patients with hyperthyroidism

Hyperthyroidism	Elective Surgery	Urgent Surgery
Subclinical/Mild Hyperthyroidism	Proceed with surgery Start oral thionamides if appropriate • Perioperative b-blockade may be considered at least 7 d before noncardiac surgery	Proceed with surgery Start oral thionamides if appropriate • Perioperative b-blockade may be considered at least 7 d before noncardiac surgery
Overt hyperthyroidism	• Delay surgery until adequate control of thyroid function test	• Initiate treatment as soon as possible with beta blockers, thionamides and possibly potassium iodide solution 1 hour after thionamides. Can consider the addition of cholestyramine. Glucocorticoids may also be given. • Close monitoring for possible postoperative complications

beta-blockers, such as propranolol, have the added benefit of decreasing the peripheral conversion of T4 hormone to its most active triiodothyronine (T3) form.

The risk for postsurgical complications in uncontrolled hyperthyroidism needs to be balanced with the urgency of the procedure. We divide the management according to 2 levels of severity of hyperthyroidism: (1) subclinical hyperthyroidism: low TSH with normal free T4 and T3 levels or asymptomatic. (2) Overt hyperthyroidism: defined as a suppressed TSH with elevated free T4 and/or T3 concentrations or symptomatic.[54,60]

Table 5 summarizes the perioperative management recommendations in patients with hyperthyroidism depending on the severity of thyroid dysfunction and the urgency of surgery.

In the postoperative setting, for patients already taking or newly initiated on thionamides preoperatively and anticipated to be unable to tolerate oral medications beyond 1 or 2 days, rectal formulations may offer a viable alternative therapy. The decision to employ rectal methimazole postoperatively should be guided by individual clinical considerations and the accessibility of rectal preparations.[61]

ADRENAL DISORDERS
Pathophysiology

Surgery in patients with adrenal insufficiency can precipitate adrenal crisis, a potentially life-threatening complication. During times of physiologic stress, such as surgery, the hypothalamic–pituitary–adrenal (HPA) axis is stimulated to produce a surge in serum cortisol.[62] Failure of the HPA axis to produce an adequate cortisol surge can result in the refractory hypotension of adrenal crisis.[63]

Adrenal crisis can be prevented by administering a short course of higher dose corticosteroids perioperatively. This practice is known as perioperative stress dosing. Patients with primary adrenal insufficiency due to bilateral adrenal gland failure and patients with secondary adrenal insufficiency due to anterior pituitary gland failure require stress dose steroids during times of physiologic stress in order to prevent adrenal crisis.[64] Patients with secondary adrenal insufficiency due to exogenous steroid use may or may not require stress dose steroids depending on the steroid formulation, the steroid dose, and the duration of steroid therapy.

Risk for Adrenal Crisis

Based on the etiology of their adrenal insufficiency, patients can be placed into 1 of 3 levels of risk for perioperative adrenal crisis[63–65]:

- Lowest risk: Patients taking the equivalent of less than 5 mg of prednisone daily and who also have not received more than 3 weeks of higher steroid doses in the previous year or patients using inhaled, intranasal, or topical steroids.
- Moderate risk: Patients taking the equivalent of 5 to 20 mg of prednisone daily for 3 weeks or longer
- Highest risk: Patients with an established diagnosis of adrenal insufficiency or taking the equivalent of more than 20 mg of prednisone daily for 3 weeks or longer.

It should be noted that there are no trial data and little other evidence supporting this categorization system. There is also some evidence that conflicts with this system of categorization.[66]

Stress Dosing and Surgical Stress Definitions

Regardless of their risk for adrenal crisis, all patients taking exogenous steroids should be continued on their usual steroid dose without interruption perioperatively. How much additional steroid should be administered, if any, depends on both the patient's risk for adrenal insufficiency and the degree of physiologic stress produced by their surgery. The degree of surgical stress can be divided into 3 categories[68]:

- Mild surgical stress: Surgery under local anesthesia or surgery lasting less than 1 hour
- Moderate surgical stress: Most patients undergoing general, neuraxial, or regional anesthesia
- Severe surgical stress: Expected blood loss greater than 1500 mL or expected postoperative intensive care unit stay

Patients undergoing mild surgical stress procedures generally do not require perioperative stress dose steroids, regardless of their risk for adrenal crisis (**Table 6**). Patients at the lowest risk for adrenal crisis based on their daily steroid dose also do not generally require perioperative stress dosing, regardless of the physiologic stress produced by their surgery. Thus, stress dose steroids are only recommended for patients at moderate or highest risk for adrenal crisis who are undergoing surgeries associated with moderate or severe surgical stress (**Table 7**).

A normal preoperative adrenocorticotropic hormone (ACTH) stimulation test may help recategorize moderate risk patients into the lowest risk category, but the ability of an abnormal ACTH stimulation test to predict the need for perioperative stress dose steroids is uncertain.[66,69] Because of the unclear role of ACTH stimulation testing and the perceived low risk of a short course of higher dose steroids, patients at moderate risk for adrenal crisis may be treated similarly to patients at high risk for adrenal crisis.

The dose and duration of perioperative stress dose steroids is typically determined by the degree of surgical stress. A recommended stress dosing regimen for patients undergoing moderate stress surgery is hydrocortisone 50 mg intravenous (IV) within

Table 6
Relative potencies of commonly used steroids[67]

Medication	Glucocorticoid Potency	Mineralocorticoid Potency
Hydrocortisone (cortisol)	1	1
Cortisone	0.8	0.8
Prednisone/ Prednisolone	4	0.8
Methylprednisolone	5	0.5
Dexamethasone	25	0
Fludrocortisone	10[a]	125

[a] At typically used doses, fludrocortisone has minimal glucocorticoid activity.

1 hour prior to anesthesia induction followed by 25 mg IV every 8 hours for 24 to 48 hours before returning to the patient's usual steroid dose. A recommended regimen for patients undergoing severe stress surgery is hydrocortisone 100 mg IV within 1 hour prior to induction followed by 50 mg IV every 8 hours for 48 to 72 hours, then return to the usual steroid dose if the patient is recovering as expected.[64,65]

Choice of Stress Dose Agent

Hydrocortisone is the favored agent for perioperative stress dosing. It has a ratio of glucocorticoid to mineralocorticoid activity of approximately 1:1. This mimics the physiologic profile of endogenous cortisol and addresses the mineralocorticoid deficiency of patients with primary adrenal insufficiency due to bilateral adrenal gland failure. Patients with secondary adrenal insufficiency due to pituitary failure or the negative feedback exerted by exogenous steroids, however, would be expected to have intact mineralocorticoid production regulated through the renin–angiotensin–aldosterone pathway. Dexamethasone is a potent glucocorticoid with minimal mineralocorticoid activity. Perioperative dexamethasone administered in doses of 4 to 8 mg is a widely utilized and guideline-recommended therapy for the prevention of postoperative nausea and vomiting. This dose of dexamethasone has the glucocorticoid equivalent of 100 to 200 mg of hydrocortisone and a duration of action of 36 to 72 hours.[67] When perioperative dexamethasone is administered to patients with secondary adrenal insufficiency, additional stress dose steroids are unlikely to be necessary.

Endocrine Surgery

The medical management of patients undergoing endocrine surgery, including pituitary and adrenal operations, is complex and should be guided by an endocrinologist.

Table 7
Matrix guiding the need for perioperative stress dose steroids

	Mild Surgical Stress	Moderate Surgical Stress	Severe Surgical Stress
Lowest risk for Adrenal Crisis	Continue usual steroid regimen only		
Moderate risk for Adrenal Crisis Highest risk for Adrenal Crisis		Stress Dose	

CLINICS CARE POINTS

- Glycemic control in perioperative period:
  - Hemoglobin A1c may not be reliable in certain populations; fructosamine and continuous glucose monitoring are emerging alternatives.
  - Noninsulin agents require proper management, with most medications paused the morning of surgery, except for SGLT2-inhibitors and GLP-1 agonists requiring longer periods.
  - Long-acting subcutaneous insulin is generally continued, with potential dose adjustments for patients prone to hypoglycemia.
  - Continuous IV insulin infusion is recommended for prolonged procedures with glucose targets lower than 180 mg/dL for most patients.
- Thyroid function and surgery:
  - Perioperative thyroid screening is not recommended for asymptomatic patients.
  - Patients with a known thyroid history should be medically optimized, and thyroid hormone replacement initiated or adjusted accordingly.
  - Surgical delays are not necessary for mild hypothyroidism or hyperthyroidism, but severe cases may require specific interventions.
  - Thionamides, beta-blockers, potassium iodide, cholestyramine, and glucocorticoids may be used in severe hyperthyroidism undergoing urgent procedures.
- Steroid use in perioperative period:
  - Exogenous steroids should be continued without interruption perioperatively, and stress-dose steroids are recommended for patients at moderate or high risk for adrenal crisis.
  - Hydrocortisone is the preferred agent for stress dosing, with specific regimens outlined based on the severity of surgical stress.
  - All patients should be closely monitored for potential postoperative complications.

REFERENCES

1. Johnston LE, Kirby JL, Downs EA, et al. Virginia Interdisciplinary Cardiothoracic Outcomes Research VICTOR Center. Postoperative hypoglycemia is associated with worse outcomes after cardiac operations. Ann Thorac Surg 2017;103(2): 526–32.
2. Cook CB, Kongable GL, Potter DJ, et al. Inpatient glucose control: a glycemic survey of 126 U.S. hospitals. J Hosp Med 2009;4(9):E7–14.
3. De La Rosa Gdel C, Donado JH, Restrepo AH, et al. Grupo de Investigacion en Cuidado intensivo: GICI-HPTU. Strict glycaemic control in patients hospitalised in a mixed medical and surgical intensive care unit: a randomised clinical trial. Crit Care 2008;12(5):R120.
4. Russo MP, Elizondo CM, Giunta DH, et al. Prevalence of hyperglycemia and incidence of stress hyperglycemia in hospitalized patients: A retrospective cohort. Eur J Intern Med 2017;43:e15–7.
5. Mazurek JA, Hailpern SM, Goring T, et al. Prevalence of hemoglobin A1c greater than 6.5% and 7.0% among hospitalized patients without known diagnosis of diabetes at an urban inner city hospital. J Clin Endocrinol Metab 2010;95(3):1344–8.
6. Furnary AP, Gao G, Grunkemeier GL, et al. Continuous insulin infusion reduces mortality in patients with diabetes undergoing coronary artery bypass grafting. J Thorac Cardiovasc Surg 2003;125(5):1007–21.
7. Latham R, Lancaster AD, Covington JF, et al. The association of diabetes and glucose control with surgical-site infections among cardiothoracic surgery patients. Infect Control Hosp Epidemiol 2001;22(10):607–12.

8. Ata A, Lee J, Bestle SL, et al. Postoperative hyperglycemia and surgical site infection in general surgery patients. Arch Surg 2010;145(9):858–64.
9. Umpierrez GE, Isaacs SD, Bazargan N, et al. Hyperglycemia: an independent marker of in-hospital mortality in patients with undiagnosed diabetes. J Clin Endocrinol Metab 2002;87(3):978–82.
10. Capes SE, Hunt D, Malmberg K, et al. Stress hyperglycemia and prognosis of stroke in nondiabetic and diabetic patients: a systematic overview. Stroke 2001;32(10):2426–32.
11. Foo K, Cooper J, Deaner A, et al. A single serum glucose measurement predicts adverse outcomes across the whole range of acute coronary syndromes. Heart 2003;89(5):512–6.
12. Davis G, Fayfman M, Reyes-Umpierrez D, et al. Stress hyperglycemia in general surgery: Why should we care? J Diabet Complicat 2018;32(3):305–9.
13. Kotagal M, Symons RG, Hirsch IB, et al. SCOAP-CERTAIN Collaborative. Perioperative hyperglycemia and risk of adverse events among patients with and without diabetes. Ann Surg 2015;261(1):97–103.
14. Umpierrez G, Cardona S, Pasquel F, et al. Randomized controlled trial of intensive versus conservative glucose control in patients undergoing coronary artery bypass graft surgery: GLUCO-CABG Trial. Diabetes Care 2015;38(9):1665–72.
15. Griesdale DE, de Souza RJ, van Dam RM, et al. Intensive insulin therapy and mortality among critically ill patients: a meta-analysis including NICE-SUGAR study data. CMAJ (Can Med Assoc J) 2009;180(8):821–7.
16. Umpierrez GE, Smiley D, Jacobs S, et al. Randomized study of basal-bolus insulin therapy in the inpatient management of patients with type 2 diabetes undergoing general surgery (RABBIT 2 surgery). Diabetes Care 2011;34(2):256–61.
17. McGirt MJ, Woodworth GF, Brooke BS, et al. Hyperglycemia independently increases the risk of perioperative stroke, myocardial infarction, and death after carotid endarterectomy. Neurosurgery 2006;58(6):1066–73, discussion -73.
18. Chrastil J, Anderson MB, Stevens V, et al. Is Hemoglobin A1c or perioperative hyperglycemia predictive of periprosthetic joint infection or death following primary total joint arthroplasty? J Arthroplasty 2015;30(7):1197–202.
19. Mohan S, Kaoutzanis C, Welch KB, et al. Postoperative hyperglycemia and adverse outcomes in patients undergoing colorectal surgery: results from the Michigan surgical quality collaborative database. Int J Colorectal Dis 2015;30(11):1515–23.
20. Frisch A, Chandra P, Smiley D, et al. Prevalence and clinical outcome of hyperglycemia in the perioperative period in noncardiac surgery. Diabetes Care 2010;33(8):1783–8.
21. Committee ADAPP. 16. Diabetes care in the hospital: standards of care in diabetes—2024. Diabetes Care 2023;47(Supplement_1):S295–306.
22. Dhatariya K, Levy N, Hall GM. The impact of glycaemic variability on the surgical patient. Curr Opin Anaesthesiol 2016;29(3):430–7.
23. Mendez CE, Mok KT, Ata A, et al. Increased glycemic variability is independently associated with length of stay and mortality in noncritically ill hospitalized patients. Diabetes Care 2013;36(12):4091–7.
24. Shepard JG, Airee A, Dake AW, et al. Limitations of A1c Interpretation. South Med J 2015;108(12):724–9.
25. Danese E, Montagnana M, Nouvenne A, et al. Advantages and pitfalls of fructosamine and glycated albumin in the diagnosis and treatment of diabetes. J Diabetes Sci Technol 2015;9(2):169–76.

26. Shohat N, Tarabichi M, Tan TL, et al. 2019 John Insall Award: Fructosamine is a better glycaemic marker compared with glycated haemoglobin (HbA1C) in predicting adverse outcomes following total knee arthroplasty: a prospective multi-centre study. Bone Joint Lett J 2019;101-B(7_Supple_C):3–9.

27. Shohat N, Goswami K, Breckenridge L, et al. Fructosamine is a valuable marker for glycemic control and predicting adverse outcomes following total hip arthroplasty: a prospective multi-institutional investigation. Sci Rep 2021;11(1):2227.

28. Mayberry LS, Guy C, Hendrickson CD, et al. Rates and correlates of uptake of continuous glucose monitors among adults with type 2 diabetes in primary care and endocrinology settings. J Gen Intern Med 2023;38(11):2546–52.

29. Rajendran R, Rayman G. Serious harm from inpatient hypoglycaemia: a survey of hospitals in the UK. Diabet Med 2014;31(10):1218–21.

30. Battelino T, Danne T, Bergenstal RM, et al. Clinical targets for continuous glucose monitoring data interpretation: recommendations from the international consensus on time in range. Diabetes Care 2019;42(8):1593–603.

31. Engler C, Leo M, Pfeifer B, et al. Long-term trends in the prescription of antidiabetic drugs: real-world evidence from the diabetes registry tyrol 2012-2018. BMJ Open Diabetes Res Care 2020;8(1):e001279.

32. Pfeifer KJ, Selzer A, Mendez CE, et al. Preoperative management of endocrine, hormonal, and urologic medications: society for perioperative assessment and quality improvement (SPAQI) consensus statement. Mayo Clin Proc 2021;96(6):1655–69.

33. Mendez CE, Umpierrez GE. Pharmacotherapy for hyperglycemia in noncritically ill hospitalized patients. Diabetes Spectr 2014;27(3):180–8.

34. FDA, 2020;Available at: Pageshttp://s2027422842.t.en25.com/e/es?s=20274228 42&e=312220&elqTrackId=376c7bc788024cd5a73d955f2e3dcbdc&elq=888 05802632f4dc88dd18426307959d3&elqaid=11643&elqat=1 on 05/12/2020 2020.

35. Drucker DJ. Mechanisms of action and therapeutic application of glucagon-like peptide-1. Cell Metab 2018;27(4):740–56.

36. Drucker DJ. GLP-1 physiology informs the pharmacotherapy of obesity. Mol Metabol 2022;57:101351.

37. Maselli DB, Camilleri M. Effects of GLP-1 and its analogs on gastric physiology in diabetes mellitus and obesity. Adv Exp Med Biol 2021;1307:171–92.

38. Hulst AH, Visscher MJ, Godfried MB, et al, GLOBE Study Group. Liraglutide for perioperative management of hyperglycaemia in cardiac surgery patients: a multicentre randomized superiority trial. Diabetes Obes Metabol 2020;22(4):557–65.

39. Polderman JAW, van Steen SCJ, Thiel B, et al. Peri-operative management of patients with type-2 diabetes mellitus undergoing non-cardiac surgery using liraglutide, glucose-insulin-potassium infusion or intravenous insulin bolus regimens: a randomised controlled trial. Anaesthesia 2018;73(3):332–9.

40. Silveira SQ, da Silva LM, de Campos Vieira Abib A, et al. Relationship between perioperative semaglutide use and residual gastric content: a retrospective analysis of patients undergoing elective upper endoscopy. J Clin Anesth 2023;87:111091.

41. Kobori T, Onishi Y, Yoshida Y, et al. Association of glucagon-like peptide-1 receptor agonist treatment with gastric residue in an esophagogastroduodenoscopy. J Diabetes Investig 2023;14(6):767–73.

42. Klein SR, Hobai IA. Semaglutide, delayed gastric emptying, and intraoperative pulmonary aspiration: a case report. Can J Anaesth 2023;70(8):1394–6.

43. Anesthesiologists ASo 2023;Available at: Pageshttps://www.asahq.org/about-asa/newsroom/news-releases/2023/06/american-society-of-anesthesiologists-consensus-based-guidance-on-preoperative on 02/06/2024 2024.

44. Inzucchi SE, Bergenstal RM, Buse JB, et al. American Diabetes Association ADA, European Association for the Study of Diabetes EASD. Management of hyperglycemia in type 2 diabetes: a patient-centered approach: position statement of the American Diabetes Association (ADA) and the European Association for the Study of Diabetes (EASD). Diabetes Care 2012;35(6):1364–79.

45. Umpierrez GE, Klonoff DC. Diabetes technology update: use of insulin pumps and continuous glucose monitoring in the hospital. Diabetes Care 2018;41(8):1579–89.

46. Galindo RJ, Umpierrez GE, Rushakoff RJ, et al. Continuous glucose monitors and automated insulin dosing systems in the hospital consensus guideline. J Diabetes Sci Technol 2020;14(6):1035–64.

47. Duggan EW, Carlson K, Umpierrez GE. Perioperative hyperglycemia management: an update. Anesthesiology 2017;126(3):547–60.

48. Yogi-Morren D, Galioto R, Strandjord SE, et al. Duration of type 2 diabetes and very low density lipoprotein levels are associated with cognitive dysfunction in metabolic syndrome. Cardiovasc Psychiatry Neurol 2014;2014:656341.

49. Braithwaite SS, Clark LP, Idrees T, et al. Hypoglycemia prevention by algorithm design during intravenous insulin infusion. Curr Diabetes Rep 2018;18(5):26.

50. Sherr JL, Heinemann L, Fleming GA, et al. Automated insulin delivery: benefits, challenges, and recommendations. a consensus report of the joint diabetes technology working group of the european association for the study of diabetes and the american diabetes association. Diabetes Care 2022;45(12):3058–74.

51. Davis GM, Hughes MS, Brown SA, et al. Automated insulin delivery with remote real-time continuous glucose monitoring for hospitalized patients with diabetes: a multicenter, single-arm, feasibility trial. Diabetes Technol Therapeut 2023;25(10):677–88.

52. Yen PM, Young AS. Review of modern insulin pumps and the perioperative management of the type 1 diabetic patient for ambulatory dental surgery. Anesth Prog 2021;68(3):180–7.

53. Mendez CE, Umpierrez GE. Management of type 1 diabetes in the hospital setting. Curr Diabetes Rep 2017;17(10):98.

54. Palace MR. Perioperative management of thyroid dysfunction. Health Serv Insights 2017;10:1–5.

55. Pronovost PH, Parris KH. Perioperative management of thyroid disease. Postgrad Med 1995;98(2):83–98.

56. Stathatos N, Wartofsky L. Perioperative management of patients with hypothyroidism. Endocrinol Metab Clin North Am 2003;32(2):503–18.

57. Komatsu R, You J, Mascha EJ, et al. The effect of hypothyroidism on a composite of mortality, cardiovascular and wound complications after noncardiac surgery: a retrospective cohort analysis. Anesth Analg 2015;121(3):716–26.

58. Himes CP, Ganesh R, Wight EC, et al. Perioperative evaluation and management of endocrine disorders. Mayo Clin Proc 2020;95:2760–74.

59. Parker JLW, Rogers WJ, Baxley WA, et al. Death from thyrotoxicosis. Lancet 1973;2:894–5.

60. Schiff RL, Welsh GA. Perioperative evaluation and management of the patient with endocrine dysfunction. Med Clin North Am 2003;87(1):175–92.

61. Nabil NMD, Amatruda JM, Amatruda JM. Methimazole: An alternative route of administration. J Clin Endocrinol Metab 1982;54:180–1.

62. Woodcock T, Barker P, Daniel S, et al. Guidelines for the management of glucocorticoids during the peri-operative period for patients with adrenal insufficiency: Guidelines from the Association of Anaesthetists, the Royal College of Physicians and the Society for Endocrinology UK. Anaesthesia 2020;75(5):654–63.

63. Seo KH. Perioperative glucocorticoid management based on current evidence. Anesth Pain Med (Seoul) 2021;16(1):8–15.

64. Freudzon L. Perioperative steroid therapy: where's the evidence? Curr Opin Anaesthesiol 2018;31(1):39–42.

65. Liu MM, Reidy AB, Saatee S, et al. Perioperative steroid management: approaches based on current evidence. Anesthesiology 2017;127(1):166–72.

66. Marik PE, Varon J. Requirement of perioperative stress doses of corticosteroids: a systematic review of the literature. Arch Surg 2008;143(12):1222–6.

67. Hupfeld CJ, Iñiguez-Lluhí JA. Adrenocorticotropic hormone, adrenal steroids, and the adrenal cortex. In: Brunton LL, Knollmann BC, editors. Goodman & gilman's: the pharmacological basis of therapeutics. 14th Edition. New York, NY: McGraw-Hill Education; 2023.

68. Donati A, Ruzzi M, Adrario E, et al. A new and feasible model for predicting operative risk. Br J Anaesth 2004;93(3):393–9.

69. Glowniak JV, Loriaux DL. A double-blind study of perioperative steroid requirements in secondary adrenal insufficiency. Surgery 1997;121(2):123–9.

Postoperative Complications

Heather E. Nye, MD, PhD, SFHM[a], Edie P. Shen, MD, FHM, DFPM[b],
Furheen Baig, MD[b],*

KEYWORDS

- Postoperative complications - Fever - Stroke - Nausea - Ileus - Urinary retention

KEY POINTS

- Postoperative complications occur in up to 20% of cases, contributing to increased patient suffering, hospital length of stay, health care costs, and readmission rates.
- To optimally prevent and treat postoperative complications, it is imperative to identify high-risk patients, monitor closely following surgery, and institute early treatment when complications are detected.
- It is important to understand key differences in management strategies for clinical symptoms such as fever, stroke, and ileus in postoperative settings versus management employed in a nonsurgical setting.

INTRODUCTION

Surgery under anesthesia poses a significant stress to the body, triggering inflammation, blood loss, hemodynamic and fluid shifts, and pain.[1] Additionally, a multitude of new medications are routinely administered in the operating room and during recovery. Together, these can destabilize comorbid conditions, introduce metabolic disturbances, disrupt homeostasis of physiologic systems, and impair organ function. Despite ideal conditions and surgical techniques, up to 20% of surgeries are plagued by complications.[2,3] Older adults, those with medical comorbidities (American Society of Anesthesiologists [ASA] physical status > 2), and those being admitted from a care facility represent a growing proportion of surgical patients and are at even greater risk for complications after surgery (odds ratio 1.36–3.0 for multiple complications).[4] Moreover, these populations are expected to increase, with projections estimating over 20% of the US population will be over age 65 years in the coming decade.[3,5]

[a] San Francisco VA Health Care System Hospital Medicine, SFVAHCS Department of Medicine, University of California, San Francisco, 4150 Clement Street, Box 111, San Francisco, CA 94121, USA; [b] Division of General Internal Medicine, University of Washington, Hospital Medicine, 325 9th Avenue, Seattle, WA 98104, USA
* Corresponding author.
E-mail address: furbaig@uw.edu

Med Clin N Am 108 (2024) 1201–1214
https://doi.org/10.1016/j.mcna.2024.04.011   medical.theclinics.com

Postoperative complications (POCs) cause not only patient suffering but are also tied to increased hospital length of stay, health care costs, and readmission rates.[3] As such, it is imperative to adopt rigorous prevention and management strategies. Effective programs should include risk assessment, risk mitigation, early recognition, and treatment components. A comprehensive understanding of possible POCs and their management is essential to optimize health care quality and cost-effectiveness.

Major POCs including cardiovascular complications, thromboembolism, acute renal injury, anemia, and delirium have been covered elsewhere in this review. This article discusses a selection of POCs frequently encountered in clinical practice whose treatment often differs in the surgical setting from that seen in nonsurgical scenarios: postoperative fever, cerebrovascular accident, nausea and vomiting, ileus, and urinary retention.

POSTOPERATIVE FEVER

Fevers are a common POC, estimated to occur in 10% to 40% of surgical patients.[6] Fever in the postoperative setting is commonly identified as a temperature greater than 38°C or 100.4°F. The presence of fever in the inpatient setting understandably raises concerns for underlying infection, often leading to a reflexive workup that may be low yield depending upon the clinical situation and timing of the febrile event.

The evaluation of postoperative fever is best undertaken with a structured approach, considering both pathologic causes and physiologic events in the context of fever timing. Postoperative fever timing is generally broken down into 4 categories: immediate (<24 hours), acute (1–4 days), subacute (<30 days), and delayed (>30 days). While postoperative fever is a common event, if it occurs soon after surgery (up to 24 hours), it has low sensitivity and specificity for predicting a serious POC. Fevers that occur in the first 4 days after surgery are less likely to represent infectious complications than fevers occurring on the fifth and subsequent days. In one study where patients developed a fever near the fifth postoperative day (POD), 90% were found to have an identifiable source such as wound infection (42%), urinary tract infection (UTI; 29%), or pneumonia (12%).[7]

The release of pyrogenic cytokines (interleukins, IL-1 and IL-6, tumor necrosis factor, and interferon-γ) is a normal physiologic response to tissue damage incurred during surgery and stimulates fever via prostaglandin release from anterior hypothalamus. Postoperative febrile events are particularly common in patients who sustained trauma or injury prior to surgery. While studies demonstrate that an infectious workup may take place in up to half of patients who are febrile within the early postoperative period, these workups are often low yield and impose unnecessary diagnostic and financial burdens.[8]

When fever occurs within hours of surgery (immediate postoperative phase), in addition to cytokine release, other potential causes include drug reactions, transfusion reactions, infections present prior to the procedure, malignant hyperthermia, necrotizing soft tissue infection (NSTI), and adrenal insufficiency (**Fig. 1**). Hypotension and rash may accompany immune-mediated reactions (drug reaction or transfusion reactions). With regard to NSTI, the classic clinical signs remain of value, including the presence of "dishwater drainage" and erythema, edema, pain out of proportion to examination findings, and bullae.

For acute fevers (PODs 0–4), the differential broadens. Infections present at the time of surgery including pneumonia can be considered, but noninfectious causes are more common, including cytokine release, venous thromboembolism, alcohol withdrawal, or myocardial infarction.[9] Despite a long-standing historical association, atelectasis

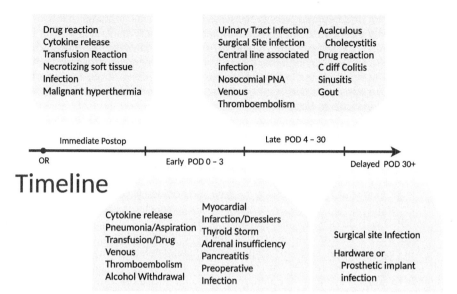

Drug reaction
Cytokine release
Transfusion Reaction
Necrotizing soft tissue
Infection
Malignant hyperthermia

Urinary Tract Infection
Surgical Site infection
Central line associated
infection
Nosocomial PNA
Venous
Thromboembolism

Acalculous
Cholecystitis
Drug reaction
C diff Colitis
Sinusitis
Gout

Immediate Postop

Late POD 4 – 30

OR

Early POD 0 – 3

Delayed POD 30+

Timeline

Cytokine release
Pneumonia/Aspiration
Transfusion/Drug
Venous
Thromboembolism
Alcohol Withdrawal

Myocardial
Infarction/Dresslers
Thyroid Storm
Adrenal insufficiency
Pancreatitis
Preoperative
Infection

Surgical site Infection

Hardware or
Prosthetic implant
infection

Fig. 1. Timeline post-op fever.

is not a cause of fever in the surgical patient.[10] Often, a thorough history and physical examination may be sufficient for workup in a patient with a benign clinical presentation. Fortunately, surgical site infection (SSI) is very rare in the early postoperative period and is unlikely before POD 4 or 5. SSI complicates 2% to 4% of surgical procedures and is defined by the CDC as an infection that occurs at or near the surgical site within 30 days of surgery or within 90 days if hardware or prosthetic material has been implanted during the procedure.[11]

The subacute or late postoperative phase is generally described as PODs 4 to 30, and in addition to venous thromboembolism, multiple infectious etiologies must be considered (see **Fig. 1**). These include UTI, pneumonia, blood stream infection, and SSI. SSI is the most common cause of fever presenting after POD 3. Early consultation with the surgical team can help to narrow the differential considerably and suggest appropriate options for judicious imaging based on surgery-specific concerns. In addition to a thorough history and physical examination, it may be reasonable to initiate a workup with blood and urine cultures, urinalysis, and chest radiographs. Empirical antibiotic therapy should be reserved for patients with a high pretest probability of infection or those in whom there are concerns for clinical instability.[12] Antibiotics should be limited to a brief course (∼48 hours) while a workup is undertaken and discontinued if no source is found.

Fever after the first 30 days should prompt consideration of a delayed SSI. Any recent prosthetic implants should be suspected as the source of a possible complicated SSI. These infections can be indolent in nature and present much later than the usual time course, even weeks to months following the surgery.

POSTOPERATIVE CEREBROVASCULAR ACCIDENT

Perioperative stroke is defined as any ischemic or hemorrhagic cerebral infarction with sequelae lasting 24 hours or more that occurs either intraoperatively or within 30 days of surgery.[13] Stroke is a well-recognized complication of cardiac surgery, carotid endarterectomy, and neurosurgical procedures due to specific features of these surgeries, including direct vascular and central nervous system manipulation. The incidence of stroke following other types of surgeries, however, is much lower, between 0.1% and 1%,[14] though the risk of clinically unrecognized strokes is perhaps as high as 7% in older adults.[15] Although the risk of perioperative stroke is overall low, given that 300 million adults undergo noncardiac surgery worldwide each year, the absolute number of patients impacted and resultant disability and mortality are significant.[16] In addition to advanced age, other common risk factors for perioperative stroke include prior TIA or stroke, atrial fibrillation, myocardial infarction within past 6 months, diabetes, renal disease, and chronic obstructive pulmonary disease.

Data are mixed, but in a large prospective study, patients undergoing noncardiac elective surgery who sustained a silent cerebral infarct on MRI had nearly double the risk of dementia at 1 year following surgery.[13] In addition to potentially devastating effects on cognitive health, independence and functional status, perioperative stroke is associated with 30 day mortality rates of up to 25%.[17]

Strokes are most commonly ischemic in the perioperative period, and the majority occurs in the first 7 days following surgery. When antiplatelet or antithrombotic medications are held perioperatively, cardioembolic stroke may result. There is insufficient evidence to support initiation of pharmacotherapy for stroke risk reduction in the immediate perioperative period, but in the weeks or months leading up to surgery, it is reasonable to optimize atherosclerotic risk factors as per guidelines pertaining to nonoperative standards of care for health care maintenance.[16]

One potentially modifiable risk factor in the setting of elective noncardiac surgery is the timing of the procedure following a history of recent stroke. A 2014 Danish cohort study examined the risk of major adverse cardiovascular events (ischemic stroke, acute myocardial infarction, and cardiovascular mortality) and found that elevated risk stabilized with timing surgery 9 months or more after an ischemic stroke.[18] A 2022 US cohort study of over 5 million surgical patients subsequently reported findings which suggest that the risk of stroke and death leveled off when over 90 days elapsed between a previous ischemic stroke and elective surgery.[19] The most recent 2021 American College of Cardiology/American Heart Association guidelines recommend that elective noncardiac surgery be deferred at least 6 months after a prior stroke but were published prior to the most recent US cohort study.[13] A reasonable approach is to take these recommendations into account in shared decision-making with the patient which balances urgency (both from a surgical and patient experience perspective) with the risks of recurrent stroke.

Interestingly, one prospective cohort study observed that patients with strokes that occurred in-hospital were significantly less likely to receive thrombolytics and were more likely to experience delays in time to appropriate imaging and treatment.[13] It is estimated that up to 60% of strokes that occur in inpatients are perioperative or periprocedural, and a significant portion (between 30% and 50%) occur in the 24 hours following surgery. The postoperative state likely contributes to confounding factors which may delay diagnosis, including recovery from general anesthesia and administration of opioids or other psychoactive medications for analgesia, which could mask newly developing neurologic deficits. Of note, in one case series of 39 patients, 15% of patients diagnosed with perioperative stroke presented with mental status changes only and were noted to have no appreciable focal deficits.[19] Hospitalists should keep a high index of suspicion for stroke in the differential for new postoperative neurologic deficits, altered mental status, and altered speech or language. Given unavoidable diagnostic challenges imposed by the perioperative period, whenever the index of suspicion for stroke arises, timely neurology consult and workup should be initiated by the activation of an institutional code stroke. For suspected large-vessel occlusion, guidelines from the Society of Neuroscience in Anesthesiology and Critical Care recommend urgent computed tomography (CT) angiography and diffusion/perfusion imaging for consideration of endovascular therapy.[20]

If acute postoperative ischemic stroke is diagnosed, decision regarding treatment with intravenous alteplase or mechanical thrombectomy will rely upon multidisciplinary collaboration between neurology, surgery, interventional, and perioperative teams.[20] High postoperative bleeding risks must be balanced with risk of long-term neurologic deficits. Of note, spine or intracranial surgery within the past 3 months is an absolute contraindication to intravenous alteplase infusion. Patients with large-vessel occlusion should be considered for mechanical thrombectomy.

POSTOPERATIVE NAUSEA AND VOMITING

Nausea and vomiting occur commonly after surgery, with an incidence of approximately 30% overall and up to 60% to 80% in high-risk populations.[21,22] Postoperative nausea and vomiting (PONV) causes significant distress to patients, limits oral intake, and may lead to unplanned admissions and prolonged hospital stays. While typically seen in the first 24 to 48 hours after surgery, PONV can persist for several days and result in dehydration, nutritional compromise, respiratory complications, and even wound dehiscence with severe retching.[21,23–25] Substantial negative impact on patient experience and cost burden to health care systems necessitate aggressive treatment and prevention protocols. The pathophysiology of PONV is multifactorial. Most PONV can be attributed to anesthesia and other medications administered in the perioperative period, though delayed gastric emptying, postoperative ileus, elevated intracranial pressure, pain, and anxiety may also contribute in specific scenarios.[26]

Nausea and vomiting are generated via a host of neurochemical pathways. Several areas within the central nervous system mediate the complex process, such as the chemoreceptor trigger zone (drug and toxin detection), cerebral cortex (pain and anxiety response), and vestibular nuclei in the brainstem and inner ear (motion sickness). Additional input from gastric mucosa (chemotherapy, non-steroidal anti-inflamatory drugs), gut stretch receptors, cardiac ischemia, or kidney disease can elicit symptoms via the vagus and splanchnic nerves.[27,28]

Numerous neurotransmitters and receptors mediate signals in these complex pathways and are key targets for pharmaceuticals in the prevention of PONV. These include D2 (dopamine), 5HT3 (serotonin), NK-1 (neurokinin-1, substance P), H1 (histamine), and M1 (muscarinic cholinergic) receptors[27,28] (**Fig. 2**).

Consensus guidelines published on the management of PONV recommend risk assessment with a validated tool.[21] This can be done through the use of tools such as the Apfel score, which calculates risk based on cumulative criteria that increase likelihood of PONV, such as prior history of PONV, female sex, nonsmoker, age less than 50 years, and opioid use after surgery.[21,22] The use of inhaled anesthetics, longer duration of anesthesia, and specific surgery types (cholecystectomy, gynecologic, and laparoscopy) further increases the risk. In highest risk patients, management strategies should consist of avoidance of opioids and nitrous oxide, minimizing inhaled anesthesia in favor of intravenous (eg, propofol), use of regional blocks and multimodal techniques for pain to reduce postoperative opioid use, and preoperative administration of prophylactic antiemetics.[21,24,25] Strong evidence exists for the efficacy of corticosteroids and several receptor antagonists in reducing PONV. These include D2 (eg, droperidol, metoclopramide), 5HT3 (eg, ondansetron, granisetron), NK-1 (eg, aprepitant), muscarinic (M1; eg, scopolamine), and histamine (H1; eg,

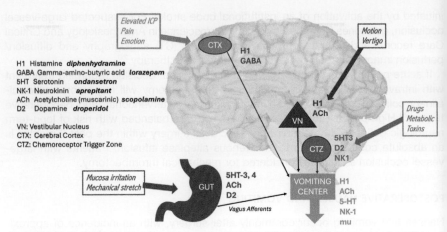

Neurochemical pathways in the central nervous system and periphery that mediate nausea and vomiting. Figure depicts various types of stimuli that can evoke nausea and vomiting through neural pathways with associated neurotransmitters. Examples of antiemetics targeting specific receptor pathways are noted within figure.

Fig. 2. Neurochemical pathways of nausea and vomiting.

diphenhydramine) receptor antagonists. Drugs may be used alone or in combination with others from different classes, which can produce a more robust antiemetic effect.[28] Higher risk patients may receive up to 4 prophylactic agents before, during and after the operation, while low-risk patients require only one or two (**Fig. 3**). A typical regimen might be single dose of dexamethasone prior to induction followed by scheduled ondansetron every 8 hours for 24 hours. Despite excellent efficacy, the use of some agents (NK-1 antagonists) is restricted due to high cost, while most other agents are inexpensive and readily available. Antiemetics are reasonably well-tolerated, but when side effects occur they can range from mild (headache, constipation, sedation) to more serious (ileus, QT prolongation, arrhythmias). While some

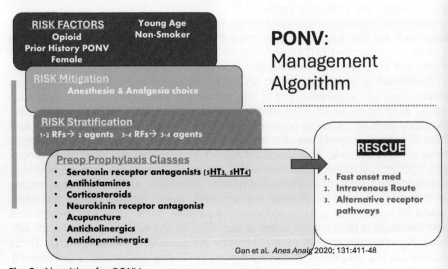

Fig. 3. Algorithm for PONV.

concern may exist for administration of steroids in the perioperative period increasing infection, a Cochrane review of the literature found that with a single dose of dexamethasone, this is unlikely.[29]

Patient comorbidities and characteristics should govern the choice of drug class with these side effects in mind.[21,28] Other approaches to reducing PONV after general anesthesia have shown mixed benefits. While a recent meta-analysis reported dexmedetomidine may be effective,[30] administration of higher percentages of supplemental O_2 intraoperatively or low-dose propofol infusions were not beneficial in other studies.[31,32]

Despite preventative measures, up to 30% of patients still experience breakthrough PONV, making rescue strategies an essential part of care. While limited studies are available on specific strategies, rescue treatment for PONV generally requires a knowledge of agents already administered and selection of a complementary drug that will work through an alternative pathway[23] (see **Fig. 3**).

Additionally, several nonpharmacologic strategies to reduce PONV have been studied, with favorable effects noted with aromatherapy, acupuncture, listening to music, and oral ginger intake.[33,34] While data are limited, these techniques in combination with standard pharmacologic strategies may achieve more a robust response.

POSTOPERATIVE ILEUS

Postoperative ileus is defined as a temporary state of bowel dysmotility after surgical intervention that results in ineffective transit of intestinal contents and poor tolerance of oral intake.[35] This process is due to a variety of nonmechanical factors and is typically self-limited, though it has notable implications in clinical care. Patients with postoperative ileus experience increased length of stay, and with the incidence estimated to be around 20%,[36] this has a significant impact on patient outcomes and health care costs.[37]

The etiology of postoperative ileus is multifactorial (**Box 1**). In the healthy adult, a migrating motor complex of electrical activity starting at the stomach and progressing through the small bowel induces intestinal contraction.[38] This process is inhibited by incision of the peritoneum or bowel manipulation.[39] Surgical intervention also causes notable sympathetic nervous system activation that inhibits peristalsis, as well as activation of proinflammatory cytokines that lead to release of nitric oxide and prostaglandins that inhibit smooth muscle contractility.[35] Intestinal edema, often related to excess perioperative volume resuscitation, has been shown to contribute to ileus, due to a combination of mechanical effect and pathways causing release of nitric oxide.[40] Observational data have suggested that hypokalemia may also contribute to

---

Box 1
Postoperative ileus

Suspected mechanisms

Disruption of the usual migrating motor complex of electrical activity in the gastrointestinal tract via peritoneal incision or bowel manipulation

Inhibition of peristalsis via sympathetic nervous system activation and/or activation of μ-opioid receptors

Reduced smooth muscle contractility via activation of proinflammatory cytokines, hypokalemia, and/or intestinal edema

Partial mechanical obstruction in setting of intestinal edema

ileus, theoretically in relation to potassium's effect on voltage-dependent calcium channels in smooth muscle contraction.[35] Last, pharmacologic factors, particularly opioid analgesics, have been shown to slow perioperative gut motility, specifically via μ-opioid receptors.[35,41]

Risk factors for developing postoperative ileus include older age, male sex, peritoneal incision, open surgical approach, prolonged operative time, perioperative opioid use, nasogastric tube use, excess blood loss or need for volume resuscitation, and bowel wall edema (**Table 1**).[35] Presenting symptoms include nausea, vomiting, abdominal pain, distension, absence of flatus, and inability to tolerate oral intake. Symptoms lasting beyond the expected duration (typically 4 days postoperatively), or that resolve and then recur, should prompt investigation into other underlying processes contributing to dysfunction, such as obstruction or infection.[35] Abdominal plain films can be used in initial evaluation for ileus and to help distinguish from obstruction, though with low sensitivity compared to CT. If plain films are inconclusive, or if infection is suspected, CT imaging should be pursued.[42,43]

Several approaches to prevention of postoperative ileus have been studied. In preoperative planning for abdominal surgery, less invasive laparoscopic approaches should be considered. Mitigating use of opioids by utilizing multimodal analgesia (including mid-thoracic epidural anesthesia, intravenous lidocaine, and/or nonsteroidal anti-inflammatory drugs) has also been shown to be beneficial.[35] A randomized controlled trial investigating celecoxib initiation preoperatively showed reduced rates of postoperative ileus in groups with similar opioid utilization; it is theorized that the drug's effect in inhibiting prostaglandin release may contribute, in addition to its potential for being opioid sparing.[44] Maintaining euvolemia and avoiding excess intravenous fluid administration is also of likely benefit.[45]

Regarding pharmacologic options for treatment of postoperative ileus, opioid receptor antagonists appear to be of greatest utility. Alvimopan, a peripherally acting μ-opioid receptor antagonist, has shown benefit in accelerating gastrointestinal recovery without reduced analgesic effect, given minimal crossing of the blood–brain barrier.[41,46] Other pharmacologic treatment options that have been theorized but have not shown reliable benefit include nonspecific beta-blockers such as propranolol, metoclopramide, and neostigmine.[47] The routine use of these agents is not recommended.

Various nonpharmacologic interventions have also been studied. Early oral nutrition has demonstrated low adverse event rates and favorable effect in time to first flatus and first stool postoperatively.[35,38,48] "Sham feeding," such as chewing gum, to

Table 1	
Risk factors and risk mitigation strategies for postoperative ileus	
Risk Factors	**Potential Mitigation Strategies**
Older age Male sex	Have higher index of suspicion in these populations for early diagnosis
Peritoneal incision Open surgical approach Prolonged operative time	Consider less invasive laparoscopic surgical approaches when able
Perioperative opioid use	Pursue multimodal analgesia
Nasogastric tube use	Avoid routine placement of nasogastric tubes preoperatively
Excess blood loss Need for volume resuscitation Bowel wall edema	Target euvolemia preoperatively; avoid excess intravenous fluids

stimulate the cephalic vagal axis has also been shown to reduce time to passage of first flatus and first defecation in several randomized controlled trials.[49]

Nasogastric tubes have historically been utilized in the management of postoperative ileus. Prophylactic placement of nasogastric tubes for decompression in the postoperative state was previously studied but found to have no benefit in shortening time to return of bowel function. In fact, the study populations with nasogastric tubes in place experienced increased time to passage of first flatus. Routine nasogastric tube placement is therefore not recommended.[50] In patients with significant vomiting or abdominal distension, nasogastric decompression can still be considered for symptomatic benefit.

POSTOPERATIVE URINARY RETENTION

Postoperative urinary retention (POUR) is seen following many different types of surgery. It can cause significant discomfort and places patients at higher risk for infection, delirium, unplanned admissions, and prolonged hospital stay.[51–53] POUR comes at a great cost to health care systems as a result of these complications and increased length of stay and, if untreated, can result in permanent detrusor dysfunction and kidney injury. Mainstays of management include (1) risk assessment and risk reduction; (2) monitoring and early recognition; (3) addressing reversible causes (medications or clinical conditions); and (4) bladder decompression.

The incidence of POUR ranges anywhere from 2.1% to 79% in the literature, with the highest rates observed after total joint arthroplasty, colorectal, and pelvic procedures.[51–55] Even some ambulatory procedures such as hernia repair are complicated by meaningful rates of POUR (5.8%–9.1%).[56] While criteria used to classify POUR are inconsistent, the inability to void despite a full bladder (urine volumes >400 cc) in the first week after surgery is a generally accepted definition. Potential contributors to the development of urinary retention may be anatomic variants, disruption in neuronal pathways, or muscle dysfunction. In the healthy adult, micturition is governed by a series of afferent and efferent neural pathways communicating signals between the brain, bladder, and spinal cord. Parasympathetic (acetylcholine) and sympathetic (norepinephrine) systems modulate bladder contraction and sphincter relaxation, respectively, and are impacted by a myriad of medications during the perioperative period.[54,57] A wide variety of drug classes can potentiate urinary retention, including anticholinergics (atropine, oxybutynin), antihistamines (diphenhydramine), antipsychotics (haloperidol), antidepressants (tricyclics and selective serotonin reuptake inhibitors), calcium channel blockers, opioids and alpha-adrenergic agents (pseudoephedrine).[57,58] The most common offenders causing retention in the postoperative period are typically opioids and anticholinergic drugs (or drugs with anticholinergic properties). Frequently cited risk factors for POUR include male gender (experiencing roughly twice the incidence of POUR), advanced age (odds ratio 2.11 if >60 year old), pre-existing benign prostatic hypertrophy (BPH) (odds ratio 2.83), neurogenic bladder, and pelvic floor anomalies.[59] Certain comorbidities (diabetes, depression, paralysis) and significant constipation also appear to be associated with increased risk.[51] Procedures requiring neuraxial anesthesia and longer operative times (>120 minutes), excessive intraoperative IV fluid, nonsupine operating room positioning, or pelvic and spinal cord manipulation likewise confer higher risk of POUR.[57,59,60]

Research on preventative measures for POUR has largely focused on alpha-antagonist use and preoperative catheterization. Alpha-1 antagonists have been shown to improve urine flow in both men and women through smooth muscle relaxation in the bladder neck and prostate and are also commonly used in treatment of POUR.[52] Evidence is mixed, however, on the benefits of these drugs as a class for POUR prevention. A recent meta-analysis focusing on tamsulosin (a selective alpha-1A blocker) suggested that this drug may be effective if administered preoperatively in reducing rates of POUR following total joint arthroplasty, though a separate trial showed no benefit in elective abdominal surgery.[61,62] Although evidence for prophylactic administration is lacking, a general rule of thumb in the preoperative setting, is to ensure that alpha-1 antagonists for BPH are continued perioperatively. Preemptive short-term placement of urinary catheters prior to surgery has also been explored as a way to reduce POUR, though most studies do not show benefit and catheter use may introduce unnecessary risks.[63,64] However, if operative time is expected to exceed 3 hours, a short-term Foley is generally recommended. Thoughtful postoperative medication management to reduce POUR risk includes avoiding or limiting drugs known to potentiate urinary retention to the extent possible. Initiation of tamsulosin as treatment of POUR postoperatively can be effective.

Vigilance in monitoring urine output and postvoid residuals (PVRs) is important postoperatively for all patients but is essential in those at higher risk for POUR. Early detection of urinary difficulties is key to avoid prolonged periods of bladder distention and initiate early treatment.[51–54] It is generally recommended that a PVR bladder scan be obtained 4 hours after surgery or after Foley removal.[53,54] When a patient is unable to urinate or empty the bladder completely (PVR > 400 cc), bladder decompression via catheterization should be performed (either intermittent catheterization or indwelling catheter placement). If retention is noted, or a patient is high risk, monitoring should be extended for up to 24 hours by checking PVRs every 6 hours and performing decompression when necessary. If two or more catheterizations are required, it is acceptable to place an indwelling catheter and start an agent to promote voiding such as tamsulosin. There is not a single strategy around timing of catheter removal and subsequent voiding trials, but 2 to 3 days is often needed for medications to have an effect. The use of indwelling catheters may cause urethral trauma and come with risk of catheter-associated UTIs, which increases with each day of additional use. As such, clean intermittent catheterization may be preferable for POUR management when symptoms persist. Urology follow-up should be arranged for all patients being discharged with an indwelling catheter, to determine timing of removal and whether further urodynamic studies are needed.

CLINICS CARE POINTS

- The evaluation of postoperative fever is best undertaken with a structured approach, considering both pathologic causes and physiologic events in the context of fever timing.

- Strokes that occur in-hospital are significantly less likely to receive thrombolytics and are more likely to experience delays in time to appropriate imaging and treatment; keeping stroke in the differential for postoperative neurologic deficits, altered mental status, and altered speech or language is of critical importance.

- Rescue treatment for PONV involves review of agents already administered and selection of a complementary drug that will work through an alternative pathway. Knowledge of mechanisms of action of various antiemetic options is essential.

- Postoperative ileus is best prevented and managed through a multimodal approach, including utilizing less invasive surgical techniques, limiting opioid burden, and initiating early oral nutrition or sham feeding. Routine nasogastric tube placement is not recommended, unless needed for symptomatic relief.

- Early detection of postoperative urinary difficulties by monitoring urine output and PVRs is key to avoid prolonged periods of bladder distension and initiating early treatment.

DISCLOSURES

The authors have nothing to disclose.

REFERENCES

1. Cusack B, Buggy DJ. Anaesthesia, analgesia, and the surgical stress response. BJA Educ 2020;20(9):321–8.
2. Anderson O, Davis R, Hanna GB, et al. Surgical adverse events: a systematic review. Am J Surg 2013;206(2):253–62.
3. Ludbrook GL. The Hidden Pandemic: the Cost of Postoperative Complications. Curr Anesthesiol Rep 2022;12(1):1–9.
4. Tevis SE, Cobian AG, Truong HP, et al. Implications of Multiple Complications on the Postoperative Recovery of General Surgery Patients. Ann Surg 2016;263(6): 1213–8.
5. The Organisation for Economic Co-operation and Development. Population projections. 2024. OECD data explorer. Available at: https://data-viewer.oecd.org/? chartId5457. [Accessed 31 January 2024].
6. Lesperance R, Lehman R, Lesperance K, et al. Early Postoperative Fever and the "Routine" Fever Work-Up: Results of a Prospective Study. J Surg Res 2011; 171(1):245–50.
7. Narayan M, Medinilla SP. Fever in the Postoperative Patient. Emerg Med Clin 2013;31(4):1045–58.
8. Petretta R, McConkey M, Slobogean GP, et al. Incidence, Risk Factors, and Diagnostic Evaluation of Postoperative Fever in an Orthopaedic Trauma Population. J Orthop Trauma 2013;27(10):558–62.
9. Wainaina JN. Chapter 34: Fever. In: Cohn S, editor. Decision making in perioperative medicine: clinical Pearls. 1st edition. McGraw Hill/Medical; 2021.
10. Hyder JA, Wakeam E, Arora V, et al. Investigating the "Rule of W," a Mnemonic for Teaching on Postoperative Complications. J Surg Educ 2015;72(3):430–7.
11. Agency for Research Healthcare and Quality. Patient Safety Primer: Surgical site infections, Available at: https://psnet.ahrq.gov/primer/surgical-site-infections, 2019. Accessed January 28, 2024.
12. Ashley B, Spiegel D, Cahill P, et al. Post-operative fever in orthopaedic surgery: How effective is the 'fever workup? J Orthop Surg 2017;25(3):1–9.
13. Benesch C, Glance L, Derdeyn C, et al. Perioperative Neurological Evaluation and Management to Lower the Risk of Acute Stroke in Patient undergoing Noncardiac Nonneurological Surgery. Circulation 2021;143:e923–46.
14. Glance L, Benesch C, Holloway L. Association of Time Elapsed Since Ischemic Stroke With Risk of Recurrent Stroke in Older Patients Undergoing Elective Nonneurologic, Noncardiac Surgery. JAMA Surg 2022;157(8):e222236.
15. NeuroVISION Investigators. Perioperative covert stroke in patients under- going non-cardiac surgery (NeuroVISION): a prospective cohort study. Lancet 2019; 394:1022–9.
16. Marcucci M, Chan M, Smith E. Prevention of perioperative stroke in patients undergoing noncardiac surgery. Lancet Neurol 2023;22:946–58.

17. Mpody C, Kola Kehinde O, Awad H, et al. Timing of Postoperative Stroke and Risk of Mortality After Noncardiac Surgery: A Cohort Study. J Clin Med Res 2023;15(5):268–73.

18. Jorgensen M, Torp-Pedersen C, Gislason G, et al. Time Elapsed After Ischemic Stroke and Risk of Adverse Cardiovascular Events and Mortality Following Elective Noncardiac Surgery. JAMA 2014;312(3):269–77.

19. Vlisides P, Mashour G, Didier T, et al. Recognition and Management of Perioperative Stroke in Hospitalized Patients. A&A Case Reports 2016;7:55–6.

20. Vlisides P, Moore L, Whalin M, et al. Perioperative Care of Patients at High Risk for Stroke During or After Non-cardiac, Non-neurological Surgery: 2020 Guidelines From the Society for Neuroscience in Anesthesiology and Critical Care. J Neurosurg Anesthesiol 2020;32:210–26.

21. Gan TJ, Belani KG, Bergese S, et al. Fourth Consensus Guidelines for the Management of Postoperative Nausea and Vomiting. Anesth Analg 2020;131(2):411–48.

22. Apfel CC, Läärä E, Koivuranta M, et al. A simplified risk score for predicting postoperative nausea and vomiting: conclusions from cross-validations between two centers. Anesthesiology 1999;91(3):693–700.

23. Gan TJ, Jin Z, Meyer TA. Rescue Treatment of Postoperative Nausea and Vomiting: A Systematic Review of Current Clinical Evidence. Anesth Analg 2022;135(5):986–1000.

24. Rajan N, Joshi GP. Management of postoperative nausea and vomiting in adults: current controversies. Curr Opin Anaesthesiol 2021;34(6):695–702.

25. Schlesinger T, Meybohm P, Kranke P. Postoperative nausea and vomiting: risk factors, prediction tools, and algorithms. Curr Opin Anaesthesiol 2023;36(1):117–23.

26. Zhong W, Shahbaz O, Teskey G, et al. Mechanisms of Nausea and Vomiting: Current Knowledge and Recent Advances in Intracellular Emetic Signaling Systems. Int J Mol Sci 2021;22(11):5797.

27. Horn CC, Wallisch WJ, Homanics GE, et al. Pathophysiological and neurochemical mechanisms of postoperative nausea and vomiting. Eur J Pharmacol 2014;722:55–66.

28. Weibel S, Rücker G, Eberhart LH, et al. Drugs for preventing postoperative nausea and vomiting in adults after general anaesthesia: a network meta-analysis. Cochrane Database Syst Rev 2020;10(10):CD012859.

29. Polderman JA, Farhang-Razi V, Van Dieren S, et al. Adverse side effects of dexamethasone in surgical patients. Cochrane Database Syst Rev 2018;11(11):CD011940.

30. Zhao W, Li J, Wang N, et al. Effect of dexmedetomidine on postoperative nausea and vomiting in patients under general anaesthesia: an updated meta-analysis of randomised controlled trials. BMJ Open 2023;13(8):e067102.

31. Markwei MT, Babatunde IO, Kutlu-Yalcin E, et al. Perioperative Supplemental Oxygen and Postoperative Nausea and Vomiting: Subanalysis of a Trial, Systematic Review, and Meta-analysis. Anesthesiology 2023;138(1):56–70.

32. Kutlu Yalcin E, Kim D, Mao G, et al. Effect of intraoperative subhypnotic infusion of propofol on postoperative nausea and vomiting: A retrospective analysis. J Clin Anesth 2022;78:110672.

33. Arslan HN, Çelik SŞ. Nonpharmacological Nursing Interventions in Postoperative Nausea and Vomiting: A Systematic Review. J Perianesth Nurs. 2024;39(1):142–54.

34. Asay K, Olson C, Donnelly J, et al. The Use of Aromatherapy in Postoperative Nausea and Vomiting: A Systematic Review. J Perianesth Nurs 2019;34(3): 502–16.

35. Bragg D, El-Sharkawy AM, Psaltis E, et al. Postoperative ileus: Recent developments in pathophysiology and management. Clin Nutr 2015;34(3):367–76.

36. Stephenson C, Mohabbat A, Raslau D, et al. Management of Common Postoperative Complications. Mayo Clin Proc 2020;95(11):2540–54.

37. Vather R, Trivedi S, Bissett I. Defining postoperative ileus: results of a systematic review and global survey. J Gastrointest Surg 2013;17(5):962–72.

38. Miedema BW, Johnson JO. Methods for decreasing postoperative gut dysmotility. Lancet Oncol 2003;4(6):365–72.

39. Luckey A, Livingston E, Taché Y. Mechanisms and treatment of postoperative ileus. Arch Surg 2003;138(2):206–14.

40. Shah SK, Uray KS, Stewart RH, et al. Resuscitation-induced intestinal edema and related dysfunction: state of the science. J Surg Res 2011;166(1):120–30.

41. Ludwig K, Enker WE, Delaney CP, et al. Gastrointestinal tract recovery in patients undergoing bowel resection: results of a randomized trial of alvimopan and placebo with a standardized accelerated postoperative care pathway. Arch Surg 2008;143(11):1098–105.

42. Frager DH, Baer JW, Rothpearl A, et al. Distinction between postoperative ileus and mechanical small-bowel obstruction: value of CT compared with clinical and other radiographic findings. AJR Am J Roentgenol 1995;164(4):891–4.

43. Frager D, Medwid SW, Baer JW, et al. CT of small-bowel obstruction: value in establishing the diagnosis and determining the degree and cause. AJR Am J Roentgenol 1994;162(1):37–41.

44. Wattchow DA, De Fontgalland D, Bampton PA, et al. Clinical trial: the impact of cyclooxygenase inhibitors on gastrointestinal recovery after major surgery - a randomized double blind controlled trial of celecoxib or diclofenac vs. placebo. Aliment Pharmacol Ther 2009;30(10):987–98.

45. Chowdhury AH, Lobo DN. Fluids and gastrointestinal function. Curr Opin Clin Nutr Metab Care 2011;14(5):469–76.

46. Zeinali F, Stulberg JJ, Delaney CP. Pharmacological management of postoperative ileus. Can J Surg 2009;52(2):153–7.

47. Holte K, Kehlet H. Postoperative ileus: progress towards effective management. Drugs 2002;62(18):2603–15.

48. Boelens PG, Heesakkers FF, Luyer MD, et al. Reduction of postoperative ileus by early enteral nutrition in patients undergoing major rectal surgery: prospective, randomized, controlled trial. Ann Surg 2014;259(4):649–55.

49. Fitzgerald JE, Ahmed I. Systematic review and meta-analysis of chewing-gum therapy in the reduction of postoperative paralytic ileus following gastrointestinal surgery. World J Surg 2009;33(12):2557–66.

50. Nelson R, Edwards S, Tse B. Prophylactic nasogastric decompression after abdominal surgery. Cochrane Database Syst Rev 2007;2007(3):CD004929.

51. Wu AK, Auerbach AD, Aaronson DS. National incidence and outcomes of postoperative urinary retention in the Surgical Care Improvement Project. Am J Surg 2012;204(2):167–71.

52. Darrah DM, Griebling TL, Silverstein JH. Postoperative urinary retention. Anesthesiol Clin 2009;27(3):465–84.

53. Baldini G, Bagry H, Aprikian A, et al. Postoperative urinary retention: anesthetic and perioperative considerations. Anesthesiology 2009;110(5):1139–57.

54. Choi S, Awad I. Maintaining micturition in the perioperative period: strategies to avoid urinary retention. Curr Opin Anaesthesiol 2013;26(3):361–7.

55. Cha YH, Lee YK, Won SH, et al. Urinary retention after total joint arthroplasty of hip and knee: Systematic review. J Orthop Surg 2020;28(1):2309499020905134.

56. Croghan SM, Mohan HM, Breen KJ, et al. RETAINER I Study Group of the Irish Surgical Research Collaborative. Global Incidence and Risk Factors Associated With Postoperative Urinary Retention Following Elective Inguinal Hernia Repair: The Retention of Urine After Inguinal Hernia Elective Repair (RETAINER I) Study. JAMA Surg 2023;158(8):865–73.

57. Kowalik U, Plante MK. Urinary Retention in Surgical Patients. Surg Clin 2016; 96(3):453–67.

58. Verhamme KM, Sturkenboom MC, Stricker BH, et al. Drug-induced urinary retention: incidence, management and prevention. Drug Saf 2008;31(5):373–88.

59. Mason SE, Scott AJ, Mayer E, et al. Patient-related risk factors for urinary retention following ambulatory general surgery: a systematic review and meta-analysis. Am J Surg 2016;211(6):1126–34.

60. Koseoglu E, Acar Ö, Kılıç M, et al. Urinary retention after non-urological surgeries: Management patterns and predictors of prognosis. Continence 2022;3:100507.

61. Baysden M, Hein D, Castillo S. Tamsulosin for prevention of postoperative urinary retention: A systematic review and meta-analysis. Am J Health Syst Pharm 2023; 80(6):373–83.

62. Papageorge CM, Howington B, Leverson G, et al. Preoperative Tamsulosin to Prevent Postoperative Urinary Retention: A Randomized Controlled Trial. J Surg Res 2021;262:130–9.

63. Crain NA, Goharderakhshan RZ, Reddy NC, et al. The Role of Intraoperative Urinary Catheters on Postoperative Urinary Retention after Total Joint Arthroplasty: A Multi-Hospital Retrospective Study on 9,580 Patients. Arch Bone Jt Surg 2021; 9(5):480–6.

64. Weintraub MT, Yang J, Nam D, et al. Short-Term Indwelling Foley Catheters Do Not Reduce the Risk of Postoperative Urinary Retention in Uncomplicated Primary THA and TKA: A Randomized Controlled Trial. J Bone Joint Surg Am 2023;105(4):312–9.

UNITED STATES POSTAL SERVICE®

Statement of Ownership, Management, and Circulation
(All Periodicals Publications Except Requester Publications)

1. Publication Title	2. Publication Number	3. Filing Date
MEDICAL CLINICS IN NORTH AMERICA	337 – 340	9/18/2024

4. Issue Frequency	5. Number of Issues Published Annually	6. Annual Subscription Price
JAN, MAR, MAY, JUL, SEP, NOV	6	$336.00

7. Complete Mailing Address of Known Office of Publication (Not printer) (Street, city, county, state, and ZIP+4®)

ELSEVIER INC.
230 Park Avenue, Suite 800
New York, NY 10169

Contact Person
Malathi Samayan

Telephone (Include area code)
+91 42994507

8. Complete Mailing Address of Headquarters or General Business Office of Publisher (Not printer)

ELSEVIER INC.
230 Park Avenue, Suite 800
New York, NY 10169

9. Full Names and Complete Mailing Addresses of Publisher, Editor, and Managing Editor (Do not leave blank)

Publisher (Name and complete mailing address)

Dolores Meloni, ELSEVIER INC.
1600 JOHN F KENNEDY BLVD. SUITE 1600
PHILADELPHIA, PA 19103-2899

Editor (Name and complete mailing address)

TAYLOR HAYES, ELSEVIER INC.
1600 JOHN F KENNEDY BLVD. SUITE 1600
PHILADELPHIA, PA 19103-2899

Managing Editor (Name and complete mailing address)

PATRICK MANLEY, ELSEVIER INC.
1600 JOHN F KENNEDY BLVD. SUITE 1600
PHILADELPHIA, PA 19103-2899

10. Owner (Do not leave blank. If the publication is owned by a corporation, give the name and address of the corporation immediately followed by the names and addresses of all stockholders owning or holding 1 percent or more of the total amount of stock. If not owned by a corporation, give the names and addresses of the individual owners. If owned by a partnership or other unincorporated firm, give its name and address as well as those of each individual owner. If the publication is published by a nonprofit organization, give its name and address.)

Full Name	Complete Mailing Address
WHOLLY OWNED SUBSIDIARY OF REED/ELSEVIER, US HOLDINGS	1600 JOHN F KENNEDY BLVD. SUITE 1600 PHILADELPHIA, PA 19103-2899

11. Known Bondholders, Mortgagees, and Other Security Holders Owning or Holding 1 Percent or More of Total Amount of Bonds, Mortgages, or Other Securities. If none, check box ▶ ☐ None

Full Name	Complete Mailing Address
N/A	

12. Tax Status (For completion by nonprofit organizations authorized to mail at nonprofit rates) (Check one)
The purpose, function, and nonprofit status of this organization and the exempt status for federal income tax purposes:

☒ Has Not Changed During Preceding 12 Months
☐ Has Changed During Preceding 12 Months (Publisher must submit explanation of change with this statement)

PS Form **3526**, July 2014 (Page 1 of 4 (see instructions page 4)) PSN: 7530-01-000-9931 PRIVACY NOTICE: See our privacy policy on www.usps.com.

---

13. Publication Title				14. Issue Date for Circulation Data Below
MEDICAL CLINICS IN NORTH AMERICA				JULY 2024

15. Extent and Nature of Circulation			Average No. Copies Each Issue During Preceding 12 Months	No. Copies of Single Issue Published Nearest to Filing Date
a. Total Number of Copies (Net press run)			240	228
b. Paid Circulation (By Mail and Outside the Mail)	(1)	Mailed Outside-County Paid Subscriptions Stated on PS Form 3541 (Include paid distribution above nominal rate, advertiser's proof copies, and exchange copies)	160	143
	(2)	Mailed In-County Paid Subscriptions Stated on PS Form 3541 (Include paid distribution above nominal rate, advertiser's proof copies, and exchange copies)	0	0
	(3)	Paid Distribution Outside the Mails Including Sales Through Dealers and Carriers, Street Vendors, Counter Sales, and Other Paid Distribution Outside USPS®	55	62
	(4)	Paid Distribution by Other Classes of Mail Through the USPS (e.g., First-Class Mail®)	17	15
c. Total Paid Distribution (Sum of 15b (1), (2), (3), and (4))		▶	232	220
d. Free or Nominal Rate Distribution (By Mail and Outside the Mail)	(1)	Free or Nominal Rate Outside-County Copies included on PS Form 3541	7	7
	(2)	Free or Nominal Rate In-County Copies Included on PS Form 3541	0	0
	(3)	Free or Nominal Rate Copies Mailed at Other Classes Through the USPS (e.g., First-Class Mail)	0	0
	(4)	Free or Nominal Rate Distribution Outside the Mail (Carriers or other means)	1	1
e. Total Free or Nominal Rate Distribution (Sum of 15d (1), (2), (3) and (4))		▶	8	8
f. Total Distribution (Sum of 15c and 15e)		▶	240	228
g. Copies not Distributed (See Instructions to Publishers #4 (page #3))		▶	0	0
h. Total (Sum of 15f and g)		▶	240	228
i. Percent Paid (15c divided by 15f times 100)		▶	96.74%	96.49%

* If you are claiming electronic copies, go to line 16 on page 3. If you are not claiming electronic copies, skip to line 17 on page 3.

16. Electronic Copy Circulation	Average No. Copies Each Issue During Preceding 12 Months	No. Copies of Single Issue Published Nearest to Filing Date
a. Paid Electronic Copies	▶	
b. Total Paid Print Copies (Line 15c) + Paid Electronic Copies (Line 16a)	▶	
c. Total Print Distribution (Line 15f) + Paid Electronic Copies (Line 16a)	▶	
d. Percent Paid (Both Print & Electronic Copies) (16b divided by 16c × 100)	▶	

☒ I certify that 50% of all my distributed copies (electronic and print) are paid above a nominal price.

17. Publication of Statement of Ownership

☒ If the publication is a general publication, publication of this statement is required. Will be printed in the NOVEMBER 2024 issue of this publication. ☐ Publication not required.

18. Signature and Title of Editor, Publisher, Business Manager, or Owner		Date
Malathi Samayan - Distribution Controller	*Malathi Samayan*	9/18/2024

I certify that all information furnished on this form is true and complete. I understand that anyone who furnishes false or misleading information on this form or who omits material or information requested on the form may be subject to criminal sanctions (including fines and imprisonment) and/or civil sanctions (including civil penalties).

PS Form **3526**, July 2014 (Page 2 of 4) PRIVACY NOTICE: See our privacy policy on www.usps.com.

Moving?

Make sure your subscription moves with you!

To notify us of your new address, find your **Clinics Account Number** (located on your mailing label above your name), and contact customer service at:

Email: journalscustomerservice-usa@@elsevier.com

800-654-2452 (subscribers in the U.S. & Canada)
314-447-8871 (subscribers outside of the U.S. & Canada)

Fax number: 314-447-8029

Elsevier Health Sciences Division
Subscription Customer Service
3251 Riverport Lane
Maryland Heights, MO 63043

*To ensure uninterrupted delivery of your subscription, please notify us at least 4 weeks in advance of move.

ELSEVIER

Printed and bound by CPI Group (UK) Ltd, Croydon, CR0 4YY
08/05/2025
01864752-0002